The human rights, ethical and moral dimensions of health care

French edition:

La santé face aux droits de l'homme, à l'éthique et aux morales

ISBN 92-871-3054-X

Cover: Graphic Design Workshop of the Council of Europe

Council of Europe Publishing
F-67075 Strasbourg Cedex

ISBN 92-871-3055-8
© Council of Europe, March 1998
Printed in Germany

Table of contents

List of cases

Preface

by Daniel Tarschys,
Secretary General of the Council of Europe

One of the Council of Europe's primary tasks is the everyday defence of human rights, for which the organisation has established four broad lines of work:
– strengthening European solidarity in respect of the individual, their civil and political freedoms, and their social, economic and cultural rights, through setting up effective monitoring and protection mechanisms;
– identifying new threats to human rights and human dignity;
– raising public awareness of the importance of human rights;
– developing education in and information on human rights in schools and universities and in certain professions.

The Council of Europe's main instrument in the field of human rights is the European Convention on Human Rights, signed in Rome on 4 November 1950.

The rights and fundamental freedoms guaranteed by the Convention and its protocols are:
– the right to life, the right to liberty and security of person;
– the right to a fair trial in civil and criminal cases;
– the right to freedom of thought, conscience and religion;
– the right to freedom of expression (including freedom of the press).

The Convention prohibits:
– torture or inhuman or degrading treatment;
– the death penalty;
– discrimination in the enjoyment of the rights and freedoms protected by the Convention;
– expulsion or turning away by a state of its own nationals;
– collective expulsion of foreigners.

There has been spectacular progress in medicine and biology in recent decades, bringing considerable benefits to people's health and welfare. But this progress has given rise to new problems because it has brought the risk of excesses. It was therefore felt necessary to monitor developments in these fields to ensure that science remains in the service of the individual. It is to this end that the Council of Europe is pursuing two main lines of work:
– the organisation of forums, such as the Standing Conference of European Ethics Committees and various symposia, to permit the different actors (health professionals, researchers, associations, decision-makers and parliamentarians) and the various currents of thought to express their opinions and exchange views. It is in fact only through dialogue and debate that acceptable solutions can be reached in democratic societies;

9

– the drafting of normative principles, the main achievement of which was the publication in June 1996, by the Steering Committee for Bioethics, of the draft Convention on Human Rights and Biomedicine. This text contains rules concerning in particular patients' rights, medical research, medically assisted procreation, gene therapy and organ transplants. It is the first international normative text in this field and will be completed by a number of protocols establishing more detailed rules on specific subjects.

The European Network for Scientific Co-operation, "Medicine and Human Rights", created under the auspices of the Council of Europe's Parliamentary Assembly, a member of the European Federation of Scientific Networks (FER), set up an interdisciplinary and European team of researchers which worked untiringly on this study analysing the problem of medicine and human rights.

The fresh contribution that the originators of the project wanted to make was to analyse the possible responses of health professionals faced with situations giving rise to ethical problems. The authors studied the action that these professions might envisage in order to be in line with international legal standards, ethics and the major religious and lay moral principles.

The outcome of this endeavour is an important contribution to the teaching of ethics in the faculties of medicine and pharmacy, nursing colleges and other establishments training health professionals. This work is directly connected with the Council of Europe's fundamental objectives and as such has been of the greatest interest to me and received my full support.

Preface

by Jean-Pierre Massué,
Secretary General of the European Federation of Scientific Networks

Europe has set its seal firmly upon the concept of human rights and the way it is taken into account in the constitutions and laws which govern us. Human rights are for Europe its *Geisteshaltung und Lebensform*. Professor René-Jean Dupuy writes on this subject:

"The advent of such a system of thought was possible only after a prodigious revolution which took place in Antiquity and consisted of a transfer of the sacred. Then everything in matter was sacred, or could be – springs, rocks, clouds, mountains. Everything in nature was sacred except man.

Socratism, Judaism and then Christianity had the effect of reversing this order of things and desacralising everything but man. The way was now open. The Epistle to the Colossians breaks down the discriminations on which ancient society was based: 'Neither Greek, nor Jew, (...) Barbarian, Scythian'. The part played by Protestantism in the struggle for civil and political rights is well known, as is that of the Age of Enlightenment and Freemasonry and, today, the witness of the Catholic Church, which after having held aloof, because of its links with the *ancien régime*, from a doctrine which was nevertheless of Christian essence, finally joined it with solemn acts: the Encyclical of Pius XI condemning nazism *'mit brennender Sorge'*; *'Pacem in terris'* of John XXIII and Vatican II; the messages of Paul VI and John Paul II (...) These diverse sources finished by joining together and, after the second world war, which had stained them with the blood of the innocent, they gave birth to a movement which led to the European Convention on Human Rights and Fundamental Freedoms of 1950. It is the richness of this doctrinal foundation which explains the technical superiority of the system of guarantees it has put in place."

Human rights affirm the principle of the safeguard of life and are thus directly concerned when we analyse the problems posed by therapeutics, namely the use of the methods made available to us by science, and in particular medical science, in the service of human health.

It is in this context that in 1981, in the context of the Parliamentary Assembly exercise on scientific co-operation, the study group on human rights and medicine chaired by Professor G. Gerin was created. This has now become the European Scientific Co-operation Network on Human Rights and Medicine within the European Federation of Networks.

Religions and philosophies in general have been playing a major role for a very long time in the establishment of basic rules for codes of medical ethics. We have only to remember the Hippocratic Oath:

"I will prescribe regimen for the good of my patients according to my ability and my judgment and never do harm to anyone. To please no one will I prescribe a deadly drug, nor give advice which may cause his death. (...) In every house where I come I will enter only for the good of my patients, keeping myself far from all intentional ill-doing and all seduction."

Similarly, the prayer composed in the twelfth century by Moses Maimonides, a Talmudic doctor, says:

"Support the strength of my heart so that it will always be ready to serve the poor and the rich, the friend and the enemy, the good and the bad. Let me see only the man in he who suffers."

The interest in determining an international deontology has developed since the end of the second world war.

One of the first texts dealing with ethical problems in the field of experimentation was a work published in Prussia in 1900 entitled *Instructions to the administrators of hospitals*, in which it was stipulated that research other than for diagnostic, treatment or immunisation purposes should be excluded, and there must be no experimentation on subjects who are not legally capable.

The Nuremberg Code of 1947 is the first declaration on experimentation on human subjects. This code, stemming from the trial of doctors who conducted experiments during the war against the will of the subjects, stipulates the necessity for the free consent of the subject submitted to biomedical experimentation.

Then come the texts adopted by the World Medical Association (WMA): the Declaration of Helsinki, giving recommendations to guide the doctor in the field of biomedical research, adopted by the 18th World General Assembly (Helsinki, 1964), amended by the 29th World General Assembly (Tokyo, 1975) and the 35th World General Assembly (Venice, 1983).

The Conférence internationale des ordres de médecins et des organismes d'attributions similaires, together with the World Medical Association and the World Health Organisation put forward international guidelines on experimentation in Manila in 1981. These guidelines are mainly concerned with population groups not in a position to give informed consent who are subjected to research (children, pregnant women, prisoners, the mentally ill, etc.).

In 1977, the World Psychiatric Association adopted the Hawaii Declaration, concerned with psychiatric research and stressing the patient's freedom to renounce voluntary treatment or participation in a research programme for any reason and at any time.

In the report drafted for the Council of Europe by Maître H. Anrys of Brussels on the problem of medical deontology in the protection of patients' rights, he sums up very well the special relationship which exists between doctors and patients:

> "Frightened by the mystery of death in the face of which they are helpless, patients know they have no choice but to give themselves up to the knowledge and conscience of the doctor, which are their only hope. Trust and conscience come face to face. But the greater the doctor's conscience, the greater the patient's trust, to which a reputation for integrity and skill will contribute. Efforts to guarantee these qualities may take two forms: either they may be imposed from outside, or doctors may be conditioned to have an acute personal awareness of the requirements of their ministry."

The rapid development of research in the field of genetic engineering has made relations between doctors and patients even more complex. As Professor F. Gros points out: "Since the advent of genetic engineering, we are able to analyse the human genome just as the chemist can analyse a molecule. We can read the encoded message and predict certain physiological consequences. What is more, man has become capable of rearranging the genes of all species, including his own." The biologist can discover the keys to certain extremely complex hereditary diseases and detect the precursors of a genetic disease with great precision during pregnancy. It will soon be possible, on the basis of work on experimental somatic transgenosis, to remedy the biological destiny by means of gene therapy.

Genetic engineering includes the human genome project, aimed at establishing the sequence of the three-and-a-half thousand million chemical "characters" which constitute the complete genetic code hidden in man's forty-six chromosomes.

The colloquy on "Genetic heritage and human rights" held between 25 and 28 October 1985 in Paris led to the publication of a white paper of recommendations. In the synthesis prepared by Gérard Hubert, the ethical choices in genetic engineering are presented as follows:

> "Living beings cannot be assimilated to mechanical devices such as clocks. Just as there is a qualitative leap between the mineral and the living world, because of the architecture and the dynamics of the relations between its constituent parts, so there is a qualitative leap between the rest of the living world and man.

13

This observation justifies the existence of ethical choices, but in no way permits us to say what they should be.

In philosophical terms, the ethical enunciation may take the following form: act and intervene in the genetic code in order to free what, in its language, makes possible more creativity and freedom, in the modes of speech and action."

The creation of national consultative ethics committees represents a big step forward. In France, for example, the National Consultative Ethics Committee was created by decree in 1983. It deals with subjects which were long considered taboo, such as the problem of sterilising the mentally handicapped. The French newspaper *Le Monde* published a series of articles on this subject on 19 April 1996, showing that:

– non-voluntary surgical sterilisation has been very widely practised throughout the world, especially in the first half of the twentieth century. It has often been practised on people labelled as "socially inadequate" (the poor, criminals, alcoholics, the mentally ill). These measures were based on the conviction that a certain number of conditions and behaviours were hereditary pathologies.

– up to the eve of the second world war, these measures were supported by reputed scientists, especially in France. In Germany, after Hitler came to power, a law of 14 July 1933 instituted voluntary or even compulsory sterilisation for certain people afflicted by hereditary defects.

– certain countries today have legislation authorising such practices. This is the case in particular in South Africa (since 1975) and China, which in November 1994 passed a law intended to "improve the quality of the new-born population".

Mental deficiency alone cannot justify this practice. Furthermore, the question of the free and informed consent of mentally handicapped persons for any kind of medical or surgical intervention whatever gives rise to problems.

For the French National Consultative Ethics Committee "the specific problem that arises is that of defining the parameters for the decision on a case-by-case basis, with due regard to the circumstances in which the contraceptive choice is to be made. This choice must necessarily take account of the constraints imposed by medical and/or biological arguments, as well as the particularities of the history, behaviour and environment of each mentally handicapped person".

From whom does the request for contraception emanate and what are the real reasons? "It is not always clear that this request corresponds to a desire for an active sex life, expressed by the mentally handicapped person. Attention should therefore be directed primarily at the desires of this person and being sure of his or her agreement", as the committee prudently points out.

Another topical example of the problems encountered by doctors is the limitation on medical aid to illegal immigrants. The French Secretary of State for

Emergency Humanitarian Action, Dr Xavier Emmanuelli, sums up the position of medical ethics very well:

> "No serious doctor can take this seriously. I shall simply recall Pasteur's doctrine: 'I do not ask who you are or where you come from, I ask only what is the matter'. This is all our tradition, all our ethic: when somebody is sick we treat him, full stop. This is what my father, a doctor, instilled in me, and this is what I taught my son, also a doctor. Afterwards, when the person is cured, then and only then, can you consider his administrative situation. There is nothing more to say."

Research into possible treatments for Aids and the application of the findings raises many ethical questions. It is known for example that in order to multiply, the Aids virus (HIV) transforms its RNA genetic material into DNA by means of an enzyme with reverse transcriptase. This is the operation which is countered by the association of two drugs, AZT and DDC or DDI. Another important stage in the multiplication of the virus is that in which the injected cell produces a protease specific to the virus which plays a major role in the multiplication process. There are now antiproteases which prevent the protease from acting. This is the aim of drugs like Ritonavir, Indinavir, etc. It has been observed that through associating these three types of drug – AZT, DDC or DDI and an antiprotease – a very significant quantity of the virus is destroyed. But this raises a number of questions:
– what are the secondary effects of this triple therapy?
– is the treatment less effective in the longer term?
– when can patients start benefiting from this treatment? In the meantime, given the limited production of the drugs, how should the recipients be chosen: through drawing lots? Selection by means of money?
These are some of the ethical and deontological problems which need to be addressed.

In a first stage, the Council of Europe's European Network of Scientific Co-operation on Medicine and Human Rights, made up of European researchers concerned with these questions, embarked upon a major concerted research programme, co-ordinated by Professor G. Gerin, President of the International Institute for Human Rights Studies in Trieste (Italy). Several years of research led to a work of 1485 pages, *Le Médecin face aux droits de l'homme* ("The doctor and human rights", in French only), published by Cedam in June 1990.

This publication comprises:
a. the inventory of legal, ethical, deontological and moral texts, national and international, existing in Europe which concern the problem of medicine and human rights;

15

b. a set of 146 case sheets describing typical situations encountered by the doctor in the exercise of his functions;

c. an evaluation of these cases from the standpoint of legal, deontological and ethical reference texts and that of various moralities.

One of the main aims of this research project was to provide medical and paramedical staff with an aid to decision-making and to produce a tool for use in the teaching of ethics in medical schools and other institutions involved in the training of health professionals. We felt it was important to produce this second, more condensed work in the form of a paperback, entitled *The human rights, ethical and moral dimensions of health care.*

This book is essentially based on the inventories contained in the main work. The number of cases analysed was set at eighty-two, plus a further thirty-eight corresponding to the everyday concerns of nursing care. To represent the different moralities we have taken the Catholic, Protestant, Jewish, Muslim, Buddhist and agnostic views.

I again sincerely thank all the authors who made the original work possible, those who agreed to revise their contributions for the present work, and also the new authors:

Maître H. Anrys (Brussels)

Dr F. Ben Hamida, assisted by Dr G.H. Hadj Eddine Sari Ali (Paris)

Maître H. Caillavet, assisted by Dr J. Brunschwig, Dr G. Payen and Prof. P.C. Ranouil (Paris)

Prof. J.-F. Collange (Strasbourg)

Prof. P. Cüer (Strasbourg)

the late Dr J. Farber (Brussels)

Prof. G. Gerin (Trieste)

Chief Rabbi A. Guigui (Brussels)

the late Prof. R. Leray (Paris)

Dr J. Martin, assisted by Dr C. Chevassut and Dr M.-A. Pratili (Paris-Marseilles)

Miss M.-Th. Mangin (Neufchâteau-Vittel)

Mrs C. Pierre-Evrard (Paris)

Prof. A. Piga Rivero, assisted by Prof. T. Alfonso Galán, (Madrid)

Prof. M. Scalabrino (Milan)

Mgr. Prof. E. Sgreccia, assisted by Dr. A. Spagnolo (Rome)

Dr. A. Wynen (Brussels)

As this book goes to press, a work produced by the European Network of Scientific Co-operation on Medicine and Human Rights of the European Federation of Scientific Networks, we have already returned to our loom to carry out research on the theme of ethics and disaster medicine in co-operation with the European Centre for Disaster Medicine (CEMEC) (San Marino) and the Higher

Institute of Emergency Planning (ISPU) (Florival, Belgium), both created under the Council of Europe's EUR-OPA Major Hazards Agreement.

Preface

by Professor Guido Gerin,
Head of the International Institute for Human Rights Studies,
and the International Centre for Bioethics Studies, Trieste,
Chairman of the European Network for Scientific Co-operation
"Medicine and Human Rights"

The Institute for Human Rights Studies has been asked by the scientific community to look in detail at the ethical problems that arise in medicine and research.

Human beings have human rights from the day they are born. "Human rights" refer, of course, to the whole human being and include, therefore, human dignity, liberty and health.

The right to life is inherently one of the fundamental human rights. Indeed, all international texts, whether conventions or charters, state that the right to life is our first and most important fundamental right.

Since it is doctors who are responsible for looking after human life, the institute has published a vast study at the request of the Council of Europe on *Le médecin face aux droits de l'homme* ("The doctor and human rights", in French only). This study contains all the international texts and national legislation on the medical profession and research in this field, as well as provisions governing state responsibility; it also includes professional codes of ethics and examines moral and religious problems encountered not only by doctors but also patients. Finally, a series of case studies answers questions asked by doctors in specific circumstances that arise, for example as regards the right to have children, medical secrecy, sterilisation, organ transplants, etc.

The publication therefore comprises comprehensive documentation on the sources of the various texts, but it is intended above all for use by universities, doctors and health workers in general. The European working group which helped produce the study also decided to publish a shorter text, which summarises existing relevant documentation. The summary updates the larger publication and also examines new problems such as Aids.

It was decided to publish this new updated version in English, as well as French, owing to the numerous requests for the text in that language. In publishing the work, the institute hopes that it will be of use to all health workers and all those responsible for hospitals and health services in general.

Furthermore, the Conférence internationale des ordres de médecins et des organismes d'attributions similaires, meeting on 14 January 1980, likewise defined a series of deontological standards imposing on doctors a kind of behaviour that ensures the respect of human rights and the rights of the patient. However, it should also be borne in mind that doctors are very often faced with legal, ethical or religious problems which need to be solved on the spot. They must sometimes decide whether to apply national legislation, an international

19

convention, a professional code of ethics, or whether account must be taken of certain moral considerations.

It is for this reason that the institute, which I have the honour to head, has tried to provide answers to specific cases, particularly in the present context of diseases such as Aids which raise serious doubts concerning the limits fixed with regard to the doctor's action and responsibility. The extremely rapid progress of scientific research, with its positive results – which necessitate constant change – together with technological development, mean that it is impossible to find solutions that will remain valid in the longer term.

The tremendous pace of scientific activity might incite scientists to declare that they are also philosophers. This would be a dangerous step, because it might lead to a form of "scientism" that is completely sterile and unacceptable given the criteria of universality which a critical analysis of science needs to be able to satisfy. Science has certain tasks that it must fulfil, but it also has certain limits that it must respect.

Through scientific research, opinions are expressed and answers are provided that have a relative value, limited sometimes only by time. Very often, however, the value of the answers provided will depend on the kind of scientific discipline concerned.

The institute considered the creation of the European working group on ethical questions to be very important, since scientific discovery cannot be confined to one university alone, nor can it be contained within the boundaries of one country. Research can and must be co-ordinated within a much wider framework, even extending beyond Europe. The scourge of Aids has already compelled the International Academy of Sciences to co-ordinate the work of numerous laboratories seeking a vaccine against this terrible disease. The modest activity carried out by the institute in this field leads to just one conclusion: everybody – scientists, lawyers, philosophers and religious leaders – must work closely together so that our points of reference as regards ethics and, in particular, as regards scientific information, may be our right to life and the right of the human race not to suffer irreparable harm.

Nonetheless, the principal aim of this publication, as with the previous work, is much simpler – to supply information to all those working in the health sector, whether in the field of medicine, biology, the environment or the administration of scientific institutes or hospitals. In so doing, we hope to provide a certain minimum of data that will enable new requirements to be met as and when they arise, also taking the emergence of new and even more serious diseases into consideration.

We must hope that the work undertaken by the institute is successful. Since the Council of Europe has requested our co-operation, already well-established in other fields, I have the honour, as Head of the Institute, of presenting this study

20

which, though modest, has been drafted and updated by specialists in the different fields.

One final comment: in addition to gaining considerable ground in universities, the question of bioethics is also beginning to be a cause of concern for governments. France was the first country to set up a national ethics committee, but both Denmark and Italy have now also formed similar committees. Likewise, in the United Kingdom, the Warnock Commission has drawn up a set of principles to be observed. Nonetheless, it seems that ethics committees are much more helpful as they can provide answers on a day-to-day basis as new situations arise.

We can only hope that the Council of Europe itself will also react to this problem by setting up a European ethics committee, followed on a worldwide level by Unesco. A sick person remains a human being, and, while the results obtained from scientific research have led to a considerable rise in average life expectancy, we have also witnessed the emergence of serious problems of an ethical nature closely connected with both the beginning and end of human life and also with the "dignity" which should characterise the life of each and every one of us.

Initiation to bioethics

by Pierre Cüer,
Professor, Co-Director of the European Training Centre
"Médicine, ethique et droits de l'homme"
at the Université Pierre et Marie Curie – Paris VI,
Co-ordinator of the bioethics training of the European Network
"Médicine et droits de l'homme"

This book, interdisciplinary, European in vocation, is addressed to teachers, members of ethics committees, researchers in the human sciences, doctors, pharmacists, dentists, biologists, jurists and students of these disciplines, nurses, care personnel, and patients. Through its introductory statements and 120 representative cases, mostly clinical, it seeks to present international and European legal rules, ethical standards and reference points on which there is an international consensus, and the standpoints of religious and agnostic moralities. It can serve as a guide for professional activity, or as an initiation to ethics, in conformity with the rights, duties and dignity of man and his convictions.

For pedagogical and practical reasons, after a number of introductions intended to inform the reader about the foundations and consequences for the health field of these legal rules and these religious and agnostic ethical standards, the core of the book takes the form of case studies, classified according to the type of problem involved.

An experimental fascicule preceding this book, drafted by members of the network in 1990 on the initiative of Dr J.-P. Massué, then Head of the Higher Education and Research Division of the Council of Europe, served as the basis for training in bioethics and human rights implemented by the network. This fascicule contained 50 cases considered to be very representative and raising questions of particular interest, selected out of the 146 actual cases proposed by the late Dr Farber, then Chairman of the World Medical Association, contained in the reference manual of the network, a work of 1 500 pages published by Cedam (Padua) under the aegis of the International Institute for Human Rights Studies in Trieste and the Council of Europe. Eight new cases were added, at my suggestion, on genetic manipulation, transplants, Aids and transsexualism. These 58 cases (numbered 1-58 in this book) have been the subject of studies, discussions and arguments in the training sessions initiated by the network. The replies to the questions involved have recently been updated by the authors.

This fascicule was translated into Russian and Italian and is at present being used in many training courses in Europe, notably in France, in several eastern European countries, and in Lebanon.

In order to take account of the questions most frequently raised by participants in training courses and the rapid progress in therapies and biotechnologies, I drafted a further 22 cases (59 to 80 in this book), which were submitted for examination and approval to Dr L. René, Honorary Chairman of the French Medical Council (*Ordre des médecins*), member of the National Consultative Ethics

Committee, and Professor B. Hoerni, Chairman of the "Ethics and Deontology" section, Vice-Chairman of the National Council of the French Medical Council, both active contributors for the past five years to our pilot training scheme at Pierre et Marie Curie, whom I thank most warmly. Maître A. Garay, barrister-at-law, was kind enough to propose several specific cases concerning the replacement of blood transfusions, for Jehovah's Witnesses, by recombinatory human erythropoietin, an important example of which was selected and dealt with in the same way as the other cases (case 82).

However, these 82 cases, essentially based on medical progress, scarcely correspond to the everyday concerns of nursing care. Mrs C. Pierre-Evrard, *infirmière générale*, Chair of the *Mouvement associatif des infirmières de la Seine-Saint-Denis*, organiser of three European colloquies on nursing care, was kind enough to select and write an introduction to 38 cases (cases 83 to 120 in this book) representative of everyday nursing from a total of 120 situations submitted by Belgian, Spanish, French and Greek nurses and by Miss M.-Th. Mangin, Co-ordinator of Ethics Training at the Neufchâteau-Vittel Centre supported by the network.

The legal rules and ethical guidelines put forward are international and European and the prescriptions of the religious moralities are in principle transcendent and universal.

This work is not intended to be a systematisation in case study form of ethics and the religious moralities, based either on universals emanating from human rights and human dignity or from revealed teachings on the nature of man; but it is likely that considerations of principle would remain relatively inaccessible to teachers, researchers, practitioners and patients if ethical or moral recommendations were not capable of giving a clear indication, for each important act, of the way the care decision should go, at the risk of creating conflicts of values to be discussed and if possible ranked in a spirit of interdisciplinary pluralism.

This book thus sets out to make a contribution to the understanding, teaching, practice and harmonisation of bioethics at the European level. Society, its representatives and decision-makers, whose attitudes to, and knowledge of, the subject are largely drawn from sensational media presentations of therapeutic or biotechnological "breakthroughs" – often shocking, always over-simplified – are seeking fuller information or even education which can give a better understanding of the reasons for the decisions taken in the increasingly sensitive field of health care.

Certain scientists and practitioners, egged on by the media, have sometimes raised most regrettable false hopes. Many media, even those involved in scientific popularisation, still refuse to adopt a deontology and an ethical code, despite pressure by a number of bodies, including on several occasions the Council of Europe. This is the case in France in particular, where an unconditional right to information is invoked. Respect of the human dignity of others and acceptance of responsibility for the consequences of certain types of information for society as a whole should nevertheless take precedence over objective truth at any price and the obsession with ratings and sales figures.

From this standpoint, in addition to an independent consultative body with equal representation of scientists and the media, of recognised moral authority, like that set up in certain European countries and recommended by the French National Consultative Ethics Committee, would it not be desirable to make efforts to raise media awareness of ethical issues?

Because of the concise nature of this work, we are not presenting here, as was the case in the reference manual, an inventory of international conventions, binding United Nations resolutions or those of European ministers stemming from the European Parliament or the Council of Europe. Nor do we present the Geneva Oath, the European Code of Ethics, the Declarations of the World Medical Association, the CIOMS, Unesco, the WHO declarations on the promotion of patients' rights, nor the International Nursing Code of Ethics, nor the national Codes of Deontology, nor bodies of case-law on health matters. The rich literature on ethics, the list of journals, reports, the many meetings on the subject, none of these are mentioned.

Because of the vital importance of information and documentation in this rapidly changing field however, any research and any initiation into bioethics has to use these resources. All countries have one or more readily accessible documentation centres in this field. In France, training courses, and in particular those of our network, have the benefit of the diligent services of the Ethics Documentation and Information Centre of the National Consultative Ethics Committee and the National Institute for Health and Medical Research.

The Council of Europe has been a vector for human rights ever since its creation in 1947, co-opting its new members according to their application of these rights. For some years now the Council's Steering Committee for Bioethics, whose members are designated by individual states, had been working on a draft convention for the protection of human rights and dignity of the human being with regard to the application of biology and medicine, known as the "Convention on Human Rights and Biomedicine". This draft, which has now been adopted, contains several explicit appendices dealing with matters which are still the subject of controversy in Europe, such as experimentation on vulnerable persons and embryos, but it will not become a binding convention until after ratification by signatory states.

International emergence of biomedical ethics
Emergence of a certain distrust of scientific progress, causing the World Medical Association (WMA) to issue rules of good conduct

After Hiroshima and Nagasaki, it was the shock of the Nuremberg trials in 1947 which made people realise that scientific progress was by no means synonymous with human progress. Twenty German doctors were condemned for crimes against humanity for having put reasons of state before the Hippocratic Oath in their dangerous experimentation on human beings. These doctors nevertheless belonged to the only European country in which strict directives on new therapies and scientific experimentation on humans had been promulgated as early as 1900 and 1931.

The ten articles of the historic code established by the Nuremberg judges stress in particular: "the well-informed consent of the volunteer, the scientific and animal experimentation prerequisites, the absence of risk, the qualifications of the experimenters and the possibility of stopping the tests at any moment". The Geneva Oath and the International Code of Medical Ethics, amended in Sydney in 1968 and Venice in 1983 of the World Medical Association (WMA), founded in 1947, updating the Hippocratic Oath, take account of this code. After some regrettable American experiments, notably that of Tukesgee, the WMA's Declaration of Helsinki in 1964, on biomedical research on human subjects, amended in Tokyo in 1975, Venice in 1983 and Hong Kong in 1989, details the methods and conditions of experimentation, stipulating in particular that the association of research with care is justified only by its diagnostic or therapeutic usefulness for the patient and affirms the primacy of the subject's welfare over the interests of science and society.

Extension of the medicalisation of human activity

Since medicine became rational in the eighteenth century, the efforts made in the field have tended to save more and more lives, that is to increase the average age or life expectancy.

After Pasteur and the eradication of most infectious diseases in children, a trend which accelerated after the introduction of vaccination, after the discovery of antibiotics by Fleming, the fight against the major scourges such as cancer by means of radiotherapy, the goals of medicine seemed to have been achieved with the doubling of life expectancy in the space of a hundred years.

This being so, after Nuremberg and the birth of the first ethical principles, and in the general euphoria of the post-war period, the WHO in 1947 greatly extended the scope of medical care, defining health as being "a state of complete physical, mental and social well-being, which does not consist solely in an absence of disease or infirmity". The care person is no longer a simple healer, but is encouraged to help palliate anomalies in the functioning of the family and society which impair the individual's quality of life. Biotechnicians, hospital staff and carers now have to contribute to the "happiness" of their patients through allowing them to benefit, among other things, from contraception, abortion, medically assisted procreation and tranquillisers; they also have to ensure informed consent, take preventive action, ease the situation of the dying, all this while the training of practitioners is moving ever more towards highly effective, but dehumanised, scientific technique.

Despite this incitation to pay more attention to the spiritual and human needs of the patient, the many-faceted and rapid developments in medicine and biotechnology, treating diseases rather than patients, have deliberately moved away from holistic care. They have sometimes even taken a competitive path, typically "scientific", extending life but leading to a number of excesses calling into question a medical reliability which had been intact since Hippocrates. The purely scientific teaching of health care, neglecting the art, has become even more marked, subdividing the study and specialised treatment of parts of the human body, and casting aside psychology and other human sciences.

The rapid progress of molecular biology associated with sophisticated physico-chemical methods and computerised techniques, notably in the field of human genetics, has made it possible to discover medical conditions stemming from a perturbed personal genetic make up. This has led to very promising developments in preventive and predictive medicine, but also to a search for genetic factors affecting behaviour, thus threatening the secret of the identity of the human being. Genetic engineering permits the welcome production of essential substances such as insulin, hitherto derived from man, and the appearance of gene therapy, a real hope for the treatment of cancer. But the beginnings of a curative genetic medicine could, in uncontrolled and unscrupulous hands, threaten the human genetic stock through interference with the germ cell line.

In the United States, pioneers in this field under the impulsion of two Catholic theologians labelled as "liberal", D. Callahan and A.E. Hellegers, two now well-known ethical research centres were set up: the Hastings Centre in 1969 and the Kennedy Institute of Ethics in 1971. After J. Fletcher had called for real autonomy for the patient in 1954, F. Ramsey, also a Protestant theologian, published his celebrated *The patient as person* in 1970.

In Europe, *ad hoc* committees, colloquies, seminars and then training courses, following the example set by the United States and Canada, emerged some fifteen years ago in the United Kingdom, Spain, Belgium, the Netherlands, Denmark, Germany and Italy, often emanating from religious or lay centres.

In France, after the setting up of the multidisciplinary National Consultative Ethics Committee in 1983, initiatives multiplied in Lyons, Strasbourg, Lille, Paris, Marseilles and Toulouse.

Birth and evolution of bioethics

Bioethics, a term coined in 1970 by the American cancerologist V.R. Potter in order to express an approach for surviving and "living better" in a natural environment thanks to progress, has, like ethics, been defined in many ways and is still the subject of argument.

Concerned essentially with the human being in relation to his environment – nature, culture, society – bioethics covers a broader and much more interdisciplinary field than biomedical ethics, which is more limited to matters concerning carers and patients. Like ethics, it is not a transcendent morality of Good and Evil, nor an academic discipline like medicine to be passed on and applied. Regulatory in nature through its interdisciplinary prescriptions of reasonable and humane behaviour in research, therapy and the application of biotechnologies, it contains more than the legal rules governing citizens and society, and more than enforceable deontological standards primarily concerned with codes of good conduct between carers and patients.

Bioethics is to a large extent the experimental ethics laboratory in the field of life, and as such it embraces a rational metabioethics of principles and a normative bioethics oriented towards action. As with ethics, some commentators restrict bioethics to the basic principles guiding a morality for action. Others by contrast endow it with a very wide scope encompassing broad areas of human behaviour and the living world. Scientific rationality which, in the name of objectivity, sets aside subjectivity, feelings, tradition and morality, obviously does not constitute a sufficient basis or preparation for bioethics, despite the claims made by certain "scientists". In addition to honesty, scientific rigour and the search for truth, which form the basis of a good scientific training, bioethical thinking draws broadly on human qualities which are neither taught nor tested in university courses, and are sometimes even cast aside by researchers caught up in the fierce national and international rivalry orchestrated by certain media. These personal qualities, essential to any evaluation and any action, are by contrast given a high place in religious, and indeed agnostic, moralities, to which we have therefore turned in order to better guide the action of the scientist and the carer, with a view to ensuring better respect of the patient's beliefs.

The arrival of medically assisted procreation is inducing a medical ethics of principles and standards

Since the introduction and mastery of the techniques of medically assisted procreation, the many problems arising – legal, ethical, moral and social – have catalysed the emergence of multidisciplinary ethics committees with the task of translating moderation and prudence into ethical standards to replace what are considered to be outmoded moralities.

This approach, recalling that of Aristotle's prudent and virtuous man in his teleological quest for Good through a morality minimising the Bad, has promoted an "ethical" commitment and behaviour which better supplement the Hippocratic Oath than transcendental moralities now deemed inadequate for the many human problems raised.

The richness of the two aspects of the Greek etymology of the word "ethics" adds to the scope of the attributes whose usual definitions, too often pragmatic, are still numerous and sometimes contested. The *ethos* provides the rational, objective, universal, consensual bases, issued from the preservation of human dignity in the face of the technological advances that motivate ethical prescriptions. The *ethos*, made up of personal virtues such as compassion, love of art and humanity, "the clothing of the soul" (Jean Bernard), essential for any human behaviour implementing the *ethos*, is still sometimes assimilated to morality.

Attributes of human dignity
In the field of health, what are the consensual values, complementary to human rights and stemming from human dignity, which are to motivate the *ethos*? The human being, unique and non-exploitable subject, is the only living creature which has independent powers of reflection, decision and action and a sense of responsibility. He is guided by his reason, his prudence, his respect of the humanity of others.

For a micro-ethics of the carer-patient relationship, full information adapted to the patient, free choice for the patient and a search for a form of partnership are necessary. In a care team, this means information, concertation and the taking into account of a plurality of opinions.

Respect of the humanity of others and of human rights induces a striving for equity, solidarity and benevolence in a macro-ethics of public health.

The implementation of these values is effected through the intervention of the personal *ethos*. Spinoza tells us that "souls are not conquered by arms but by love and generosity".

These human values have issued from various sources – religious, cultural, philosophical – which long remained formal. They were sometimes contested, but they are now subjected to the supreme test of therapeutic and biotechnological progress.

Hinduism, Taoism, Confucianism, Buddhism, Judaism, Christianity and Islam all admit the primacy of the human being, his unicity, his involvement in a divine plan, and require the respect of his life and condemn his murder. The Old Testament, for example, affirms the pre-existence, for any law, of the fundamental alliance of standards between God and his people, which imposes duties. Jesus of Nazareth proclaimed the equality of all men in the eyes of God, in whose likeness they were created, which is the basis for their dignity.

In the name of their particular gods, three men – Hippocrates, fifth century BC, a Greek physician from Cos; Avicenna, born in 980, an Arab physician and philosopher (Ibn Sina), in his famous *Canon of medicine* and Maimonides, a Jewish physician and philosopher born in Cordoba in 1135, in his *Aphorisms of medicine* –

promulgated in the Greco-Roman civilisations and those stemming from them, and in the Arab and Jewish civilisations, certain solemn recommendations for carers: absolute respect of patients and their lives; never do them any harm; maintain confidentiality; respect the masters.

. These traditional human values, personal and common, thus contribute to a bioethics which regulates biotechnologies and new therapies, and not as some people fear, a bioethics stemming from and dependent upon biotechnologies.

Philosophical foundations of ethics and bioethics

Protagoras, a Greek sophist of the fifth century BC, already advocated agreed standards for conduct with man as the measure of all things.

Hippocrates, shortly afterwards, abandoned the supernatural conception of medicine and recommended systematic, clinical and holistic observation of disturbed vital functions in order to restore the natural conditions and defences of the sick person.

Aristotle, the founder of ethics twenty-four centuries ago, a partisan, like the Greek world of that time, of a heteronomic conception of Man, the external motor no longer being God but nature, recommended a prudent and harmonious development of the human being towards the good. This working towards good through a prudent rational approach is what motivates most members of ethics committees; more interested in resolving contentious cases and conflicting values by reaching a consensus than in imposing prohibitions.

However, while Aristotle may be considered the father of ethics, it is Immanuel Kant, an eighteenth-century German philosopher, who formulated the principles now accepted for the *ethos*. Confident in the resources of enlightened eighteenth-century man, he proposed an autonomic approach rooted in human reason and free of any metaphysical influence. These principles concern a human being above and beyond any material evaluation, not to be used as a means, but treated as an end. His sovereign reason endows him with a dignity rooted in the human and ensures his free will. His rational thought leads to universal principles to be respected as laws of nature, inciting a deontological approach which in fact accords with most religious moralities and the codes of conduct of health organisations. The essential distinction between people and things, which has extended to jurisprudence, the unconditional condemnation of all forms of slavery, all forms of torture, the respect of the embryo as a potential human being, all bear the mark of Kant.

The German Kantian J. Habermas, initially influenced by Marx and his dialectic, rejected Kant's innate rationality and postulated an essentially communicational rationality which seems in fact to be present in the multidisciplinary deliberations and pluralist opinions of ethics committees and interactive ethics training courses.

30

In sociology, this means an approach uniting solidarity and justice – very evident in humanitarian actions.

The well-known Harvard Kantian J. Rawls stresses the great influence for ethical formulation of the process of establishing equitable social justice, leading for example to being able to manage a plurality of beliefs and even to positive discrimination in favour of the most vulnerable patients.

In order to properly safeguard the factors protecting life, H. Jonas of Frankfurt proposes using a heuristic method based on the fear engendered by the present and foreseeable excesses of certain biotechnologies in order to arouse awareness in each person of his own responsibility, both here and now and *vis-à-vis* future generations. The formal prohibition of human chimera by all national, European and international authorities, the present concern with germ cell therapy and the affirmed will to conserve the human genetic stock appear indeed to be manifestations of this fear and this sense of responsibility.

R. Hare, a contemporary successor of the celebrated British utilitarian school of Jeremy Bentham and John Stuart Mill, has developed the concept of consequentialist utility, making it possible for example to treat, in a fashion acceptable to the society concerned, the greatest number of patients with limited resources. This concept led eight years ago to the introduction of "Qualys" (Quality Adjusted Live Years), sometimes recommended in order to be able to treat individuals and groups in the most cost-effective way for the society as a whole. A certain implementation of this concept permits the United Kingdom to treat each patient at a cost half that in France, but with very questionable ethical criteria, such as a ban on any dialysis after the age of 65 and of any transplantation over 70. It should be pointed out, however, that pragmatic utilitarian arguments are often put forward in ethics committees to try to achieve a consensus on the "least bad solution" in a given case.

H.F. Engelhardt, a post-Kantian, influential in the United States and in the ethical thinking of a western world grappling with a multitude of cultures and moralities which are hard to reconcile, advocates complete autonomy of thought and action for the conscious rational being, in the respect of pluralism of opinion and under the aegis of the principle of benevolence. The evolution in the United States of the carer-patient relationship towards a kind of written contract and the promotion of well-informed consent, notably taking account of all the risks, clearly appear to stem from this view. But the attribution of an absence of dignity in the case of the unconscious, the severely handicapped, those in vegetative coma and embryos, and the fostering of a geo-ethics in place of the universality of the Hippocratic Oath and the Geneva Oath are not attractive features.

E. Levinas stresses alterity and the respect of others as the basis of an ethics of proximity (micro-ethic). According to him, relations with others and with the community (macro-ethic) depend on a deontological process analogous to that of establishing justice. This dualism, sometimes the victim of divergent interests, is found in the preservation of certain interests of the patient despite public health service imperatives.

The search for a symbiosis in the discussion of cases within ethics committees, between deontological prescriptions and a teleology beneficial for the patient, seems indeed to generate an ethic of attestation combining conviction and responsibility, as desired by the contemporary French philosopher P. Ricœur.

How is an ethical approach to be guided in practice? We cannot simply advocate here a strictly scientific process consisting of the experimental application to each situation of principles derived from human rights and human dignity by a procedural method based on a descending order of priorities, since such an approach comes up against numerous particular cases and conflicts of values. In order to illustrate this approach we have therefore taken many examples in this book of situations in which no binding legal or deontological norms have yet been promulgated, thus permitting a specifically ethical approach. The ethical debate often begins in fact with a series of questions raised by a situation which is unforeseen or which presents a conflict of values to which due priority must be given in each case; the aim is to seek an optimum solution based on the least harm or the least ethical cost, in accordance with a consensus in acceptance of the various standards. Several members of ethics committees have observed that an interdisciplinary consensus on a given objective could be achieved by the practice of a very explanatory and open dialectic and concertation in association with a very Aristotelian *phronesis* (practical wisdom). The fundamental ethical step is, after all, as the well-known Kantian philosopher K.O. Apel put it, a full and equal recognition of the argumentation of each speaker and of its specificity.

However, agreement on the bases, essential to any training in bioethics, necessitates not only long confrontations of uncertain outcome, often connected with unshakeable convictions, but above all requires a truly "horizontal" interdisciplinary immersion which is very difficult to achieve in a "vertical" interdisciplinary culture which advocates specialisation. Thus it is scarcely possible for any complete training in bioethics to be dispensed solely by health actors, who are as yet unprepared for this interdisciplinary culture, despite the recent introduction, in France at least, of human sciences in first-year medical studies.

In the often difficult choice of obligations, sometimes contradictory, between an individualistic micro-ethic, favoured hitherto by medical deontologies and the opinions and recommendations of European and international organisations, and a macro-ethic of public health sought by those responsible for health services, certain forms of behaviour weigh heavily. Professor A. Fagot-Largeault, philosopher and psychiatrist, member of the French National Consultative Ethics Committee and a bioethics pioneer in Europe, reminds us, for example, that the health of the healthy

person who volunteers for biotechnological experimentation is much better protected than that of a sportsman or soldier, sacrificed for the team or the army without even the otherwise sacrosanct informed consent. In addition to pointing out the
risk of reducing living human material to the status of a mere "thing", she raises the
thought-provoking question as to whether this traditional ethic of individual autonomy will long remain compatible with the meteoric rise in the use of biological
"spare parts", assimilating the human body to a "public good" as has been recommended by adherents of agnostic morality.

Can we aid and guide this ethical approach by teaching, by giving an initiation
to and training in bioethics? A controversy having arisen over the feasibility of
bioethics teaching or training after the WMA Declarations of Madrid in 1987 and
Malta in 1991, and considering it essential for doctors to have a good training in
ethics, our network, on the initiative of Dr J.-P. Massué, decided to try to introduce
some pilot training courses at different levels, based on its two works and the voluntary contributions of its multidisciplinary members.

Training courses initiated by the network

There is an interdisciplinary training course of seventy-two hours spread over two
months, entitled "Medicine, ethics and human rights". It is given by some thirty high-
level European specialists: philosophers, jurists, doctors, researchers, theologians,
sociologists and members of national ethics committees and of international organisations such as NGOs, WHO and Unesco. Very interactive, the course follows a
methodology inspired by the approach of the practitioner, who, after having clearly
defined all the scientific aspects, the clinical options and the risks, seeks in the first
place to identify the legal constraints of the situation and his possible liability, then
tries to adopt an ethical approach, which is likely to be influenced by his convictions
and those of his patients. Three modules following this methodology are offered:

A. legal and deontological norms;

B. ethical standards and Catholic, Protestant, Jewish, Muslim, Buddhist and
agnostic moralities;

C. ethics, sociology, state, socioeconomic constraints, patients' rights, international solidarities. There are also a number of round tables or open debates on subjects such as: the status of the embryo; Aids and society; the patentability of the
human genome; experimentation on vulnerable persons; palliative care; dying
with dignity; ethics in the face of socioeconomic constraints.

This training has been offered since 1991 at the Centre for Medical Ethopsy-
chology and Human Ecology of the Université Pierre et Marie Curie – Paris VI. The
directors of studies are Professor J.M. Alby and myself, at the European Unit for
Training in Biomedical Ethics. The students come from many fields: members of
ethics committees, health system administrators, doctors, jurists, philosophers,

scientists, nurses, midwives. Courses are even open, like the round tables, to interested outsiders. The acceptance of a dissertation by the directors of studies leads to the award of a certificate.

Among the score of dissertations on current ethical problems presented so far, four have been rewarded by prizes, notably Médi-Futur: Ethical problems raised by organ transplants; Ethics, biology and the future. What humanity do we want?; Catholic and Buddhist morality and the problem of palliative care; agnosticism and medical bioethics.

A course in bioethics and human rights, compulsory and leading to an examination for students, but also open to interested outsiders, was organised during the synthesis term of the fifth year as early as 1992 in the Faculty of Pharmacy and Biological Sciences of the Université Descartes – Paris V, under the direction of Mrs D. Guillat-Demonchy, lecturer in this faculty.

This course was organised with the aid and under the aegis of our network, interested in the proper implementation of a second cycle university course of a dozen hours on this subject. A dozen high-level interdisciplinary contributors took part in the sessions and answered the questions raised by the students, who received our network's book as a textbook for the course.

This pilot course at the European level has aroused the sustained interest and questioning of the students and has been successful beyond all expectations. A number of theses have been submitted dealing with ethical aspects of such concrete problems as: Gene therapy; Medically assisted procreation; Preventive medicine; Palliative care for terminal cancer patients.

At our suggestion, the National Pedagogic Committee for Pharmaceutical and Biological Studies in France has made the study of bioethics and human rights compulsory in the official programme of preparation for a doctorate in pharmacy and biological sciences. Mrs D. Guillat-Demonchy has just been appointed to a specially created post in pharmaceutical bioethics and has been invited by several countries to help them set up similar courses.

There has been training in ethics since 1991 at the nursing training institute in Neufchâteau-Vittel, and study sessions for external teachers are organised. Those in charge are Miss M.-Th. Mangin, nursing teacher, and Mrs M. Jh. Bougard, Head of nursing at the Neufchâteau Hospital (Vosges).

A number of nursing training institutes in France – Bar-le-Duc, Chaumont, Nancy, Remiremont, Saint-Dié – have recently introduced similar training in ethics, and are using the works produced by our network.

The experimental training manual is also used by the ANIG (*Association nationale des infirmières générales*), the UNASIIF (*Union nationale des associations et syndicats infirmiers and infirmières de France*), and the Institutes of Angers, Grenoble, Rouen, Val d'Aoste (Italy) and Alcalá de Henares (Spain).

The network has helped organise a number of awareness-raising seminars and training courses in bioethics and human rights in several countries, in particular Lebanon.

This book contains contributions by twenty-two authors from four European countries and five disciplines.

Mrs M. Scalabrino, Associate Professor of International Law at the Sacred Heart University in Milan, despite the great dispersion of sources of international law, her many commitments and very limited help, has been kind enough to pursue her research which began back in 1985 for the manual and the fascicule, and write detailed replies to the cases in a limited time. She also contributes to our training courses at the Université Pierre et Marie Curie, for which we owe special thanks.

Some commentators, in particular a number of English-speaking colleagues, thought that the opinions of non-interdisciplinary medical organisations were more deontological than ethical, as is the case with the rules of medical councils, which are often binding and carry disciplinary penalties. Henry Anrys, former legal adviser to the World Medical Association, author of the introduction on "Medical Ethics and human rights" and answers to the first fifty-eight cases, also a contributor at Pierre et Marie Curie, points out, however, that the opinions of the WMA, duly concerted, are, like those of ethics committees, only recommendations on which member associations and ethics committees may draw, without any obligation. These opinions are therefore genuinely ethical in nature.

We benefited from the great experience of Dr A. Wynen, an experienced practitioner and former very active General Secretary of the WMA, who was kind enough to continue Maître Anrys' work and write the answers to the new cases. He too makes a valuable contribution to our courses at Pierre et Marie Curie.

Professor A. Piga Rivero, formerly Head of the WHO Regional Office for Europe, Director of the Health and Medico-Social Sciences of the University of Alcalá de Henares (Madrid), WHO correspondent and regular lecturer at Pierre et Marie Curie, was kind enough, together with Professor T. Alfonso Galán, to present a broad historic and international view of patients' rights.

Monsignor E. Sgreccia, Professor of Bioethics at the University of the Sacred Heart in Rome, General Secretary of the Vatican Committee for the Family, Vice-President of the Pontifical Academy for Life, assisted by Dr G. Fasanella and Dr A.-G. Spagnolo, made his valuable contribution despite his new responsibilities.

Despite the fact that Protestant morality focuses essentially on conscience and individual responsibility, and is made up of several not always convergent trends, Professor J.-F. Collange of the Faculty of Protestant Theology in Strasbourg, recently elected Vice-Chancellor of the University of Human Sciences and Dean of the Faculty of Protestant Theology, was kind enough, in collaboration with P.-E. Panis, theologian, to fill a gap deplored by us all when the reference manual appeared,

35

and also to make a much appreciated contribution to our courses at Pierre et Marie Curie.

We are very grateful to Chief Rabbi A. Guigui of the Central Jewish Consistory of Belgium for having been good enough, despite the absence of a magisterium in the Jewish religion, to set out the essential aspects of its morality and its impact on health. We also thank him for his faithful contribution to our courses at Pierre et Marie Curie.

Dr F. Ben Hamida, Honorary Director of Research in Molecular Biology at the CNRS and former member of the French National Consultative Ethics Committee, kindly gave us the benefit of his twin scientific and Koranic culture, pointing out the essential points of Muslim morality and participating very actively, for five years now, in our courses at Pierre et Marie Curie. On his initiative, the replies to the cases concerned with nursing care were written by Dr G.H. Hadj Eddine Sari Ali, a theologian of repute, adviser to the Muslim Institute of the Paris Mosque and also a teacher in our courses.

It is often said that moral reactions in Europe are entirely inspired by the Judaeo-Christian tradition. We were therefore aware of the interest of a comparison of Judaeo-Christian and Muslim religious prescriptions with those of a wholly different tradition. The considerable development of Buddhist trends in Europe, the moral authority of the Dalai Lama, the highly specific basis of this philosophy and its oriental origins convinced us of the interest of presenting the Buddhist replies. Dr J. Martin, Chairman of the Buddhist Union of France, kindly provided these in consultation with his specialist colleagues, in particular Dr C. Chevassut, trainer in palliative care, and Dr M.-A. Pratili, gynaecologist and cancerologist, who lectures on this morality in our courses. Apart from organ transplants, where the continued presence of the spirit in the lifeless body calls for a wait of three days, except in the case of accident, the replies are similar to those of the other religious moralities which, moreover, agree on many essential values.

However, many jurists, scientists, members of the care professions, teachers and students do not wish to make use of any religious references. We have therefore tried to include the motivations of a lay, rationalist morality, which we have called with due reserve an "agnostic morality". After a number of attempts, we found in the late Professor R. Leray, former Grand Master of the Grand Orient of France and member of the French National Consultative Ethics Committee, someone willing to set out the main lines of such a morality, namely a resolute faith in man and human solidarity. At our request, representatives of the Grand Orient of France and the Rationalist Union of France have contributed to our training courses each year. Thanks to the constant efforts of Dr J. Brunschwig, faithful and active participant in our training, and despite the prevalence of personal choice in this morality, Mr H. Caillavet, former minister, Vice-President of the Rationalist Union, member of the

French National Consultative Ethics Committee and active promoter of associations advocating the application of the prescriptions of agnostic morality, was kind enough to consult with his colleagues and provide us with some essential elements, for which we express our sincere thanks.

As can be seen, there is a substantial base of "invariants" common to these moralities and to ethics, which can be used in this procedural approach. This is very encouraging from the standpoint of the international promotion of common values concerning human dignity. On the other hand, the recommendations of normative ethics should naturally be adapted to cultures.

A philosopher familiar with the medical world, C. Canguilhem, wrote indeed in his early work, when presenting his thesis in Strasbourg in 1943, that the standard for all standards in this field remained convergence.

Nursing practice and ethics

by Clette Pierre-Evrard,
Head of Nursing Services, France

Nursing has particular characteristics, namely:
– round-the-clock activity, meaning that nurses may find themselves alone with no doctor present, especially at night;
– the specific nature of nursing care, which is concerned with satisfying the patient's basic needs, means that at times the nurse's role *vis-à-vis* the patient closely resembles that of parent, spouse, child, sister or brother, grandparent or confidante, a type of relationship which is rare among doctors, who are perceived more as technicians, "idols" or friends.

All this means that nurses are confronted every day with situations which present dilemmas and force them to take decisions, and they have to live with the consequences of these decisions. The ethical questions with which nurses are regularly confronted seem to increase proportionally with the progress of health care technology, without there being any parallel development of awareness of the ethical implications of the care process.

Thus all nurses find themselves obliged to try to develop a rational base and a system of values to guide them when taking ethical decisions which will promote the aims of their profession and enable them to live and act according to their conscience.

In this regard it may be asked whether nurses' values and ethical standards will prevent them from participating in certain types of intervention, and if so what the consequences of such decisions will be. Will they lose money, or their job, or suffer some other loss?

The ethical dimension of the profession was concomitant with its creation

Published in 1893 by Lystra Gretter, Florence Nightingale's Oath was the first ethical code for nurses, recognised first in the United States, then in the rest of the world:

"I promise before God and in the presence of this assembly to live properly and to faithfully exercise my profession.
I shall abstain from anything which is harmful and I shall neither take nor knowingly administer any harmful drug.
I shall do everything in my power to raise the level of my profession and I shall keep in confidence all personal information confided to me and all family business which I may come to know through the practice of my calling.

I shall loyally help the doctor in his work and I shall devote myself to the service of all those entrusted to me for care."[1]

This oath remains in fact the basis of the nurse's commitment and the fundamental component of their code of conduct.

The Trained Nurse and Hospital Review, the first American journal of nursing practice, which appeared in the 1880s, ran a series of articles on nursing ethics.

Since it first appeared in the first decade of this century, the *American Journal of Nursing* has published hundreds of articles focused on ethical issues.

Between 1900 and 1960 over sixty works on nursing were devoted to this subject, the first being that published by Isabel Hampton Robb in 1900, entitled *Nursing ethics: for hospital and private use.*

The foundations of the nursing profession

In 1850 Florence Nightingale published a study devoted to hospital organisation and administration: *Notes on hospitals.*

In 1860 she realised her ambition: the creation of the first school for nurses at St Thomas Hospital. She wrote the basic textbook *Notes on nursing* in 1859.

Florence Nightingale's main lines of thought

Florence Nightingale had two main ideas in mind, both still valid today: nursing care for the sick and nursing care for health.

She said that correct nursing for the sick consisted of helping the patient to live, while nursing care for health consisted of maintaining the health of a human being at a stage where it did not develop any sickness.

A very moving quotation from Florence Nightingale's diary at the height of the Crimean War read: "I am close to the altar of these dead men and as long as I live I shall defend their cause."

Attention should also be drawn to the values substituted by Florence Nightingale for the religious values in nursing activity: promotion of health and preventive action; and defence of the quality of care and the rehabilitation of women in nursing practice.[2]

The concept of "care" has been associated with the nurse since Florence Nightingale wrote her *Notes on nursing,* in use from 1860:

---

1. Florence Nightingale's Oath was drafted by a special committee nominated by the board of the Farrand School of Harper Hospital in Detroit in 1893. The name was chosen because Florence Nightingale represents the highest level of nursing and an ideal. Quoted from the editorial of the *American Journal of Nursing,* 11 (10) 777, 11 July 1893, USA.
2. *Les infirmières,* Syros, Paris 1992.

"An essentially interpersonal philosophy of therapeutic care puts the accent on the nursing role as that through which the nurse helps the patient to establish more comfortable interpersonal relations. It is through obtaining this comfort and through the fact that the nurse shows herself to be capable of controlling her feelings that she increases her capacity to care for patients. It also helps to see the patient in a holistic fashion and to abandon the traditional role, which simply authorises the satisfaction of the patient's physical needs, for a more active role which encourages her to use her health potential and become a real agent for health."

Peplau (1952) says that: "If a patient has difficulties with the fact of living, it is then the nurse's function to help him with this experience of living his full life."[1]

Constant concern for ethics
Right from its creation in 1899, the International Council of Nurses (ICN) has been concerned with the ethical and legal aspects of nursing practice.

Thus on the ethical plane nurses now have in addition to Florence Nightingale's Oath the International Code of Ethics adopted by the Grand Council of the ICN in São Paulo, Brazil, on 10 July 1953, subsequently revised in May 1973 and finally drafted in its present form and adopted by the Council of National Representatives of the ICN in Mexico City. Used all over the world, it is based on traditional ethical principles and sets out general guidelines adaptable to all cultures and deals with all aspects of a nurse's life as a professional.

In Europe, the best known national nursing code is that of the Royal College of Nursing in the United Kingdom, translated into several languages, including French, by the ICN. It was published in 1978 in an ICN work intended for nurses throughout the world entitled *The nurse's dilemma: considerations of professional deontology in nursing practice.*

At each advance in the reflection and work on the ethics of nursing practice at international level, the national associations belonging to the ICN, totalling 112 countries at the time, were invited to make the latest work known to the nurses and nursing schools of their respective countries. In addition, nurses were encouraged to inform the ICN directly of any problems of professional ethics, resolved or otherwise, which they themselves had experienced.

The moral, human and ethical constants which govern the nursing function are sometimes confused with the actual concept of nursing practice, defined in France as follows by Article 1 of Decree 93-345 of 15 March 1993 on professional acts in the exercise of the nursing profession:

---

1. I. Graham, *Vaincre la douleur*, Paris 1990, *Mouvement associatif des infirmières de la Seine-Saint-Denis.*

"Nursing care, preventive, curative or palliative, is of a technical, relational and educative nature. Its practice takes account of the evolution of science and techniques. The purpose is, while respecting the professional rules of nurses, including professional secrecy in particular:
– to protect, maintain, restore and promote the health of persons or the autonomy of their vital physical and mental functions, taking account of the psychological, social, economic and cultural components of the personality of each of them;
– to foresee and evaluate people's suffering and distress and to help relieve them;
– to contribute to the collection of information and methods which will be used by the doctor to establish his diagnosis;
– to participate in the evaluation of people's degree of dependence;
– to administer the medical prescriptions and treatments established by the doctor;
– to participate in the clinical monitoring of patients and the development of therapies;
– to favour the maintenance, insertion or reinsertion of people in their family and social environment;
– to comfort terminal patients, and where necessary their families."

Reasons why nurses have contributed to this work
If we are asked why nurses are interested in such a work, the answers are already to be found in the other introductions:
– the discovery that certain questions have no answer in terms of law, as pointed out by Mrs Scalabrino;
– the discovery that there are many questions to which there are answers but which are experienced in everyday life as having no answer or one which is too uncertain. In this sense, the inclusion of actual nursing cases in this book will help bring answers to nurses through another channel than that of their corporation, thus facilitating exchange and decision-making
– the discovery that, as Professor Guido Gerin puts it: "'Human rights' refer, of course, to the whole human being, and include, therefore, human dignity, liberty and health";
– the discovery that through using this work common to different socioprofessional categories, nurses find themselves on the same wavelength as the other health care professionals as regards ethics.
It is only right that nurses should make their contribution to the construction of this work, but it is also true that having joined the project when it was already under way they cannot do so as freely as would have been the case in other circumstances. Thus a work of reflection produced by our Greek colleague Afroditi Raya

is marked with the seal of orthodox belief, but it has to be observed that the standpoint of orthodox morality does not appear in this work.

This in no way diminishes the European value of the work, nor that of the cases more particularly concerned with nursing practice. The references proposed are of a nature to rally nurses to the main objective pursued by the work, namely that of guiding them in their professional activity and in their choices in accordance with human rights and dignity, for as Professor P. Cüer says: "it is likely that considerations of principle would remain relatively inaccessible to teachers, researchers, practitioners and patients if ethical or moral recommendations were not capable of giving a clear indication, for each important act, of the way the care decision should go, at the risk of creating conflicts of values to be discussed and if possible ranked".

The participation of nurses in this work bears witness to their reflection on man and their contribution to giving him all the means of advancement and enjoyment of his own dignity as R. Leray says in his introduction.

The objectivity of the information in this book is a prime necessity to nurses who by virtue of their numbers constitute the essential force for the generalisation of its content, hence the need today to alert, inform and educate all health professionals about ethics.

The cases

The cases we collected came from Greece, Belgium and France. They were very numerous: seventy-one for the three countries. Since many of them overlapped with cases already treated in the book, we considered it advisable to proceed to a selection before going on to collect data in other European countries, so as to be able to give more details to the professionals called upon so that they can submit cases specifically concerned with nursing.

The cases received were often accompanied by numerous queries on different aspects of a single question; others were concrete cases expressing fears about crossing the administrative and legal boundaries of the exercise; others again were presented as textbook examples richly documented and commented and supported by evidence from foreign studies and personal reflections.

It is obvious that judgments will probably be made on the situations or cases presented by the nurses, but such was the risk and it was gladly accepted. For the rest, a deliberate choice was made not to move outside the general standpoint of the book.

Lastly, the presentation of the nursing cases under four headings – migrants, family, human rights and satisfaction of the individual's basic needs – appears to us acceptable.

43

Rules and principles of international law in the field of health

by Michelangela Scalabrino,
Associate Professor of International Law,
Catholic University, Milan

It is unfortunately impossible in such a short introduction to discuss the rules and principles of international law now in force, concerning health in general and the doctor-patient relationship in particular as thoroughly as these subjects deserve.

This is not only due to the complexity of the problems raised, but also because these problems are discussed and dealt with at international level by a fairly large and ever-increasing number of normative and quasi-normative, binding and non-binding, enforceable and non-enforceable legal instruments.

In addition to the conventions and outline treaties of a universal nature (for example the United Nations Covenant on Civil and Political Rights, the United Nations Covenant on Economic, Social and Cultural Rights) or of a "regional" nature (the European Convention for the Protection of Human Rights and Fundamental Freedoms, the Inter-American Convention on Human Rights, the African Charter on Human and Peoples' Rights) aimed at protecting human rights and fundamental freedoms, there are in fact several sectorial conventions as well as a considerable number of decisions adopted by the IGOs,[1] in particular the resolutions and recommendations of the Committee of Ministers and the Parliamentary Assembly of the Council of Europe; the resolutions of the United Nations General Assembly; the resolutions and recommendations of the WHO; the regulations and directives of the EEC[2] and the resolutions of the European Parliament.

In addition to these instruments there is also the case-law of the international legal bodies, namely the Commission and Court of Human Rights (Council of Europe) and the International Committee of Human Rights, instituted by the Optional Protocol to the United Nations Covenant on Civil and Political Rights.

The decisions of the Commission, the judgments of the Court and the observations of the Committee, while applying the European Convention on Human Rights and the Covenant, have in fact in the course of time become occasions for evolutive and even innovative interpretations of these texts, thus enriching international law through the effects of living jurisprudence, once exclusively known to common law.

Despite its multiple sources, international law today in force is not yet capable of solving all the legal problems raised by the most recent applications of

---

1. IGO: Intergovernmental organisation.
2. EEC: European Economic Community (European Union).

biotechnology and medical science, and by the new frontiers of biomedical research. There are several reasons for this.

First we must take account of the fact that the entire legal universe has been put to the test by unforeseeable events, difficult to deal with in terms of traditional categories and concepts. But while each national legal system makes its own choice with reference to, and in the context of, a given society, pluralistic though it may be, international law must be able to be referred to by a multitude of states and individuals with rather diverse characteristics.

Several questions stemming from advances in medicine and biology may in fact have different, or even conflicting, legal solutions, depending on the religious, philosophical, moral or ethical ideas imposed or adopted.

Moreover, it must not be forgotten that states always jealously guard their decision-making powers, which both makes the process of consent necessary for the adoption of any new international act or instrument very slow, and makes it difficult at times to adapt domestic law to international requirements.

The path taken by international law, in particular in the field of human rights, is irreversible however, the demand for common solutions, worked out from the standpoint of respect for the human being, being increasingly strongly voiced by national, professional and legal circles.

Proof of this is the Convention for the Protection of Human Rights and Dignity of the Human Being with regard to the Application of Biology and Medicine: Convention on Human Rights and Biomedicine, drafted by the Council of Europe's Steering Committee on Bioethics, and adopted on 4 April 1997.

Reference has been made to this convention in the cases presented below.

Since these pages are addressed principally to non-jurists, it is useful to give an overview, even if brief, of the sources of international law referred to in this work.

International law, as is known, imposes on states duties and obligations which are intended to be applied to domestic law.

Nevertheless, the degree of penetration of the international provisions in to national systems varies according to the legal nature of the rules concerned, that is whether they are compulsory or not.

In the first case, states are bound to comply with the engagements freely agreed upon or decided by the decision-making organs of the IGOs, in the second they remain free to implement or not the international provisions, which then appear to be more guidelines than legal provisions.

As regards the obligatory legal provisions, a distinction has to be made between binding and non-binding rules, according to whether they stipulate duties or obligations.

As regards the former, there may be no exception or delay in the adaptation of national law; as a result, the violation of one of these standards entails the international liability of the defaulting state.

As regards the latter, any, the obligation is fulfilled once the states take the steps they deem appropriate to achieve the goals set, without there being any time limit. In fact, states cannot be forced to accelerate the process of adapting domestic law to the international law, nor even to start this process, if they invoke other priorities or a lack of economic or financial resources. As a result, violation by default of one of these rules does not entail the liability of the state at international level.

Having set out these principles, let us now look more closely at the classification of international acts and instruments according to their nature and legal effects:

a. International treaties and conventions (including supplementary protocols), the primary source of modern international law, are obligatory for member states from the date of signature and ratification when requested.

Member states are thus bound to conform domestic law to such international instruments, which namely means to abrogate incompatible previous domestic laws and to enact laws necessary for these instruments to be fully complied with.

Moreover, treaties and conventions which put upon states the duty to abstain from undermining the human rights of individuals (for example the prohibition of torture, inviolability of the person and of personal freedom) are binding, and even immediately binding.

The same is true when the state can fully comply with its obligations only through the promulgation of domestic laws, as in the case of several international provisions relating to human rights and fundamental freedoms (for example Articles 2, 8 and 10 of the European Convention on Human Rights). These tend – it is true – mainly to protect individuals against arbitrary interference by public authorities, but the effective respect of the rights and freedoms involved cannot be achieved if states do not take measures to permit those concerned to fully enjoy the rights they derive from these provisions.

As a result, according to the established case-law of the European Court of Human Rights, states are constrained by the "positive obligation" to enact appropriate law for this purpose, as well as to undertake any other necessary activity.

Various options are open to states in these cases, but legislation which does not provide effective respect of one of the fundamental rights or of the positive obligations related thereto infringes against the international provisions concerned and entails the international liability of the defaulting state.

On the other hand, where the international treaties or conventions impose on states obligations involving economic resources (which is the case in particular of the Covenant on Economic, Social and Cultural Rights), the provisions are obligatory, but not binding.

However, to avoid a lack of resources depriving these provisions of any practical effect and hence preventing the implementation of the rights concerned, the United Nations Economic and Social Council watches carefully to ensure that states conform, even if only gradually, with the obligations that concern them, notably through international co-operation with other member states and the specialised agencies of the United Nations.

International treaties and conventions concern not only states, but also, more frequently than it might be thought, individuals, nationals and/or foreigners legally present or domiciled in the territories concerned.

The obligatory and binding rules, conventions and treaties are enforceable by individuals, if they are concerned, as soon as ratified; conversely, obligatory but non-binding legal rules, even if signed and duly ratified by member states, are not enforceable by individuals, even when they are concerned.

It is worth pointing out at this stage that the principle of sovereignty still allows states to enact the laws of their choice, including laws incompatible with obligatory and binding international provisions signed and duly ratified.

The state's international liability is in this case involved: nevertheless, individuals being subject to domestic law legislation, the rights they derive from the international provisions are negated.

In order to avoid this consequence the constitutions of several states now stipulate the primacy of international conventional law, and in particular international conventions on human rights, over domestic law, so that no subsequent national law can void obligatory and binding international provisions actionable by individuals.

b. Besides international treaties and conventions, which involve protracted preliminary work, contemporary international law has other instruments which enable it to evolve more rapidly. This is the field of the law-making and quasi-law-making instruments adopted by the IGOs.

First, the resolutions adopted by the United Nations General Assembly, the Committee of Ministers and Parliamentary Assembly of the Council of Europe, and by the European Parliament, by virtue of the constitutive treaty and the statutory obligations, are obligatory for member states, and sometimes even binding.

Violation of a resolution by default or by a subsequent incompatible law entails the international liability of the state *vis-à-vis* the IGO.

Since resolutions are exclusively addressed to states, they are not actionable by individuals (nationals or foreigners), even if they are concerned. However, IGO resolutions are, nevertheless, being increasingly applied by courts, if not as a source of law, at least as criteria for the interpretation of national laws.

Recommendations are not obligatory for member states, nor *a fortiori*, actionable by individuals.

Experience shows, however, that states are more inclined to adopt domestic laws to recommendations than to sign an international convention, which would not only oblige them more strictly, but would often submit them to control by *ad hoc* bodies, as it is the case for example with the committees set up by the two

Conventions for the Prevention of Torture and Inhuman or Degrading Treatment or Punishment.

   c. The law-making instruments formulated within the European Union, in particular the regulations and directives, deserve a special mention.

   Regulations, obligatory and binding for both member states and individuals (persons and legal entities), constitute an exception, indeed the only exception, to the general principle of the necessity for national laws to give effect to the legal instruments adopted by the IGOs.

   They are in fact directly and immediately applicable within member states as soon as they are published in the *Official Journal* of the European Union, and also actionable in courts by individuals concerned.

   In addition, European regulations have primacy not only over existing national laws but also over subsequent laws, if these conflict with the regulations.

   As for directives, these are addressed to member states, making them responsible for obtaining results.

   The objectives indicated are obligatory and binding, though the states remain free to choose the ways and means by which they are to be achieved. The deadline set by the directives is also obligatory and binding.

   Violation of a directive by default entails the liability of the state *vis-à-vis* both the European Union and other member states.

   According to the established case-law of the European Court of Justice, directives are actionable by individuals, when their rights are concerned.

   d. Lastly, mention must be made of the case-law of the European Commission and Court of Human Rights[1] of the Council of Europe and the United Nations Committee on Human Rights.

   As regards the European system, the Commission and the Court have the task of ensuring the respect of the commitments resulting for member states from the European Convention on Human Rights and its protocols, in particular Protocols Nos. 1, 4, 6 and 7.

   For this purpose the Convention stipulates that any person, any non-governmental organisation or group of individuals claiming to be the victim of a violation of the Convention by a member state may submit an individual application to the Commission in the case where the state concerned has declared that it recognises the competence of the Commission in this matter.

   The application may be addressed to the Commission only after all domestic remedies have been exhausted, member states being bound in the first place to conform domestic laws to the provisions of the Convention and to apply it.

---

1. Our analysis of the case-law of the Court goes up to March 1996.

After having established the facts, and, where appropriate, tried to arrive at an amicable settlement, the Commission drafts a report and expresses an opinion on the point of whether the observed facts reveal on the part of the state concerned a violation of the obligations incumbent upon it under the terms of the Convention. This report is transmitted to the Committee of Ministers.

Within three months of this transmission the case may be brought before the Court, which settles it by means of a judgment, with which member states are obliged to comply. It is for the Committee of Ministers to ensure compliance.

If the Court judgment holds that a decision taken or a measure ordered by a legal authority or any other authority of a member state is partly or wholly in opposition with the obligations stemming from the Convention, and if the relevant domestic law permits only the partial remedy of the consequences of this decision or this measure, the Court judgment, where appropriate, grants fair compensation to the injured party.

It should be noted that individual application to the European Commission of Human Rights (and, after the coming into force of Protocol No. 9, referral of a case to the Court by an individual, after a decision by the Commission on admissibility) constitutes the very first example of access of individuals to an international legal authority and a notable exception to the international default of *locus standi* in the case of the individual.

The exception shall became even more remarkable after the entering into force of Protocol No. 11, signed in Strasbourg on 11 May 1994, because individuals will apply directly to the Court, without going through the stage of the prior examination by the Commission on admissibility.

As regards complaints addressed to the UN Committee of Human Rights, findings of violation of the Covenant on Civil and Political Rights are not binding for member states. It is thus for the defaulting state to conform spontaneously or not to the points of law in the finding.[1]

Having briefly outlined the international system, it remains to evaluate what is the attitude of the international law today in force towards health problems, notably from the standpoint of the respect of the person, his rights and his fundamental freedoms.

The interest of the IGOs, and in particular the Council of Europe, in this connection clearly emerges from reading the texts, whether it be a matter of protecting

---

1. The problem of "double decisions" of the European Court of Human Rights and findings of the UN Human Rights Committee was settled by Resolution (70) 17 of the Committee of Ministers of the Council of Europe: the complaint may be taken to the Committee in the case of rights not guaranteed in the European Convention or where the state is not a party to this Convention or has not yet accepted the competence of the European Commission of Human Rights as regards individual applications.

prisoners or persons with mental disorders placed as involuntary patients, the rights of women and of children born inside and outside marriage, the rights of migrant workers and their families, and also the removal and transplantation of organs from persons capable or not capable of consent, medical databanks and, more recently, the use of human embryos and foetuses for diagnostic, therapeutic, industrial and commercial purposes, and in scientific research, or again the protection of Aids patients or prenatal genetic screening and diagnosis.

The High Contracting Parties to the Treaty of London would never have dared prophesy in May 1949 that the decisional organs of the Council of Europe would have managed to embark on an activity on such a large scale, nor even those who drafted the European Convention on Human Rights at the time of its signature in Rome on 4 November 1950.

But the same is true of the San Francisco Charter and the United Nations General Assembly with respect to a great many of the resolutions adopted, which have since become international conventions.

This being said, the fact remains that both the Council of Europe and the United Nations protect the individual in the health field mainly by means of quasi-normative legal instruments (resolutions) or non-normative instruments (recommendations).

A few passages of Judgment No. 232 C of 25 March 1992 handed down by the European Court of Human Rights in the case of *B. v. France*, explain this fact very well:

> "According to the applicant, science appears to have contributed two new elements to the debate on [the problem concerned] (...). As regards the legal aspects of the problem (...) the differences which still subsisted between the member states of the Council of Europe as the attitude to be adopted towards transsexuals were counterbalanced to an increasing extent by developments in the legislation and case-law of many of those states. This was supported by resolutions and recommendations of the Assembly of the Council of Europe and the European Parliament. Finally, the applicant stressed the rapidity of social changes in the countries of Europe, and the diversity of cultures represented by those countries which had adapted their laws to the situation of transsexuals. The government did not deny that science had in the twentieth century, especially in the last three decades, made considerable advances in the use of sexual hormones and in plastic and prosthetic surgery (...). National laws were also evolving and many of them had already changed, but the new laws thus introduced did not lay down identical solutions. In short, things were in a state of flux, legally, morally and socially. The Court considers that it is undeniable that attitudes have changed, science has

progressed and increasing importance is attached to the problem of trans-sexualism. It notes, however, in the light of the relevant studies carried out and work done by experts in this field, that there still remains some uncertainty as to the essential nature of transsexualism and that the legitimacy of surgical intervention in such cases is sometimes questioned. The legal situations which result are, moreover, extremely complex: anatomical, biological, psychological and moral problems in connection with transsexualism and its definition; consent and other requirements to be complied with before any operation; the conditions under which a change of sexual identity can be authorised (validity, scientific presuppositions and legal effects of recourse to surgery, fitness for life with the new sexual identity); international aspects (place where the operation is performed); the legal consequences, retrospective or otherwise, of such a change (rectification of civil status documents); the opportunity to choose a different forename; the confidentiality of documents and information mentioning the change; effects of a family nature (right to marry, fate of an existing marriage, filiation), and so on. On these various points there is as yet no sufficiently broad consensus between the member states of the Council of Europe to persuade the Court to reach opposite conclusions to those in its Rees and Cossey judgments."

Where the differences of view between member states – and even within member states – are still considerable, the activity of the decision-making bodies of the IGOs working towards solutions which, allthough not immediately acceptable to all members and all milieux, are likely to impregnate the legislation to come, must necessarily use flexible instruments, capable of being modified and amended over time, following the advance and/or evolution of science.

The capacity to propose itself, nevertheless, as an inspirer of principles is becoming the "strong point "of international law today, whereas it seems to be (and to some extent is) the "weak point".

While quasi-normative and non-binding international legal instruments continue along the path of protecting the health of the human being – as well as the human being in the field of health – from the "positive" standpoint, the fact remains that interference in the exercise of rights and fundamental freedoms remains the prerogative of obligatory and binding instruments, namely international treaties and conventions.

International law has in fact no hesitation on this subject, and the same is true as regards the case-law of the international organs of justice.

To be convinced of this, it suffices to recall the established case-law of the Court with respect to Article 5 of the European Convention on Human Rights, as regards not only persons arrested or detained, but also persons with mental disorders:

"The Commission likewise stresses that there must be no element of arbitrariness; the conclusion it draws is that no one may be confined as 'a person of unsound mind' in the absence of medical evidence establishing that his mental state is such as to justify his compulsory hospitalisation (...) The Court fully agrees with this line of reasoning. In the Court's opinion, except in emergency cases, the individual concerned should not be deprived of his liberty unless he has been reliably shown to be of 'unsound mind'" (Judgment No. 33).

In addition, the Convention for the Protection of Human Rights and Dignity of the Human Being with regard to the Application of Biology and Medicine shows us that the time has come for the adoption of an obligatory and binding international convention concerned with human rights and fundamental freedoms in the field of health.

The constant emphasis in international legal instruments on respect of the integrity and identity of the person, as well as his dignity, in particular with respect to the weakest and most disadvantaged, has in fact already had beneficial effects on national legislations, so that national law granting individuals less extensive protection than that provided by the acts and instruments of international law are no longer conceivable.

The fact remains, however, that serious problems can arise at any moment in the doctor-patient relationship, for example the problems associated with the fuzzy boundaries between the administration of due treatment and relentless prolongation of life, and between relentless prolongation of life, due treatment and what is known as "passive" euthanasia, in particular with respect to patients in the terminal phase. These problems are still unresolved, and probably will remain so for some time, especially if detailed and precise answers are expected, stipulated by obligatory and binding provisions.

Perhaps international law will show all its limitations in this respect, but can blame be attached to international law for not succeeding where the philosophical, ethical and moral debates have been raging for two thousand years?

Nobody doubts indeed that the law, all the law, can sometimes do no more than stop at the boundaries of conscience, and that at this stage each one of us, in his turn, can do no more than continue on his own along the paths and ways indicated by it.

In conclusion, permit me to evoke the memory of my father, a generous and knowledgeable physician, who would have liked to introduce me to the art of healing, and to associate with him the memory of Doctor Joseph Farber, with whom I worked so much on the first version of this work, "for a thousand years in thy sight are but as yesterday when it is past, and as a watch in the night" (Psalms 90, 4).

Medical ethics and human rights

by Henry Anrys,
Legal Adviser to the World Medical Association

Ethics and human rights

Whatever the legal or social context, a medical intervention, that is, diagnosis and treatment of a patient, takes place in private. The doctor is alone and the patient is alone.

The patient has a host of rights, but what he expects of the doctor is ultimately that he should do his best, that he should give him conscientious, diligent care in keeping with the latest state of medical knowledge. This dialogue, which has been described as an encounter between trust and conscience, is safeguarded by the ethics of the doctor, whose conduct must be governed by the interests and wishes of the patient. Ethics and human rights merge: respect for the patient's free and informed decision, but also respect of his choice of doctor and freedom of treatment, which give meaning to informed consent since these choices suppose an alternative, respect for life, respect for human dignity, respect for privacy and professional secrecy.

Ethics encompasses human rights as a whole, when, in its Declaration of Venice (1983), the World Medical Association states that "a physician shall respect the rights of patients". But ethics goes beyond rights, for a right is satisfied by respect for the rule in its strict interpretation. Ethics requires of the doctor that he should also be good, honest and disinterested, in the broadest sense of the word, which is something no right can guarantee.

Ethics confers obligations and rights on patients before ever they are written down. The World Medical Association and other international professional bodies made up of organisations representing doctors reached a consensus on the rules to be followed in fields where the law remained silent and where morality hesitated before the uncertainty of new technology. They have clarified the contents of the human rights claimable by patients vis-à-vis the ethical obligations accepted by doctors.

This is not the place to set out all the declarations on medical ethics, which have guided medical attitudes and positive legislation in so many countries, but among the major declarations of the WMA we cannot fail to mention the Declaration of Helsinki (1964), amended in Tokyo in 1975, designed to guide doctors in biomedical research, which still serves as a guideline in matters of human experimentation; the Declaration of Tokyo (1975) forbidding participation by doctors in torture and cruel and degrading treatment, the Declaration of Brussels (1985) on in vitro fertilisation and the Declaration of Venice (1983) on terminal illness. I would also mention the Declaration of the World Psychiatric Association on the abuse of psychiatry (Hawaii, 1983), that of the International Council of Prison Medical Services on the care of prisoners (Athens, 1979) and all the declarations of the Standing Committee of Doctors of the EU, the International Conference of Medical Councils, the European Union of Medical Specialists, the European Committee of Private Hospitals, etc.

What emerges from the obligations imposed on doctors in all the declarations of the international medical organisations is intransigence when it comes to the respect of medical ethics.

The dilemma

Medical ethics impose on doctors not only respect of patients' rights but their defence against possible infringements, ranging from flagrant violations such as inhuman treatment or abusive experimentation to limitations on care for purely economic reasons.

And this is precisely the doctor's dilemma: ethics and human rights combine to impose on him the defence of patients' interests. This requires of the doctor a rare force of character and personal courage, but above all it requires recognition of practitioners' medical independence in the face of threats to their patients, while the media, public opinion, public authorities and even sometimes some patients' associations, which have taken issue with the wrong opponents, combine forces to weaken medical authority. We cannot ask doctors to defend their patients, and still less to defend their rights against all comers, if we want them to be at the bidding of the authorities and the health service, mere executors of instructions issued to them under a policy in which the system has taken over the exercise of patients' rights.

The doctor's defence of human rights depends on his independence. A context of care provision which grips the doctor-patient dialogue in an administrative vice, renders the problem particularly acute.

The institution of systems for health care provision and cover in Europe has undoubtedly improved considerably the citizen's chances of asserting his right to access to care. But this is a social right, and, as such, limited by the resources available to states. By laying down the conditions for intervention, states have involved themselves in the medical dialogue and to a certain extent taken over patient's rights. It is the paying authority which claims to be able to authorise the attending doctor to give treatment, rather than the patient, or which authorises payment for drugs. Because it pays, the authority wants to have access to the patient's medical record in his place and there is violation of the patient's private life which he, being resigned, abandons in exchange for the benefits of organised care. The protection of individual rights, particularly in a health care system which considers doctors to be its employees or organs and not the spokesmen for the patients, represents the biggest challenge in medical ethics today.

Ethics and progress

Scientific progress throws up new ethical problems every day: genetic manipulation, *in vitro* fertilisation and research on foetuses carry as many risks as hopes, and the doctor must find the narrow path between the enormous potential advantages to humanity and the possible abuses and excesses.

Furthermore, the funding crisis has been concomitant with an increase in costs caused by greater longevity, the survival of incurable or fragile individuals and the explosion of technological possibilities in the diagnostic and therapeutic fields. The greater possibility of obtaining results and being effective increases costs and at the same time the doctor's responsibility in making a conscientious choice of methods of treatment, and the cuts in public spending limit the extent to which he can use new technologies for the benefit of his patients. Rationing is close to rationalisation.

The doctor is faced with the authorities' temptation to control health care expenditure by rationing it. The political difficulty of deliberately calling into question the principle of free access to and free provision of care gives rise to the need to find a way of denying the necessity of certain forms of care under the cover of an ethical justification. Arguments based on the problems of limits to therapeutic efforts, euthanasia, costly sophisticated care given to the elderly (dialysis, pacemakers) and rationalisation in the use of scientific progress are open to the suspicion of seeking an ethical alibi for an economic problem. For doctors, ethics is not an alibi, but the pursuit of the patient's interest in his free choice between the values to be respected. This is today's second major challenge.

The age-old challenge

The Aids epidemic exposes all the contradictions between the right to health and the limited resources available for the collective implementation of this right. Attitudes are dictated as much by the inadequacy of the resources as by scientific impotence.

Aids also raises the acute problem of the confrontation of two rights and two interests: those of the carrier of the virus, who counts on the respect of medical secrecy, and those of the threatened partner, or even the community at large, if because of his or her profession – prostitution, for instance – the patient constitutes a public danger. The sensitive nature of this disease has prompted keener calls for respect of the individual sufferer's rights, while in a thousand other areas, the public authority has had no difficulty in imposing the right to the most private information in the name of the general interest. The doctor is in the front line, torn between the needs and rights of the different parties and a choice determined by his individual

57

mission to provide care and to protect the interests of society as a whole. Professional secrecy, so decried, violated to permit insurance companies to limit their intervention, or to defend society, remains the keystone for the patient's confidence. This is what brings him to entrust himself to the doctor. This is the age-old challenge.

The problem is compounded by the general changes in people's moral and ethical values and their distancing from traditional ethics. The public authorities are endeavouring to modify medical ethics in parallel with the ethics of society through setting up committees made up of thinkers and moralists of different currents of thought in order to seek a consensus reflecting the changed attitudes according to time and place. An Islamic ethic and a Christian ethic come together in this new morality. Muslim, African or European human rights are confronted with the corresponding morality; the acceptation of pluralism or not. Taking account of these factors, the evolution of professional medical ethics requires very serious thought, for which a place of pluralist consensus, such as the World Medical Association, is essential.

The Catholic Church and the exercise of the medical profession

by Elio Sgreccia,
Professor of Bioethics,
Catholic University of the Sacred Heart, Rome[1]

The history of health care in the Catholic Church

Care of the sick has always been a field of particular commitment for the Catholic Church: the doctrinal basis for this commitment is the teaching and example of Christ himself.

The theological significance of Jesus' healing activity, as deduced from the evangelical texts, is twofold: Jesus wants to give a "sign" of his messianic nature, that is his divine mission which has the value of salvation, and in addition he wants the Disciples to understand his desire to serve suffering mankind (diaconal value). The two aspects are well illustrated in the parable of the good Samaritan, reported in the gospel according to St Luke (Chapter 10, v. 29-38), a parable which ends with an order: "Go, and do thou likewise". This order is given explicitly by Jesus to his Disciples: "And he sent them to announce the Kingdom of God and to heal the sick" (Luke, 9, v. 2), "And as ye go, preach, saying, The Kingdom of heaven is at hand. Heal the sick, cleanse the lepers, raise the dead, (...)" (Matthew, 10, v. 7).

The Catholic Church draws from these words of Jesus the motivation for organising places of shelter for the sick. In the period of the persecutions, these were set up in the houses of some of the faithful, and later, from the fourth century onwards, they were in monasteries in both the east and the west. The religious orders of hospitallers and charitable organisations have kept health care active in the church in all evangelised areas.

Even after the secularisation of hospitals, which began in Europe with the French Revolution, the Catholic Church still continued its presence in the service of the sick in various ways, through members of religious communities working in civil hospitals and through its own institutions.

In fact presence at the side of the sick has been considered within the Church not so much as a substitute form of service as a way of bearing witness through service to the sick person, who represents Christ himself: "I was sick and ye visited me (...) Inasmuch as ye have done it unto one of the least of these my brethren, ye have done it unto me" (Matthew, 25, v. 35-40).

The ethical conception of medicine

From the doctrinal point of view, the Catholic Church has always respected the beneficial breakthroughs and therapeutic resources of medical science, and has

---

1. With the collaboration of Dr A. Spagnolo for cases 83 to 120.

used them for its hospitals. It has also seen in the doctor a kind of sacred official, invested with a "life ministry" (Paul VI), since he is called to help life, to care for the sick and to alleviate pain.

Medical morality within the Catholic Church has adopted the standards of Hippocratic ethics, enhancing them with the concept of the sacredness of life as a gift of God and of the sick person as the son of God and the embodiment of Christ himself. Within the Catholic Church, crimes against life have always been condemned since the Church's early days, among them, abortion (Didache, early second century), homicide, suicide, desertion of children and any violent treatment.

When moral theology was systematised in the medieval *summae* and in the treatises of the Renaissance and those of our times, these points of medical ethics found their place in commentaries on the Fifth Commandment: "Thou shalt not kill", or in treatises on justice.

Moral doctrine has been enriched above all under the most recent popes – Pope Pius XII (1939-59), in his addresses to doctors, and his successors in response to three concomitant phenomena: the crimes against life, even the lives of innocents, during the last war, developments in thinking on "human rights", to which the Church has adhered and made its own contribution, particularly from Pope John XXIII (1959-64) onwards, and the progress of medical science and technology in the biomedical field.

The great debates on birth control, sterilisation, legalisation of abortion, genetic engineering, artificial reproduction, organ and tissue transplants, euthanasia and "relentless prolongation of life", and the health needs of developing countries, have prompted the Catholic Church to issue a succession of doctrinal replies and statements. Thus all biomedicine has been considered from the ethical point of view. Given the special nature of the Pope's doctrinal authority (magisterium), the complex collection of official documents constitutes, within the Catholic Church, the sole and compulsory reference.

Fundamental values and principles

Like any other morality, medical morality within the teaching of the Catholic Church refers to an anthropology which is part of Christian revelation. Medical morality is therefore a morality based on the inherent and objective dignity of the human person. On the basis of this conception, man is not only placed at the acme of the material universe and at the centre of society, but he is also endowed with eternal value, given his transcendence in relation to the world and history and the spirituality which makes him what he is. The respect owed to the human person is therefore based on the respect we owe to God and to the immortal spirit of each individual. Consequently, Christian morality cannot countenance a utilitarian concept of ethics or a system in which freedom is absolute, be it pure biologism or naturalistic sociobiologism.

We derive from the original anthropocentric nature of Christian revelation the following essential points: human corporality is conceived in a personalist sense, that is the body forms a unity with the personal self. From the Catholic point of view, one can say not only "I have a body", but "I am my body", because the body is substantially linked to the spirit in such a way as to constitute a "single whole".

On the basis of this value of corporality, physical life is considered as a fundamental value in relation to other values, even those superior in dignity (freedom, solidarity, etc.), because all the other personal values presuppose the individual's physical existence. Hence the Catholic Church's opposition to deliberate abortion and euthanasia on the basis of the concept of physical life as a sacred and fundamental value.

Consequently, the healing principle or the principle of totality, on the basis of which any medical or surgical (or genetic) intervention is allowed so long as it is necessary to save or restore the health of the whole person, occupies a central place in medical ethics. Any intervention in the medical field must also be based on the principle of freedom (of both doctor and patient) and must be evaluated with respect to responsibility towards life and health. It is on this principle that the patient's rights and duties, and in particular his right and duty of informed consent, as well as the doctor's rights and duties, are based.

Finally, we should note the sociality-subsidiarity principle, a necessary corollary of the preceding, whereby health assistance is both a citizen's right and a duty of the community, and health is a common good. Therefore greater aid should be given – including in terms of allocation of resources – to the person in greater need.

As regards the magisterium of the Catholic Church, we make reference to the following documents:

Humanae Vitae
(Paul VI, encyclical, 25 July 1978)
Taking up what had already been affirmed in the Pastoral Constitution *Gaudium et Spes* of the Vatican II Council on the nature and aims of marriage, this encyclical letter is intended to be the fundamental document on responsible procreation, where once again the constant doctrine of the Catholic magisterium on the legitimate regulation of births is presented. The entire reflection is based on the "indissoluble link that God has willed and that man cannot break on his own initiative, between the two significations of the conjugal act: union and procreation" (n. 12).

Any conjugal act, if it is to be in conformity with the truth on the person, must thus remain open to the transmission of life; as a result only methods which prescribe abstention during fertile periods and conjugal union during infertile periods, when used for serious reasons, permit harmonisation of the union of the spouses with responsible procreation. This means that contraception is illicit, whether it be mechanical, hormonal or achieved through a manipulation of the conjugal act.

Following on from this text are three documents which expand the vision of the family context as a whole; these are: the apostolic exhortation of John Paul II *Familiaris consortio* (22 November 1981); the Charter of Family Rights (22 October 1983) and the "Letter to families" by John Paul II (2 February 1994).

Declaration on induced abortion
(Congregation for the doctrine of the faith, 18 November 1974)

This document is explicitly concerned with moral judgment of induced abortion. The Congregation for the doctrine of the faith, an official organ of the Catholic Church for doctrinal questions, basing itself on the fundamental principle of the value and inviolability of all human life, renews the condemnation of direct voluntary abortion. In this document we read: "In reality, respect of human life imposes itself as soon as the process of generation begins. As soon as the egg is fertilised, a life is inaugurated which is neither that of the father nor that of the mother, but a new human being who develops for himself." The good physical life possesses fundamental value precisely by virtue of the fact that it is the necessary condition for all the other goods, which necessarily depend upon it.

Sterilisation in Catholic hospitals
(Congregation for the doctrine of the faith, 13 March 1975)

In this document, the Congregation for the doctrine of the faith examines the moral question of sterilisation as a method of contraception. Such a procedure is declared illicit, despite the disagreement of certain theologians. Sterilisation is licit when it is connected with a true treatment of the diseased part of the sex organ; treatment which cannot be avoided and which is carried out with the consent of the patient and in the expectation of a positive result.

Declaration on certain questions of sexual ethics
(Congregation for the doctrine of the faith, 29 December 1975)

This document recalls Church doctrine concerning certain points of sexual morality in order to combat certain trends inspired by subjective ethics, prevalent above all in the United States.

It confirms that there are fundamental and immutable principles which stem directly from human nature, thus transcending any historical or cultural contingency and accessible to reason because they are contained in the natural moral law inscribed by the Creator in the heart of his creature. "There can therefore be true promotion of human dignity only in the respect of the essential order of his nature."

From this standpoint questions relating to pre-marital sex, homosexual behaviour and masturbation are examined. Each of these three situations in itself constitutes, objectively, independently of any intentionality or any psychological aspect, a serious moral defect, because it betrays the true meaning of sexuality and love.

For the sexual act to be performed in a fully human fashion and thus be able to truly meet the requirements of the purpose proper to human dignity, it must be lived in the context of an exclusive and total heterosexual donation, even from the temporal standpoint, faithful and fruitful, based on mutual consent manifested on the outside and valid before society, namely sanctioned by marriage.

The conception of human sexuality in the Christian sense was taken up in the "Catechism on human love" by John Paul II (5 September 1979-28 November 1984). Two subsequent documents refer to homosexuality: the first, more general "Educational orientations for human love" is by the Congregation for Catholic education (1 November 1983), the second, more specific "Letter to bishops of the Catholic Church on the pastoral concerning homosexual persons" is by the Congregation for the doctrine of the faith (1 October 1986).

Declaration on euthanasia
(Congregation for the doctrine of the faith, 5 May 1980)

This document defines euthanasia as "an act or omission which, it itself or in the intention, gives death in order to eliminate all pain. Euthanasia is thus at the level of intentions and of the procedures employed" (Part II).

By completing the traditional distinction, made problematical and imprecise by medical progress, between "ordinary" and "extraordinary" medical resources, the document prefers to refer to the concepts of "proportionate" and "disproportionate" resources, thus focusing not on the treatment itself, but rather on the result. From this the declaration deduces certain concrete indications, among them what is known as "relentless prolongation of life", that is all interventions which (in the attempt to prolong life at any cost) lead in the extreme case to "disthanasia", increasing the suffering without effectiveness or without a proportionate result.

The other important problems considered in this document are: the licitness of painful therapies with the consent of the patient, the non-obligatory nature of extraordinary or dangerous treatments (except in the case where they are requested by the patient himself, after he has been informed), the obligatory nature of "normal treatment" and humane care.

Donum Vitae
(Congregation for the doctrine of the faith, 22 February 1987)

This instruction, the outcome of a broad consultation process, is intended to provide specific answers, through reference to the teaching of the Catholic Church, "on the conformity with the principles of Catholic morality of biomedical techniques making it possible to intervene in the initial phase of the life of the human being and in the very process of procreation".

The fundamental principles for a moral judgment on artificial procreation techniques for humans stem from the very nature of the human being, *corpore et anima una*, and are: respect for life and the dignity of the human being called into existence from the very moment of fertilisation, and respect of the dignity of human procreation which requires that it should always be the fruit and finality of conjugal love. As for the respect of the burgeoning life, central to this is the affirmation that – given the continuity of development of the human being from the moment of fertilisation – from the ethical standpoint the human embryo should be respected and treated as a person.

As regards the application of technologies to the processes of procreation, all techniques which are an aid to the conjugal act accomplished naturally and in itself fertile are declared licit; all techniques which substitute for the conjugal act, whether intra-corporal (insemination) or extra-corporal (IVF), whether within the married couple or with recourse to a donor, are declared illicit.

Associated questions are also examined, such as prenatal diagnosis and experimentation on the embryo; these being acceptable only if they are carried out for the benefit of the child to be born and do not entail disproportionate risk. The document also considers other related problems and the relationship between moral law and civil law.

Veritatis Splendor
(John Paul II, Encyclical letter, 6 August 1993)
This document is of a general nature and is addressed to the bishops who share with the pope the responsibility and commitment to preserve "sound doctrine" (Tim II, 4, 3), stipulating certain essential doctrinal aspects in order to meet what is certainly a serious crisis, a cause of confusion and difficulty for the moral life of the faithful in society and for communion in the Church.

This text therefore analyses the foundations of morality. As regards specific moral questions, the encyclical refers to the "Catechism of the Catholic Church", which contains an organic and complete exposition of Catholic moral doctrine; the document itself deals only with certain fundamental aspects of the Church's moral teaching.

In today's social and cultural context, in which the relationship between freedom and truth is often problematical and neglected, the document recalls the intimate link between conscience, truth and freedom.

Charter of health personnel
(Pontifical Council for the pastoral of health services)
This document was designed as an ethical guide for the health field; it was published by the Pontifical Council for the pastoral of health services instituted by John Paul II on 11 February 1985.

The charter is a complete and organic synthesis of the teaching of the Catholic Church regarding the defence and promotion of human life and the dignity of man in the health field.

The text, drafted in the form of a code of ethics, considers each theme of medical ethics in short enunciations. Since it is published by an official organ of the Catholic Church it has normative authority and value for Catholic health personnel.

Evangelium Vitae
(John Paul II, Encyclical letter, 25 March 1995)

This document, the fruit of long efforts in which the bishops of all countries of the world participated, synthesises the constant magisterium of the Catholic Church for the defence of human life in general and burgeoning life in particular. The text is in the form of a meditation and an announcement of the gospel of life; it refers above all to the bible, but also appeals to reason and "is thus intended to be a precise and firm reaffirmation of the value of human life and its inviolability, and at the same time an impassioned appeal addressed to each and every one in the name of God: respect, defend, love and serve life, all human life!".

The encyclical opens with the denunciation of present threats to life and the dignity of man; it dwells on this, indicating their cultural roots, essentially permissiveness and ethical relativism.

The document examines a broad spectrum of offences and crimes against life, but it condemns in particular abortion and euthanasia. It thus reiterates the teaching on topics already dealt with in other documents (artificial procreation techniques, prenatal diagnosis for eugenic purposes, birth control imposed and practised using methods contrary to nature such as contraception and sterilisation).

In this text we find an initial discussion of the theme of demography and another on the abortive nature of contratgestatives and antinidatives.

The above documents are directly concerned with medicine and medical ethics. There are, however, others which integrate the bioethical magisterium of the Catholic Church into a broader context: John Paul II, *Mulieris Dignitatem*, Apostolic letter, 15 August 1988; Pontifical Council for the family, "Ethical and pastoral dimensions of population trends", *Instrumentum Laboris*, 25 March 1994.

Bioethics and Protestantism

by Jean-François Collange,
Dean of the Faculty of Protestant Theology
of the Strasbourg University of Human Sciences,[1]
Member of the French National Consultative Ethics Committee

Protestant ethics and responsibility

Protestant ethics are primarily ethics of responsibility. When we talk of responsibility, we are talking about "response". Response to one or more calls from elsewhere, particularly that addressed by God through his Word, as witnessed by the Scriptures. To be responsible also means to be open to the Word and the call of another. It also means being attentive to the forms of this Word and this call, and making unceasing efforts towards better understanding of both the forms it takes and the demands it conveys. Responsibility is therefore to be seen not as attached to the performance or non-performance of acts defined a priori as good or bad, but as a movement, a quest, in which each individual becomes better, more responsible, as he tries unceasingly to perceive and to do better what others and the Other expect of him.

Listen, discuss and interpret

Placed under the sign of responsibility, hence listening, the Protestant ethic is also in the field of interpretation and discussion. It does not see itself as the servile executor of some edict fallen from the sky, but is forged through the patient and unremitting search for ethical truth. The search for this truth – which is a constituent part of the ethical subject himself, a role each individual has to assume on his own responsibility without any possible substitution – cannot, however, be the fruit of a solitary quest. It can only be conceived, by definition, in terms of a dialogue, as the outcome of a debate between conscience, the Word of God as witnessed by the Scriptures and the various interpretations to which it gives rise.

The role of the Churches

This being so, the Protestant Churches have no magisterium, either in terms of dogma – although the confessions of faith with their particular identities are not devoid of dogma – nor, a fortiori, in terms of ethical precepts. Nevertheless, the Churches exist as communities, that is as places for sharing and for forming the responsibility of each individual. As such, they are led to put forward "points to ponder", "considerations" of varying degrees of urgency, to clarify and direct the debate, without ever contemplating its closure. As the Protestant Federation of France said in its position on bioethical questions in March 1987: "The ethical points to

---

1. With the collaboration of Pierre-Emmanuel Panis, agricultural engineer and theologian.

ponder here (...) are addressed to everyone (...) they are humble suggestions, as the church, as a community of women and men listening to God in Jesus Christ through the biblical witnesses, can err, even though it seeks the help of the Holy Spirit. But these proposals nevertheless seek to provide a few landmarks for members of our Churches (...) in a society which is plainly in search of a bioethics, that is morality for life."[1]

The considerations or thoughts on ethical theology put forward by the Protestant Churches are therefore to be taken with the greatest seriousness inasmuch as they testify to research and work carried out with care and offered for sharing. However, they do not have any binding status and are characterised by their diversity, which is a mark of the differing options available to those who listen in order to hear and interpret the calls of men and of the very Word of God. As a result, Protestant positions are characterised as much by their desire to open and organise the debate as by any conclusions reached.

Church positions and bioethics

Protestant Churches have not failed in their duty to put forward points to ponder and ethical proposals concerning powers over life. At the present time, some 30 official stances exist on this subject and the "Church and society" department of the World Council of Churches, an organisation to which over 300 Churches throughout the world belong, put forward in August 1989 a document some 30 pages long on the issue.[2] Besides these official positions, there are numerous theological works devoted to the ethical problems posed by progress in biological sciences. A consolidated presentation of all these documents is being prepared under the responsibility of Hartwig von Schubert at the FEST (*Forschungsstätte der Evangelischen Studiengemeinschaft*) in Heidelberg.[3]

In general terms – and whatever may be the practical conclusions they reach – the overall approach of these documents is well in keeping with the tendencies outlined above for Protestant ethics as a whole. This is clearly expressed by the Bioethics Working Group of the Federation of Protestant Churches of Switzerland,

---

1. *Biologie et éthique: éléments de réflexion*, ("Biology and ethics: points to ponder"), document published by the Protestant Federation of France (47, rue Clichy, F-75009 Paris) on 19 March 1987; also published by Autres Temps 14, 1987 and Istina 32, 1987, pp. 280-283. The ethical positions of the Protestant Federation of France are now set out in a *Livre blanc* ("White book") available from the same address.
2. *Biotechnologie: un défi pour les Eglises et pour le monde* ("Biotechnology: a challenge for the Churches and the world"), World Council of Churches, 150 route de Ferney, CH-Geneva, August 1989.
3. H. von Schubert, *Evangelische Ethik und Biotechnologie*, Frankfurt/New York, Campus Verlag, 1991; J. Hübner, H. von Schubert, *Biotechnologie und Evangelische Ethik. Die internationale Discussion, ibid.*, 1992. In addition, Protestant views and reflections are to be abundantly found in J.-M. Thévoz, *Entre nos mains l'embryon. Recherche bioéthique*, Geneva, Labor et Fidès, 1990.

which writes: "Ethics involves our responsibility at several levels: professional, religious, human. Whether or not it coincides with the legal point of view, its role is not to punish but rather to guide (...) In religious ethics, the aim is not merely to clarify an argument, but to grasp the relationship between life and truth as revealed through faith. This revelation itself, like a gushing spring, is part of the time and culture in which it is perceived. Our generation is faced with the difficult task of discerning how the Church can elucidate the possibilities offered by a world in the throes of profound change, where scientific discoveries are put forward as capable of solving any problem. What, then, should we see as the place of the human being, whose form was taken by Christ, and how are we to preserve his dignity?"[1]

The main considerations we can base ourselves upon to meet this challenge are discussed under different headings below.

Ethics, science and technology

Humanity is in fact only truly human when it receives its identity from another – from God – and does not seek to manipulate itself. Science and technology cannot therefore be ends in themselves, but must be and remain tools at the service of men and their fulfilment. This is their true purpose. Technology is neither good nor evil, but it challenges humanity to accept the true responsibility which is exercised in the respect of the humblest and in the attention paid to all. Hence discernment is called for in the choice of the methods employed by scientific research and the uses made of its results and advances in knowledge. The Protestant Federation of France thus pointed out in 1987 that "there is at the same time in the Bible a promise of domination of nature and a warning against the coveting of all power. In recognising that he is not God, that his freedom and his control are limited by the love of God and the love of his neighbour, the human being is not weakened and impoverished, but is saved from disorder and vertigo".[2]

Human dignity

Protestants also stress the fact that each human being has an inviolable dignity, expressed in biblical terms by the assertion that God created man in his own image, after his own likeness (Genesis 1,v. 26ff) and confirmed by the fact that, in Jesus Christ, God himself was made man. Created in the image and likeness of God the Other, the human being still carries within him an element of mystery. This is expressed in particular in the complexity of his nature (physical, sexual, intellectual, spiritual), by his capacity to be free and by the relational reality which constitutes

---

1. *Fécondation in vitro. Possibilités techniques et perspectives éthiques* ("*In vitro* fertilisation. Technical possibilities and ethical viewpoints"), Bioethics Working Group of the Federation of Protestant Churches of Switzerland, Lausanne and Bern, 8 April 1987.
2. *Biotechnologie: un défi pour les Eglises et pour le monde*, op. cit.

him in his humanity. Being dignified, and being so "in the image and likeness" of another, is to indicate in fact that the basis of this dignity lies in a relationship. This fundamental human dignity must be respected as such, in particular for the weakest (children, the handicapped, and even embryos). Protestants thus reiterate "the pre-eminence of the human person over all systems, all rules and even over ethical principles established and confirmed for generations".[1]

While it is true that the human being has a right to particular protection, it is also true that this must never lead to immoderation and egotism, but rather to concern for others and for the future, notably when it is a matter of a child to be born, his identity and his equilibrium. The child is an original and singular being, protected by the law of God, on which the rights of the parents can but be based and with which they can but conform. The parents in fact simply transmit a life which is not their own but one which is entrusted to them as a promise and a gift:[2] a gift of God, life is transmitted by the reciprocal gift of the parents, who, being fertile, open up the future. This promise of life goes beyond affective and educative transmission and is inalienable.

The fact that it is inalienable means in particular that the child can be considered neither as an object nor as a due. There is in fact no right to the child, but rather rights of the child to be defined and safeguarded. The child has value for his own sake and cannot be subject to any alienating and reductive control, whether by his parents or by society.[3]

The child needs to be received by a father and mother living together in a relationship of union and harmony, at the heart of a responsible parental project which provides them with an affective, relational and reassuring environment favourable to the development of their personality, permitting them to become a responsible and balanced adult, open to the love of God and of others. The attention paid to these different needs thus conditions the way in which the morality of certain medically assisted procreation practices are evaluated.[4]

The human person and biological life

However, it must not be inferred from the inalienable nature of human life that this is defined essentially through its purely biological aspects; it becomes human

---

1. J.-M. Thévoz, op. cit., p. 44.
2. Thévoz, op. cit., pp. 81-84; position of the German Protestant Churches presented in J. Hübner, H. von Schubert, op. cit., I, p. 378ff and Dutch Reformed Church, II, p. 279ff.
3. The report on the work of the mixed group "The Free Church Federal Council, the British Council of Churches", 1982, presented in H. Hübner, H. von Schubert, op. cit., II, p. 201. The child cannot be demanded as the fruit of a "duty" or as a right (conjugal, parental or even societal) nor as a response to a need (Thévoz, op. cit., pp. 81-84).
4. On the way in which this subject is treated in the English-speaking countries (United Kingdom, Canada, United States), see J. Hübner, H. von Schubert, op. cit., I, p. 198ff.

only when carried by projects, exchanges, love and words which make sense and commit those who pronounce them. The foundation of human dignity – as we have seen – lies in a relationship (with God) and opens to a whole relational life, which humanises. "One cannot deal with the man in oneself without falling into abstraction", so that man must be "considered in his dynamic and relational destiny, in all his relationships, including his relationship with God".[1]

The Protestant Churches, through their conviction that in the person of Jesus Christ and through his Word, God has adopted as sons and declared brothers all men, think that dignity cannot be measured solely by its biological aspects, but integrates many aspects related to men giving and keeping their word. For this reason the essential links of kinship appear to them to be more a matter of interaction and adoption than solely being of a biological nature. From this standpoint, the document of the Protestant Federation of France stresses "the constant recourse in the Bible to the concept and image of adoption: we are finally all adopted children, adopted through parental love, which relativises the technical or natural circumstances of fertilisation" (§4).

Status of the embryo

Concerning the status of the embryo, all the Protestant Churches of western Europe, despite the internal debates on whether or not research can be carried out on the embryo, consider the human embryo to be a potential and evolving human person. For this reason it has the right to true respect right from its conception. The positions are not unambiguous, however, as regards the way in which an embryo should be treated or whether it should be considered as a human person. Opinion here breaks along the same line as in the case of the legitimacy of abortion. For a certain number of Protestant Churches, abortion is murder and the embryo enjoys the same dignity as a born child. For other Churches, however, when pregnancy appears as a situation of distress, to do nothing might be synonymous with failure to assist a person in danger. The constitution of a human being is not at all instantaneous, but results from complex processes, both on the purely biological level and on that of the establishment of relations and the possibilities of "adoption" of the embryo.[2]

Ethics and legislation

Embarking on the path of responsibility also means specifically invoking rules – or even laws – making it possible to take up the challenges thus thrown down.

---

1. Thévoz, op. cit., p. 40.
2. As regards the German Protestant Churches, see H. von Schubert, op. cit., I, pp. 365ff and 430ff; for the other Protestant Churches see ibid., II, pp.153; 276-277; 359-364. Certain theologians and certain Churches even confer on the embryo the full status of a person as for an adult right from its conception (ibid., pp. 148ff; 360ff).

These should set standards and precise limits for the development of science and technology, as a function of the purposes which this development is to serve. These laws are of course not an end in themselves, but serve as "the indicator of what has to be respected absolutely: the neighbour, others".[1]

Protestant ethics and the case sheets

It is against the background of these general observations and the more precise indications contained in one or another of the documents mentioned that we shall approach the cases presented below. It will be understood that the "case study" method presented outside the context of the actual people concerned does not really correspond to an authentic Protestant approach. But the questions raised deserve to be considered with care. This we have done, either in the light of the texts mentioned, or, where there were no such texts, in a more personal way, by sketching out the direction in which a Protestant "answer" to the question could lie.

---

1. Thévoz, op. cit., p. 43.

Jewish morality with respect to medicine and biotechnology

by Albert Guigui,[1]
Rabbi attached to the Central Jewish Consistory, Belgium,
Chief Rabbi of Brussels

Judaism – general presentation

Judaism is not only a faith, a form of religion, a code of observance and a system of moral values; it constitutes the "sum" of the experiences of the Jewish people throughout the ages. It reflects their joys and sorrows, their struggles and triumphs, their memories and aspirations, the progression of their moral ideas and their conception of the world.

The religion is intimately identified with the people, its history, its culture and its civilisation. It encompasses the totality of Jewish attitudes and practices, the style of life, the ideals and ideas, in a word, all that the Jewish creative genius has produced throughout the ages.

1. The sources of the Jewish religion

The Hebraic Bible has twenty-four books, divided into three parts: the Torah, the Neviim and the Ketuvim.

Of all the books in the bible, the Torah occupies the most eminent place. The word Torah means "teaching, doctrine".

The Torah contains five books. It begins with the account of the origins of the world and covers the period of the patriarchs Abraham, Isaac, Jacob and Moses. It contains the precepts, laws and commandments which were given to the people of Israel by God. It contains the fundamental truths about God and about man, it constitutes a guide to religious and moral life for the individual and the people, and is the guarantor of the unity and survival of the people.

The Neviim (Prophets), the second part of the bible, is divided into two parts: the Former Prophets and the Latter Prophets.

The Former Prophets comprise the books of Joshua, Judges, Samuel and Kings. The Latter Prophets comprise the books of the three great prophets Isaiah, Jeremiah and Ezekiel and the twelve minor prophets.

The Ketuvim (Hagiographa) are very varied and contain the Psalms (150 in number), Proverbs and religious and philosophical tales on the problems which have

1. The author wishes to express his appreciation to Professor J. Brotschi, Corresponding Member of the Royal Academy of Medicine in Belgium, Foreign Associate Member of the French Academy of Surgery and Member of the World Federation of Neurosurgery Societies, for all the help he gave in drafting the replies to certain cases in this work.
The author's very sincere thanks also go to Dr G. Krzentowski of Brussels, who helped him understand and reply to cases 83 to 120 submitted by the nurses.

haunted man throughout time, such as Job and Ecclesiastes.

In parallel with the Bible an oral teaching grew up to explain and clarify the written tradition. This oral Torah was at first transmitted from masters to disciples, then it was written down between the second and fifth centuries, thus giving birth to the Talmud. The Talmud is made up of the Mishnah and the Gemara. Subsequently the Midrashic collections (allegorical and symbolic commentaries) were added to the Talmud.

Thus the Bible is for us a way of becoming aware of the active presence of the One God in the universe and in history. Reading it, studying it, is thus to listen to God. Reading and studying the Bible is also to act according to divine principles. Lastly, reading the Bible is to discover the essential problems of life and death, good and evil, doubt and hope, suffering and redemption.

For all these reasons, according to the Jewish liturgy, the Bible is "a tree of life to them that lay hold upon her" (Prov., 3 ; 18).

2. *The main stages in Jewish life*

Circumcision, bar mitzvah, marriage and burial: such are the stages of Jewish religious life.

a. Circumcision

The birth of a child is awaited with great emotion in a Jewish family. Having a child is both a joy and obedience to a divine commandment. In fact, the first commandment addressed to man by God was "increase and multiply". Transmitting life therefore consists of perpetuating the indestructible chain of generations of "children of Israel".

If the child is a boy, then on the eighth day of his life he is introduced into the "Alliance of Israel" through being circumcised. This ceremony, the *berith mila*, takes place either in the synagogue or in the home.

b. Bar mitzvah

According to Jewish tradition, the father is responsible for the child's conduct until his bar mitzvah. This comes at the age of 13, when the adolescent reaches religious majority, and can fulfil his religious obligations. As from this moment he himself is responsible for his acts.

It is at the bar mitzvah that the boy puts on the *tefillah* (phylactery) for the first time and is clothed in the *tallith* (prayer shawl). It is usual to have the young bar mitzvah read a paragraph from the sabbatic section of the Torah scroll and to make a commentary on the text he has read or a general and personalised statement explaining his awareness of his responsibility within Judaism.

Girls are considered to reach majority at 12.

Bar mitzvah is the occasion for family rejoicing.

c. Marriage

Marriage is a sacred duty under Judaism and for a Jewish wedding to take place, both bride and groom must be Jews.

The marriage is generally celebrated in a synagogue. The religious ceremony proceeds to the rhythm of the two *kiddush* sung by the celebrant or the rabbi. The groom places a ring on the finger of the bride, saying "Here, you are consecrated my wife by this ring according to the law of Moses and Israel". There then follow the reading and signature of the *ketubba* (marriage contract).

After this signature the second *kiddush* is sung. This contains seven blessings on the subjects of wine, the creation of man and of Jerusalem and the joy of the couple. After the second *kiddush* the husband breaks a glass. This act is a homage to the martyrs of Israel and the sacrifice of those who died for the faith and thus permitted the people to survive.

A Jewish marriage can be dissolved in the case of serious incompatibility. In this case the husband delivers a *get* (divorce act) to his wife.

d. Death and burial

"Blessed be the Judge of Verity" is the formula which must be chanted on the death of a dear one. As he accepts life with joy, man also accepts death with resignation. Only faith in God permits man to overcome all trials. This faith is summed up by the poet Judah Hallevi in two lines: "When I distance myself from You I am already dead, even while living, and when I unite myself with You I live on, even in death."

When the Jew is close to death he confesses his sins before God and he prays. In particular he recites the *shema* (Jewish act of faith) and invokes God's mercy. If he is in a coma, the relatives and friends present say these prayers for him.

As for burial, this takes place as soon as possible. "The dead man must return to the earth from whence he came" (Ecclesiastes, 12, 7; Genesis, 3, 19). Before the burial, the corpse is ritually cleansed by one or more members of the holy brotherhood. The *kaddish* (prayer calling for the reign of God on earth) is recited by the children of the deceased. The mourning family remains in the death house for a week, saying prayers accompanied by study each night. The mourning period continues less strictly first for thirty days, then for a further eleven months. A special lamp is lit in memory of the deceased. The sabbath and festivals interrupt the mourning rites.

Medical ethics and Judaism

Since the beginning of our century, medical science has made such enormous technical progress that a large number of thinkers fear that the moral principles which govern the medical function will be overwhelmed. Technological advances,

75

the fragmentation of knowledge into separate and independent sectors placed in the hands of ever more isolated specialists and excessive use of the analytical approach are in danger of blurring the view of the patient as a person and leading to generalised solutions which are often arbitrary, unjust and inhuman and can lead to the abandonment of essential moral laws. The end of our century is marked above all by concern with immediate utility and profitability. This situation threatens the fundamental laws which govern the life of human societies, and sometimes leads to intolerable situations.

Accordingly, it is more necessary than ever to safeguard medical ethics, to restore it to its rightful place of honour in the exercise of medicine and to return to our sources to listen to God's word.

The essentially prophylactic nature of Jewish medicine

Prophylaxis elevated to the rank of a legal, national and collective institution has been the subject of a great many specialist studies. There have been many monographs on the subject and many articles in various journals and reviews. They analyse the effect of circumcision and of abstinence during and after women's menstrual periods for sexual health; the effect of the laws concerning slaughtering according to the rite, forbidden foods and combinations, the preparation of meat, the prescriptions for meals, for hygiene; the effect of the sabbath laws, the consequences and repercussions for social health; the effect of the laws concerning divine offices, sobriety and holy studies for mental health; the effect of the laws relating to married life and conjugal relations for eugenics.

There has thus been a very great effort to preserve our physical life. The same network of prescriptions which surrounds our life to sanctify it at the same protects our health. Considered from this angle, the prevention of disease thus becomes the main preoccupation of Jewish medicine, for which a whole series of measures is implemented, extending to all spheres of human activity.

The progressive nature of the halacha

The body of Jewish law is known in Hebrew as *halacha*. This term stems from the Hebrew verb HaLoCh which means "walk with, advance, progress".

This term indicates that the Jewish law is not static – it evolves to take account of technical progress.The most striking example is that of heart transplants. Twenty years ago very few grafts were successful, in particular heart transplants. At that time, certain decision-makers considered these transplants to be a double assassination. Today, thanks to the discovery of cyclosporin and the mastery of sophisticated techniques, such operations have become almost routine, and the Chief Rabbi of Israel has in recent years authorised the transplantation of the hearts of road accident victims at the Hadassah University Hospital, provided that the committee responsible for establishing the hour of death includes a delegate of the Chief Rabbinate and the victim has given his agreement in writing (see case 23 below on this subject).

A unitarian concept – the body and the mind

One of the basic principles of Jewish medicine is the unitarian concept of the human being, whose body and mind form an inseparable whole. For Judaism, the body and the soul are one and the divine commandments apply equally to body and soul. Health and morality are complementary, and anyone who poisons himself with impure foodstuffs damages both his soul and his body.

This unity must also apply to the unity of heart and spirit. Our century gives intelligence primacy over feeling. We strive to be objective, rational, cold, but this objectivity and this impassivity are in danger of destroying humanity. In Hebrew, justice is not distinguished from charity. These two words are merged in the word *tzedakah*. *Tzedakah* is synonymous neither with charity, which alone would be weak and blind, nor with justice, which would be too rigorous and harsh, it is both at once.

The unity of the conscious and unconscious is also taken into account and refuses to see man truncated above or below. Judaism takes a holistic view of man, complete with his consciousness and unconscious, his will and his dreams.

Finally, this principle concerns the unity of the individual and society. Our age is dominated by conflicts between the individual and society. Moral aspirations often seem to be in conflict with the reality of life in society. An often impenetrable barrier seems to stand between the ideal and the reality. Judaism wants to see the ideal and day-to-day reality combined. The laws of the Torah are not supposed to be in heaven or beyond the seas, but "The word is very near you ; it is in your mouth and in your heart, so that you can do it" (Deuteronomy, 30, 1.4). The Torah seeks a just society on earth. That is why Judaism has always been hated by despots who, from Pharaoh to Hitler, have always sought to eradicate it.

Primacy of life

For Judaism, respect for human life is absolute, sacred and inviolable. Human life has infinite value because it is a gift of God and because man is made in God's image. The doctor's first thought must be that the living man is the living Torah, a constant revelation.

To witness the death of a man is to see a scroll of the Torah being consumed by fire (Rashi, Moed Qatan 24a). The body of man resembles a tabernacle in the temple whence comes the divine word. It is written in Exodus, 25, 8: "And let them make me a sanctuary, that I may dwell among them." To treat the body is to enable man to continue to utter divine praise and serve God and mankind. We can easily understand the obligation to profane the sabbath to save a sick man: the breaking of one sabbath makes possible the observance of others.

Man's life gives substance to the divine work, characterises it, makes it present and eternal. This explains the Talmudic words which state that the divine presence lies upon the face of the sick. Where human words seem choked by an implacable, incurable ill, we must do our utmost to relieve this inhuman and agonising lament which, like a blasphemy, rends asunder the image of divine goodness. Hence the sight of a suffering being should inspire in us the same respect as a scroll of the Torah and we should bear witness to this before a sufferer and do all we can to give relief.

Hope of life

Hope must never be abandoned. Even when doctors have declared themselves powerless, we can always hope for a change in the situation through divine intervention. The fact is that the doctor who is imbued with this belief can be more efficacious than the cold and cynical, purely technical practitioner.

Without neglecting any technical progress, the doctor, who, faced with an apparently hopeless situation or a doomed patient, instead of giving up, keeps his faith and communicates it to the patient, is in the situation of a general who, before a difficult or even apparently desperate battle, struggles to the end, to the extreme limit. Sometimes, this general achieves a miraculous reversal of the situation and sees victory smile upon him after all.

In Jewish medicine, the doctor must defend life to the last breath, without ever giving up. This attitude is based on the idea that man is not omniscient and that his verdicts are not divine verdicts. The doctor who gives a verdict against which there is no appeal is acting as if he were God, whereas in the Jewish tradition, for a man to claim divinity is the worst of profanations and the most serious of crimes. A man who puts himself on a level with God would determine the future, whereas this future belongs only to God.

True morality can but represent a defence of life, and from this standpoint the Torah proclaims that its prescriptions are given to men that they should live. A morality which was opposed to life or harmed it would lose all justification though becoming inhuman. Jewish tradition requires of the doctor that he be *Neeman Ve Rahman*, that is a man of complete and loving trust, who must love his patient as himself and do as much for him as he would for himself. The *midrash rabba* says that when Abraham was sick after circumcision, God himself came to bring healing and consolation. This exalts the role of the doctor, who must be not only a man of science, but also a man of heart and, one might say, a man in the highest sense of the word.

The role of the doctor[1]

Jewish tradition considers disease to be a scandal, an anomaly.

In seeking to treat a sick person, man intervenes in the plan and the acts of the Creator. Where does his legitimacy lie and how to reconcile the conflicts which may appear in the respect of tradition, in particular when the law has to be infringed to save a human life?

A midrash text explicitly deals with what is involved in the conditions of practising a medical act on a man: accompanied by a stranger, Rabbi Ismael and Rabbi Akiba are walking in the streets of Jerusalem. They are accosted by a sick man who asks them to tell him what remedy will cure him. They give their advice. Their companion then asks them "Who struck this man?". "God", they reply. "So you, doctors of the law, you permit yourselves to intervene in God's plans? God struck this man and you cure him? You are violating His will!" The two masters ask what his trade is. "I till the soil, as you can see from the sickle I am carrying." They continue the conversation, "Who created the earth, the vineyard?" "It was God", he replies. "So you yourself interfere in what does not belong to you. He created the earth and you consume its fruits." The man retorts, "Don't you see this sickle? If I didn't till the land, if I didn't cut the vine, if I didn't manure and hoe the land it would produce nothing." The rabbis then replied, "Thoughtless man! Draw the lesson from your trade. Just as a tree that is not manured, weeded, hoed and watered does not survive but dies, so it is with the human body, comparable to a tree. His manure is the medicament and he who works the earth is the doctor." The farmer accepts the argument and apologises.

Just as it is given to man to intervene in the natural state of the world to transform it and grow crops, so he is enjoined to concern himself with man's health.

Rav Kook gave an opinion which has become a reference: "It seems established that we generally take the advice of doctors. But in case of doubt – because they themselves cannot claim to be infallible, since it happens that in medicine something considered absolutely certain by a doctor, or even the majority of them is refuted by the following generation – doctors' opinions can be considered as hypothetical, and if they are taken into account to breach the prohibitions of Yom Kippur (Day of Atonement) or the sabbath (Saturday) this is because even if there may be doubt that life is in danger, all the prohibitions of the Torah may be ignored."

Judaism leaves the doctor free to intervene without restraint provided the conditions justify and authorise his action. It is obvious that the main reason for going into Jewish tradition was to show the fundamental place attributed to the individual and

---

1. See the excellent article by Emmanuel Hirsch, Director of Studies at IFREM, Paris, "Judaïsme, éthique médicale et vie", in *Le Supplément*, No. 178, 1991, pp. 117-126.

hence the obligations which stem from the unconditional respect of his existence.

While it is forbidden to hasten death, it is permitted to remove any artificial element which might prolong existence.

The Gemara (Avoda Zara 18) reports the words of Rabbi Hanania Ben Teradion: "It is for Him who has given life to take it back, and man must not himself put an end to his life." This great master spoke thus when being tortured by flames. He limited himself to accepting the support of a torturer who prevented him from being kept alive longer by the application of a wet sponge on his heart, which would have prolonged his agony.

Because man is the holder of life, he owes respect to it. It is on this standpoint that the doctor should base the principles and the limits to the practices he devotes to man.

Everything in Jewish tradition contributes to make man modest and infinitely respectful to the life that is entrusted to him, without for all that inciting him to neutrality or obscurantism where his intervention is required in order to preserve it.

Islam and bioethics

Fakhereddine Ben Hamida,[1]
Honorary Director of Research at the CNRS (Paris),
former member of the French National Consultative Ethics Committee
for the Life Sciences and Health

The prodigious technological advances in biology and molecular genetics in recent years mean that biology and medicine are in a historic phase. The astounding progress in the life sciences gives man the possibility of controlling reproduction, heredity and the nervous system.

It is now possible to predict certain genetic diseases and to detect certain malformations at a very early stage in the life of the embryo. It is also possible, thanks to genetic manipulation, to integrate into the human chromosome a healthy and functioning exogenous gene (gene therapy) or correct a defective gene (mutagenesis carried out *in vitro*).

This fantastic progress in biology gives rise to great hopes for both predictive and curative medicine. But this biological revolution also threatens to give rise to formidable problems:

– medically assisted procreation threatens to confuse the notion of filiation and to engender thousands of embryos whose very existence constitutes a problem of conscience not only in the moral field but also in the legal field;

– prenatal diagnosis may tempt man into eugenism, that is selecting and providing tailor-made children for parents who desire, for example, a male child with blond hair and blue eyes;

– genetic manipulation, a veritable plastic surgery of the genes, threatens to modify the genetic heritage of individuals when the modified genes are those from the germ cells and to become a threat to freedoms and the survival of the human race;

– organ transplants may give rise to trafficking in organs and threatens to transform the human body into a stock of spare parts ready for organ transplant operations;

– relentless prolongation of life may carry the risk of creating a field of experimentation which could become an affront to human dignity. What is more, artificial methods of maintaining vital functions give rise to serious problems of conscience, as witnessed by the heated debates over euthanasia.

It has become necessary to provide safety barriers and establish a code of conduct to limit the possibility of abuses. This appears all the more necessary as science is advancing more quickly than morals and the law.

The need to define a moral attitude and to promote public awareness, if not a social consensus, *vis-à-vis* the many problems arising has given birth to a new discipline, the

---

1. The replies to cases 83 to 120 were drafted by Dr G.H. Hadj Eddine Sari Ali, adviser to the Muslim Institute of the Paris Mosque.

ethics of life science or bioethics. While the term "morals" has been commonly used for a long time, the term "ethics" was reserved for the language of philosophers.

Today ethics can be defined as being the questioning which precedes the introduction of the idea of moral law. Ethics implies a critical reflection on behaviours. It is the expression of a standard and is of internal origin. It reflects questions and is conjugated in the interrogative mood.

The morality which has emerged from ethics is all that which is concerned with the good and the bad in laws, standards, constraints and necessities. Morality is conjugated in the imperative mood. The doctor for whom the Hippocratic Oath was once the only rule of conduct is today confronted with legal, ethical and religious problems which he has to resolve here and now.

Before addressing the major principles of Muslim morality with respect to human bioethics, concerning such matters as voluntary termination of pregnancy, medically assisted procreation, organ transplants, relentless prolongation of life and euthanasia, to name only the most important problems, it may be useful by way of preamble to recall the fundamental concepts of Islam and enumerate the various sources of Islamic law and the moral principles of Islamic canon law.

In the second part of the preamble, after having demonstrated by certain citations from the Koran the notions of tolerance and the liberal spirit of Islam, all too often ignored, we define the concept of the human person and the concept of brain death – two key elements in human bioethics.

It is indeed the concept of the human person which conditions the believer's conduct *vis-à-vis* the terrible act of deliberate termination of pregnancy, *vis-à-vis* medically assisted procreation (artificial insemination, *in vitro* fertilisation, surrogate motherhood), or the prescription of the abortion pill (antiprogesterone, RU 486).

By the same token, given that current medical progress allows prenatal diagnosis at a very early stage of a large and growing number of congenital malformations and hereditary diseases (detected by means of genetic anomalies), it is again the conception the individual has of human life and the human being which determines the decision whether to proceed with or terminate a pregnancy when there is risk of malformation. It is easy to imagine the moral problems and the anguish of parents and doctors faced with such situations.

The second essential concept in bioethics is the definition of death, as it is on this definition that organ transplants depend. It is also the concept of death which conditions behaviour *vis-à-vis* relentless prolongation of life or euthanasia.

Preamble on Islam and Muslim morality
Sources of Islamic law

The *sharia*, which may be translated as the canonic laws of Islam, and which encompasses all creation, is made up of a number of texts:

a. The Koran, which is the inviolable basic text

This is the Word of God revealed to Mohammed, the envoy of God, by the Archangel Gabriel. It contains 114 Sura or Chapters. Alongside many passages speaking of religion and morality, this sacred text contains legal verses dealing with personal status and succession.

b. The *sunna*

This is the set of *hadith* (sayings of the prophet Mohammed and accounts of his acts from which legal rules can be deduced). The *hadith* are the equivalent of the Gospels. This is the second source of Islam, which completes the Koran.

c. The *ijtihad*

This is a method of creative intellectual effort to find a solution to problems not resolved or not mentioned by the Koran or the *sunna*. It is the exercise of the human reason, which may also be translated by reflection with a suggestion of "flexibility". It is an attempt to adapt to new circumstances.

The *ijtihad* includes the *qiyas* and the *ijmaa*:

– the *qiyas* is the method by which a religious, moral or legal rule can be deduced from another rule laid down by one of the first two sources (Koran or *sunna*). For convenience it is called analogical reasoning or deductive reasoning;

– the *ijmaa* is the method by which new rules are created by the *ulemas* or Muslim jurists. The *ijmaa* may be for the common benefit of the Muslim community, that is the *istislah*.

It is thanks to the *ijtihad* (*qiyas* plus *ijmaa*) that certain problems arising from recent progress in biology, for example – which is the problem which concerns us – or economic, social and political situations fundamentally new and different from those of over a thousand years ago, can now find responses which take account of the specificities of the modern world.

Moral principles of the sharia *or Islamic canon law*

The *sharia* comprises five essential principles:

1. The first principle is witness of the faith: "There is but one God and Mohammed is his prophet." This principle is the fundamental pillar of Islam.

2. The second principle concerns the respect of personal goods and the goods of others. According to this principle a person should spend of his income only what is necessary and what he needs.

While these two principles are important, it is the following three which serve as a basis for finding a solution to the present problems of bioethics and Muslim morality. These three principles are:

3. The principle of respect of man's physical integrity:

"We have created man in the most perfect form" (Koran S, XCV, verse 4);

83

"We have modelled man according to a harmonious form" (Koran S, LXIV, verses 3 and 5, XL; verse 64).

4. The principle of respect of man's mental integrity:

"Do not modify the creation of God in either the physical entity or the mental entity of the individual" (Koran S, XXX, verse 30);

"God has breathed of his spirit into man" (Koran S, XXXII, verse 9);

"The human being is a noble creature in the eyes of God" (Koran S, XV, verse 70);

"Your being both physical and mental has a right over you" (Hadith).

5. The last principle is that of respect and safeguard of genealogical perpetuity and filiation:

"Have a knowledge of your genealogies, which will allow you to pay heed to blood relationships" (Hadith);

"God has not made of your adoptive children your own sons" (Koran S, XXXIII, verse 4);

"Call the adoptive children by the name of their father" (Koran S, XXXIII, verse 5);

These Hadith recommendations and the quotations from the Koran stress the need to ensure genetic perpetuity, eliminate the risk of incest and safeguard the family heritage in Islam.

The role of the ijtihad *with respect to the problems raised by bioethics*

The biological revolution of recent decades has given rise to new and serious problems for the human conscience at the deepest level.

What should the Muslim's attitude be to these problems? The solution is all the more delicate since there is no clergy in Islam and it is for the individual believer to face up to his responsibilities and to take a decision.

Each Muslim is responsible for commanding the good and prohibiting the evil.

The *ijtihad* is a case-law-based initiative which permits reflection and eliminates any fixed solutions; it authorises the Muslim believer to adopt an evolving position in his attitude to the new problems arising from the prodigious progress being made in the fields of medicine, biology and biotechnology.

The *ijtihad*, as we have seen, makes it possible to find solutions to problems which are not resolved, or not dealt with, by the Koran or the *sunna* and which have arisen precisely from recent progress or new situations.

Freedom of spirit and the notion of tolerance in Islam

It is interesting to note that throughout the Koran the notion of tolerance is found in many Sura (Chapters). The following principles are constantly taken up by different Sura:

"God wishes man ease, not discomfort" (Sura II, verse 181);

"We will not task a soul beyond its ability" (Sura VI, verse 153);

"We will lay on no one a burden beyond his power" (Sura VII, verse 40, S 23, verse 63);

"Let there be no compulsion in religion. Now is the right way made distinct from error" (Sura II, verse 257);

"God wishes you to feel at ease, not in hardship and rigidity."

Most prohibitions are relativised in Islam.

Thus in Sura XVI, verse 117: "Forbidden to you is that only which dieth of itself, and blood, and swine's flesh (...) but if any be forced, and neither lust for it nor wilfully transgress, then verily God is forgiving."

It seems that tolerance for old customs played a role in the extension of Islam throughout the world since this religion requires only a profession of faith for a person to enter into the Muslim community.

It should be noted that the Koran imposes on Muslims friendly relations with believers of all other religions, based on sincerity, confidence and affection. They must demonstrate religious tolerance, freedom and respect of others' opinions.

These ideas of tolerance and the respect of other religions, as well as freedom of belief and the veneration of all other opinions is found in 63 Sura and 125 verses of the Koran.

As we have pointed out above, the Koran recommends the greatest tolerance in religious matters. It accepts the Christian and Jewish religions.

The Koran authorises Muslim men to marry Jewish or Christian women, without their being obliged to change their religion or adopt that of the husband (Sura V, verse 7). Furthermore, in the *hadith* the prophet Mohammed orders the Muslim to respect the religion of his wife when she is not a Muslim and facilitate the practice and freedom of belief and if necessary to accompany her to the church or the synagogue to practise her religion.

Notions necessary for discussing the solutions to the problems of bioethics in Islam

In addition to the three moral principles of Islam mentioned above, namely the respect of physical integrity, the respect of mental integrity and respect of the maintenance of genealogical perpetuity found in numerous quotations from the Koran or the Sunna, and in addition to the *ijtihad*, it is essential to define two concepts: the concept of the human person and the concept of brain death.

These two concepts are the cornerstones of bioethics and those which condition the attitude of Muslim morality with respect to the problems dealt with here.

The concept of the human person in Islam

From what stage of its development onwards can and must the human embryo be considered as a human person? This is the form most often taken by the vital question with which ethical thinking in Islam on respect for the human embryo or voluntary termination of pregnancy is confronted.

In Sura II of the Koran, verse 228, it is stated that a divorced woman must wait 90 days before remarrying, so as to avoid any confusion of paternity. A woman who has become widowed (Sura II, verse 234) must wait 4 months and 10 days, namely 130 days, before remarrying, for the same reasons.

Hence the Koran implicitly grants a margin of between 90 and 130 days, that is from 3 months to 4 months and 10 days, as the period during which the foetus takes on human form.

This period which permits the reality of the human person to be defined in Islam is also found in a *hadith* cited by Al-Nawawiya. This fourth *hadith* states that the *sharia* accords the embryo the status of man on the 120th day of pregnancy.

Through these verses of the Koran and on the basis of the *hadith* cited above in which it is said that Allah breathed the *rouh*, that is the spirit of life, into the foetus at three months and one week, we may conclude that an embryo takes on the reality of a human person on the 100th day of pregnancy.

The concept of brain death

Generally, in Muslim countries and at Islamic conferences, there is a tendency to define brain death with the same rigour as is applied in western countries, that adopted by the medical world. But it is important to add that in the case of transplantation of organs removed from the body of a dead person, death must have been established by a committee of three specialist doctors including a neurologist. The surgeon who is to perform the operation may not be a member of this committee.

Recent problems and the position of Muslim morality

What are the different problems arising from progress in biology and genetics?

After a brief description of these techniques and the new problems created, we attempt to give the Muslim moral position on the basis of the elements provided in the first part.

Artificial procreation

The various artificial procreation procedures are:

a. Artificial insemination

In this technique, the sperm is placed directly in the uterine cavity. It is used in the case of conjugal infertility, where ascension of the sperm is rendered impossible.

According to Muslim law, this technique is licit only where the sperm donor is the woman's legal spouse.

b. In vitro fertilisation and embryo transfer

In the case of women having an obstruction of the fallopian tubes, fertilisation takes place *in vitro*, outside the body; the ovule and spermatozoid are each collected and placed together in a test tube. There, the ovule is fertilised. After forty-eight hours, it becomes an egg, and this potential embryo is placed in the mother's uterus. The pregnancy then takes its normal course. Here again, in Islam, *in vitro* fertilisation is licit only when the fertilised egg comes from the union of a woman's ovule with the spermatozoid of her husband.

c. Surrogate motherhood

This takes two forms:

– if a woman cannot bear a child but still has her ovaries, one or more ovules may be taken from her. These will be fertilised *in vitro* with her husband's sperm. The embryo thus obtained after forty-eight hours will be placed in the uterus of another woman, who will return the baby nine months later.

As Islam recognises polygamy under certain conditions and this is practised in most Muslim countries other than Tunisia, the bearing or "surrogate" mother may be the second wife of the husband who has given his sperm for fertilisation of the ovule from the first wife;

– if the surrogate mother is outside the couple and the ovule does not come from the married woman, Islam prohibits this form of procreation.

To sum up, as regards the attitude of the Muslim *vis-à-vis* artificial procreation in all its forms, the following rules may not be transgressed:

– the need to restrict artificial or medically assisted procreation techniques to legally married couples while they are both alive;

– the need to know the donor of the gametes so as to exclude incest and to ensure that the child has legitimate affiliation as prescribed by Muslim law.

Genetic fingerprints or genetic identity card

The human genome comprises 50000 to 100000 genes which are DNA sequences, each of the genes possessing the blueprint for manufacturing a protein. Analysis of DNA sequences has demonstrated substantial differences between individuals.

The structure can be visually represented by bars and this makes it possible to have a specific fingerprint for each individual. What is more, each bar being the direct reflection of a segment of DNA, it is transmitted to offspring according to Mendell's law. Thus the study of the bar codes of the different members of a family may be used to establish a link of blood relationship and be used in the legal or administrative fields (case of contestation of filiation or establishment of paternity).

These identification techniques can also be used to solve problems of identity. They provide answers to questions like: to whom does a human sample (of blood, hair, tissue, nail, etc.) belong? Thus the application of genetic fingerprinting techniques in the field of criminal investigation can lead to the identification of a victim or an aggressor.

It is easy to understand that the use of genetic fingerprints calls for certain guarantees. The fact is that the consequences of these genetic tests may conflict with social ethical values and the fundamental principles of human rights.

Used in administrative life, genetic fingerprint techniques could endanger individual privacy or the principle of non-discrimination on the grounds of race or affinity.

In criminal matters their use must take account of the difficulties associated with the certain identification of the initial sample or the reliability of the results depending on the laboratory. For this reason the carrying out of identification tests by genetic fingerprinting should be carried out solely in execution of a court order and only by authorised laboratories.

In conclusion, from the standpoint of social or public life there appear to be far more risks than benefits.

Concerning the attitude of Muslim morality towards identification by means of genetic fingerprinting, its use to establish a right of filiation can but be approved with regard to the principle of maintenance of genealogical perpetuity and filiation according to the moral principles of Islam.

Concerning its use in a criminal case, its contribution as proof or absence of proof can but be approved in the context of guarantees for the defence of human rights.

Prenatal diagnosis

We now know that there are over 3000 types of congenital malformation or hereditary disease. All of them are caused by the deformation, amplification or deletion of one or more genes (this is the case with haemophilia, mucoviscidosis, drepanocytosis, beta-thalassaemia and the myopathies). There is no treatment for any of these diseases.

The decision to be taken, that is the choice between the birth of a more or less seriously handicapped child and the deliberate termination of pregnancy, depends on the conception the individual has of the reality of the human person as a function of his spiritual and religious convictions.

The oldest technique of prenatal diagnosis is cytogenetic analysis by the establishment of the foetal karyotype on cells removed by amniocentesis (removal through the abdominal wall of amniotic fluid, which contains cells from the skin of the foetus). This test cannot be performed before the fourteenth or fifteenth week.

A very recent technique which made its appearance around 1980 is trophoblast biopsy and molecular hybridisation. In this technique, a fragment of chorionic villi, which have the same genetic material as the foetus, is removed through the vagina.

This technique allows prenatal diagnosis in the fifth or sixth week and therefore constitutes a major step forward as compared with amniocentesis.

If the foetus shows a genetic anomaly, a deliberate termination of pregnancy may be envisaged in less traumatising conditions in the ninth or tenth week. We then find ourselves faced with the problem of voluntary termination of pregnancy envisaged above.

Genetic manipulation – gene therapy

Genetic manipulation – genetic engineering or genetic recombination – constitutes one of the most prodigious techniques of molecular biology. This technique can be used to modify the sequence of genes contained in the hereditary medium, the deoxyribonucleic acid or DNA. To date, some 1 000 genes have been identified. For some of them, a correlation can be seen between their structure and the nature of the corresponding hereditary characteristics.

By means of genetic engineering, it is possible to add or remove a genetic datum or even to modify an item of genetic information in the case of mutagenesis performed *in vitro*. When the final objective is to cure a disease, these modifications constitute gene therapy.

If we take the case of introduction of a gene into stem cells which reproduce themselves, there are two possibilities:

– introduction of the gene into the fertilised egg produces germ cells, and this gene will be found in all the cells, since all the cells of the organism come from the egg. This method produces an artificial modification of the human genome which is transmissible to the person's descendants. This modification of the genetic heritage by manipulation of germinal cells is utterly forbidden in Islam, as it leads to creation of an organism which differs from a divine creation;

– introduction of the gene into somatic cells, that is stem cells of an organ deficient in a given substance corresponding to the gene introduced. Examples are the stem cells of the epidermis or those of the haematopoietic series situated in the bone marrow. These somatic cells have the property of rapid self-division. They are first removed, and treated *in vitro* and then re-injected or grafted into the organism. This gene therapy technique is still of limited application.

Gene therapy has been successfully tested in two cases of cancer: melanoblastoma and cancer of the kidney (Rosenberg and Stephenson in the United States). In these cases the patients are re-injected with their own lymphocytes in which have been introduced, thanks to retroviruses, the two genes for the expression of interleukin 2 and the tumoral necrosis factor, which makes the cell lymphocytes capable of killing the tumoral cells.

Given that the purpose of this technique is essentially therapeutic, it may be tolerated in Islam subject to all the precautions necessary to avoid any abuse.

Transplants of human organs

Living donors

The organs which may be removed from a living donor are the kidney, bone marrow and liver tissue (organs which regenerate).

In these cases, the graft may be performed in Islam provided that the donor is major and enjoys his full mental faculties, his legal capacity, and has freely and expressly consented to the donation of the organ.

Dead donors

a. Dead foetuses

The only case in which removal of organs is licit is one in which a therapeutic service is rendered (graft of bone marrow, for example) or a contribution is made to cognitive science.

b. Dead adults

As we have already seen, establishment of the donor's brain death is the essential condition for authorisation to stop the procedures which are artificially maintaining respiration and circulation in the organism and to remove the organ for transplant.

In March 1990, the Second International Congress of the Society for Organ Transplants in the Middle East was held in Kuwait. At this congress organ transplants were definitely encouraged. The donation of organs from the living or dead body was considered to be a good action (*hassana*) and even a charitable one (*sadaka*).

In recent years, there has been a rapid expansion in organ transplantation in some countries, particularly Saudi Arabia, Kuwait, Turkey, Iran, Egypt, Jordan and Syria. Doctors and surgeons from Saudi Arabia, Kuwait, Turkey, Iran and Tunisia reported on several hundred kidney transplants, particularly from living donors. Pancreas grafts have been performed in Kuwait and heart transplants in Jordan, Saudi Arabia and Tunisia.

Furthermore, for some years now there has been a Council of Arab-Muslim Ministers of Health, the executive bureau of which is chaired by Dr A.R. Awadi, Minister of Public Health in Kuwait.

This council has adopted a draft law on human organ transplants containing eleven articles. These may be summarised as follows:

– transplants of organs removed from the body of a dead person may take place provided that the next of kin have given their consent and on condition:

a. that death has been established by a committee as set out above;

b. that the deceased did not object while alive to removal of any organ from his body;

– it is forbidden to sell or buy an organ or to donate an organ in return for any kind of remuneration;

– organ transplants shall be carried out in medical centres approved for this purpose by the ministry of health.

Furthermore, to prevent any manipulation of the human genetic heritage, the law prohibits the removal from living or dead persons of reproductive organs carrying heredity.

Identical laws were promulgated in Tunisia and Algeria in 1990 and 1991.

Relentless prolongation of life and euthanasia

Relentless prolongation of life is the last option open to the doctor when confronted with a patient in the terminal phase and the apparent impotence of medicine. Present progress in the field of intensive care is such that medicine is capable of prolonging the life, or rather the survival, of the patient. This leads to a tragic debate between technology and the doctor's conscience, all the more poignant in that the patient, even if conscious, is in a situation of diminished freedom.

The doctor's duty is certainly to treat the patient and keep him alive: the criminal code sanctions failure to assist a person in danger, and the Hippocratic Oath tells the doctor not to give poison to anybody. *Primum no nocere* is the *leitmotif* of the Hippocratic Oath.

In Islam, nobody is authorised to put an end to his own life or to anyone else's, even if the person concerned is suffering from an incurable disease. What is more, experience has shown that a prognosis may never be established with absolute certainty.

Lastly, the psychological state of the person who requests the aid of euthanasia when conscious cannot be taken into consideration because of his poor physical and moral condition.

Conclusion

In conclusion, we have seen that recent progress in biology and genetics give man the possibility of controlling reproduction and heredity. This power enables him to redefine life by means of artificial procreation and to shape it by means of prenatal diagnosis and genetic manipulation.

Lastly, this power permits man to redefine death through the use of organ transplants and relentless prolongation of life, thanks to progress in the therapeutic arsenal and recent intensive care techniques.

The many scientific and technical exploits arouse a certain admiration and a certain fascination, but at the same time they give rise to serious concern.

We have shown that Muslim morality is able to bring solutions to these problems. The fundamental principles, as we have seen, are the respect of physical integrity, respect of mental integrity and the maintenance of genealogical perpetuity and filiation.

91

We have also seen that the reality of the human person could be defined as being from when the embryo reaches 100 days, and that through the laws of Islam the solutions do not remain fixed; for all the problems not mentioned in the Koran or the *sunna*, the *ijtihad* constitutes a creative tool, calling upon reflection and reason, which can bring evolutive solutions taking account of recent developments.

The following table sums up the Islamic position on different aspects of bioethics

Deliberate termination of pregnancy		Possible until the 100th day of pregnancy and for medical reasons only
MAP[1]	Artificial insemination	Licit only where the donor of the sperm is the spouse legally joined by marriage
	IVF and ZIFT[2]	Licit where the fertilised egg comes from the union of the wife's ovule and her husband's spermatozoid
	Surrogate mothers	Illicit if the surrogate mother is a stranger to the couple Licit if the surrogate mother is a co-spouse, in the case of polygamy
Prenatal diagnosis		The diagnosis must be made early, so that in the case of risk a therapeutic abortion can be done before the 100th day of pregnancy
Genetic manipulation		Licit in the case of somatic cells (stem cells of the epidermis, haematopoietic cells, etc.) Illicit in the case of germ cells which carry heredity, as this would risk modifying the species
Organ transplants		Possible in the majority of Muslim countries under the legislation specific to each country
Relentless prolongation of life and euthanasia		Nobody is authorised to put an end to his own life or that of another. The doctor's vocation is to save human life and reduce suffering

---

1. MAP: Medically assisted procreation.
2. IVF: *in vitro* fertilisation; ZIFT: zygote intra-fallopian transfer.

Buddhism and the right to respect of the person in the face of risks associated with progress in biotechnologies

by Jacques Martin[1]
Chairman of the Buddhist Union of France

Fundamental elements of Buddhist thought

Introduction

It is scarcely possible to provide in a few lines a complete summary of the enormous mass of literature that makes up the corpus of the Buddha's teaching. I shall therefore restrict myself to drawing attention to the essence of Buddhism and clearing up some possible misapprehensions.

From the moment of his Enlightenment over 2500 years ago until his death around 480 BC, the Buddha taught only one thing: how to recognise suffering in order to be free of it.

What we call Buddhism is the spiritual way which he taught throughout his ministry.

In Buddhist thinking, human existence takes on a particular value in that it enables man to deliver himself from his unsatisfactory condition and to know happiness, lucidity and inner freedom. In the Buddhist approach to existence, it is the quality of the spirit which determines happy or painful experiences and which prolongs the period of becoming spent by beings on one of the six planes which characterise the cycle of rebirth. Release from the unsatisfying and painful condition which characterises all forms of existence requires first of all a knowledge of the true nature of the phenomenal world. This world, characterised by the impermanent and fleeting nature of all things born of causes and conditions, is at the origin of universal suffering. The sequence of events is not random, nor is it the result of a divine will; it depends on complex laws of causality which determine the order of things.

The being, made up of five aggregates or physical and mental constituents in close interdependence, is linked to the rest of the environment, to nature and to other living entities – human or animal.

The Buddhist way exhorts us to lucidity and individual responsibility and seeks to help people through its practice to transcend the immediate information of the senses through analysis and mastery of the perceiving subject – the spirit.

Through personal experience based on meditation, belief in tangible realities is gradually diminished. Meditation reveals the ultimate nature of the spirit, otherwise veiled by the fundamental ignorance which maintains and upholds the erroneous perception of the duality of the inner and outer phenomenal world. It is out of these

---

1. With the collaboration of Drs C. Chevassut and M.A. Pratili for the answers to the cases.

illusory perceptions that passions arise, desire which attracts, hatred which repulses and all the ensuing negative emotions.

These passions condition acts, the consequences of which determine the destiny of beings according to a chain of causation (law of *karma*) which encompasses not only this slice of life but forces the being to remain in the cycle of successive births. More precisely, negative acts – those inspired by ignorance of the true nature of the phenomena whence greed and hatred are derived – inexorably lead to unpleasant effects and keep their perpetrator within the painful cycle of existences, whereas positive acts in harmony with the highest knowledge – vision of the impermanent and insubstantial nature of phenomena – lead to happy conditions of life and to deliverance from the cycle of existence.

As for Buddhist practice proper, the quest for enlightenment takes the spiritual path described by the Buddha, a way of rightness and balance which recommends avoidance of extreme behaviour – giving free rein to sensual desires at one extreme and austere asceticism at the other – and indissolubly associates wisdom and compassion.

The guidance we may find there demonstrates the profoundly ethical dimension of Buddhism. But this ethic has no value in itself; it is part of the fundamental triad of the spiritual path – ethics or morality, meditation or concentration, and wisdom – of which it is the foundation.

The individual is constantly referred to his own responsibility, on the basis of the great principles revealed by the Buddha. It is for each individual to choose his own way without reference to prohibitions or commandments. These are foreign to Buddhist thought. This ethics is essentially an ethics of intention and may be considered differently in the light of the growing wisdom which accompanies spiritual development. This development is achieved through practices of concentration and penetrating vision which are at the heart of Buddhist tradition. Their purpose is to transform man by enlightening and pacifying the spirit and gradually eliminating the negative tendencies which arise from belief in a permanent and substantial self.

It is through development of this inward-looking attitude, which brings balance and a subtle happiness, irrespective of external circumstances, that greed, attachment and egoism can be made to fade quite naturally, giving way to lucid wisdom and compassion.

The being released from passions and mental impurities will experience no further births. He has escaped from the painful cycle of rebirths. The perfect and lasting bliss which accompanies this deliverance is beyond all description and transcends human reason: this is the Buddhist salvation.

Is Buddhism a religion or a philosophy? It is both: a religion which does not recognise the idea of a creator god with an anthropomorphic dimension, but rather speaks of ultimate truth, the non-born, the non-become, the non-conditioned, and is based upon a highly philosophical approach without speculative purpose in the service of the inner experience.

The Buddhist system of thought is free of dogmatism. The Buddhist teachings may be compared, according to a well-known metaphor, to a boat which may be used to pass from one bank to the other, from confusion to transcendent lucidity, and which must be abandoned on arrival.

It is doubtless this last aspect which gives Buddhism all its open-mindedness and tolerance and its respectful attitude towards other religious and intellectual traditions.

Essential elements of Buddhist thought

The human person is based on five physical and mental supports known as aggregates: form (*rupa*), feelings (*vedana*), ideations (*sañña*), volition (*sankhara*) and consciousness (*viññana*). All these phenomena make up the impermanent and illusory flux of personality, which exists only in a relative and conventional way. All composed things are impermanent (*anicca*).

All phenomena, living or not, are not only impermanent but also insubstantial. Born of causes and conditions, they have no existence of their own and are therefore devoid of such existence (*anatta*). Nevertheless, they have a relative existence. Phenomena are of the nature of emptiness simply because they are conditioned. Buddhism postulates a law of causality whence the process of birth and death (*paticcasamuppada*) derives.

Rebirth is explained as follows: the human being is a flow in permanent movement, a succession of births and deaths of particular states of the five psycho-physical aggregates, a series which continues without interruption. We may therefore speak of a continuum. As there is no permanent entity which subsists from one moment to the next, it is obvious that nothing permanent can subsist from one existence to the next. A being that dies and is reborn is neither the same being nor a different being but a continuum which flows along, driven by the moral force of acts. Thus, beings tied to their acts carry in themselves the potentiality of their becoming. The law of karma (or acts) and that of rebirth are therefore intimately linked: karma (acts of will) is, as it were, the energy which feeds the flow of psycho-physical phenomena, or the continuum.

Buddhist thought always moves on two planes: that of relative truth and that of absolute truth.

Buddhist ethics is based on altruism and compassion

It calls for abstention from negative acts: take no life, human or animal; refrain from theft; refrain from drunkenness; refrain from erroneous, trivial or false speech; refrain from illicit sexual relations.

95

These precepts must, of course, be adapted to circumstances of time and place. Monastic Buddhism has a host of rules (over 200) whereas lay believers are advised to comply with the five basic precepts.

The position of Buddhism *vis-à-vis* certain problems connected with biotechnology

The fundamental principle from which a number of opinions on biotechnological risks derive, is that of the supreme sanctity of human life and all forms of existence in general.

The supreme sanctity of human life takes precedence over all other considerations. In the Buddhist approach, human life is extremely difficult to achieve and is the only way of gaining release from the existential cycle.

Biology shows that an embryo is the result of fusion of sperm and ovule, but Buddhism postulates that, in addition to these two elements, a third is necessary to life, namely the continuum of consciousness.

When the genetic conditions arise in a favourable context, the psycho-mental force penetrates and sustains the embryo. The texts report the Buddha's words in this connection:

"O Monks, where the three elements are found in combination, a seed of life is planted. Thus, if the father and mother unite but the time is not right for the mother and the being to be reborn (*gandhabba*) is absent, no seed of life will be planted. Monks, if the father and mother unite and it is the time for the mother, but the being to be reborn is absent, there too, no seed of life will be planted. And if the father and mother unite and the time is right for the mother and for the being to be reborn, then by conjunction of these three elements, a seed of life will be planted" (*Sutta-pitaka, Majjhima-nikaya, I, 265-266, Pali Canon*).

At the time of death, certain physical elements dissolve: the solid and liquid elements, the element of heat and the element of air; the solid element dissolves in the liquid element and the liquid element is absorbed in the heat element, which is reabsorbed into the air element.

The dying being experiences each of these phases in a suggestive way, an impression of being heavy, getting out of depth, being immersed in a liquid. Some of these experiences have recently been associated by American and French scientists with so-called near-death experiences. The continuum of consciousness is thought to remain in the physical frame for three days from the moment of clinical death.

In conclusion, we may say that Buddhism considers that a being is more than a simple biological entity produced by union of the couple.

It exists in its physical and mental totality as, so to speak, the heir of earlier acts. It is a continuum of consciousness possessing its own "programme", which takes shape in the dividing cell. However, although determined by his past acts, the human being has choice and the possibility of changing his future.

Buddhism, while recognising the important influence of heredity and the environment on life, nevertheless emphasises the force of former acts as the essential explanation for the diversity of beings and their situations.

This is attested by the ancient texts:

"Beings are the possessors and heirs of their acts; the act is the womb whence they come, the act is their friend, their refuge. Whatever the act they accomplish, be it positive or negative, it will be their inheritance" (*Majjhima-nikaya, III, 203*).

Buddhist medical ethics stem from these essential principles of rebirth, the law of causality and compassion.

Euthanasia

The most serious negative act in Buddhist ethics is the taking of life (one's own or another's).

But euthanasia is a sensitive and complex problem and the answers depend on whether it is a case of active or passive euthanasia. Generally speaking, it is a matter of refusing acts which end life, but avoiding relentless prolongation of life, which is a form of aggression. The approach of death is essential, and it should be peaceful if possible.

The embryo

According to what we have already said, the embryo is sacred; it possesses all the potentiality of the human being.

Contraception

The use of condoms is the preferred method.

Sterilisation

To be avoided: problem of reversibility.

Abortion

Corresponds to the taking of a life, no matter the stage at which it is performed.

In vitro *fertilisation*

In Buddhism the process of birth is effected in different ways. An embryo *in vitro* is a seed of life and must be protected like a human being. People born by artificial reproduction and children born naturally should enjoy equal status in all respects.

Removal of organs

The removal of organs should be approached from the ethical standpoint, one marked by compassion and the force of a donation made to help another.

Agnostic thought and human bioethics

by Henri Caillavet,[1]
former minister, honorary parliamentarian,
member of the French National Consultative Ethics Committee

Agnostic thought, which does not accept any metaphysical system, has man for its finality, freedom for its principle and reason for its instrument.

Bioethics is the science of morality applied to the life sciences.

Agnostic thought differs from religious thought by the fact that its moral principles are not derived from revelation or tradition, but are the fruit of reason. It is not opposed to any religion because it is upstream of any engagement of that nature. In this it is secular.

Its bioethical approach is simple. An answer is sought to each new or renewed question raised by developments in human biology. It therefore proceeds to a reflection conducted in complete freedom with the one essential duty of respecting the primacy of man. Man is conceived from the universalist perspective of being free, assured of equality, while being linked to all by fraternity. Freedom always imposes the respect of his free will. The equality due to him proscribes any discrimination. Fraternity ensures his dignity and the respect due to all.

Such a clear and assured approach to the goal pursued makes it possible to establish the foundations of a bioethics. To illustrate its implementation we shall consider in this introduction the examination of the particular moral issues raised by biology and in particular the acceleration in its development, progress in genetics and in medically assisted procreation, and also the questions connected with the avoidance of suffering, euthanasia, Aids and lastly the economic consequences of technological advances in health matters.

Knowledge of the human genome is being developed on two fronts: mapping and decoding. It will thus be possible to detect genetic diseases and intervene directly on them, but also to modify individuals and thus the species.

The new prospects for predictive and curative medicine thus opened up certainly serve man and can but be encouraged.

On the other hand, the modification of the human genome must be prohibited, whether it is desired by the individual for his own convenience or imposed collectively under the pretext of social or economic necessity. The equilibrium of any society results in fact from its diversity, the fruit of free genetic mixing. Any deliberate and methodical action on the genome can but upset this equilibrium and have unforeseeable consequences for humanity. The only thing that is certain is that the

---

1. With the assistance of Dr J. Brunschwig, stomatologist, Dr G. Payne, pneumologist, and Prof. P.C. Ranouil, Professor of Law at the Université Paris XIII.

freedom and fraternity proper to man could but suffer. What is more, the dignity of each individual implies that the heredity from which he stems must not be altered, except for the eradication of genetic diseases.

However, since the human race does not stand still, should agnostic thought accept the principle of experimentation on embryonic germ cells – limited to the period up to the fourteenth day, because after this there is functional division of the cells and organisation of the individual – to obtain greater knowledge of the mechanisms of heredity?

As for medically assisted procreation, this can free man from the servitudes of nature. This is how it is practised in our advanced societies. This technique could be used to eliminate genetic diseases, but couples must not be permitted to choose from among several embryos, something which natural procreation would not permit. This again would in fact be acting on the species and upsetting its equilibrium.

As regards the questions connected with the avoidance of suffering, euthanasia, Aids and the economic consequences of technological advances in health matters, the following remarks can be made already.

In agnostic thought there is no virtue in suffering. It is therefore legitimate not to suffer and medical techniques should be used in the service of this legitimate aim.

On the grave question of euthanasia, for agnostic morality it is not impossible that it may be the ultimate degree of freedom.

In the case of Aids, fraternity has to oppose freedom. The question thus arises of whether it would not be legitimate, if the person suffering from this disease hides the fact from his entourage, to protect these people by warning them.

Lastly, agnostic morality cannot pretend to ignore the cost of medical care associated with advances in biology and new technologies. It is therefore already necessary to make choices and this will become increasingly the case. It is important that they should be made openly and in respect of human dignity.

For agnostic thought then, bioethics should guide man in the battle described by Michelet in his *Introduction à l'histoire universelle* as: "That of man against nature, of mind against matter, of freedom against fatalism."

But modern biology has given a new dimension to this combat: that of man against himself. This is why bioethics must prevent him from harming all that is most precious and irreducible in him: his freedom, the equality which is due to him and which he owes to others, and lastly the fraternity without which he would no longer be man.

An international view of patients' rights

by Antonio Piga Rivero and Teresa Alfonso Galán,
Department of Health and Medico-Social Sciences,
Faculty of Medicine, University of Alcalá de Henares (Spain),
WHO Collaborating Centre for Bioethics and Health Legislation

Medicine operates through a personal relationship based on confidence, being an inter-human activity requiring mutual consent.[1] For this reason medicine is a profession in the etymological sense of the word, a declaration of commitment. The oaths and codes of the medical profession developed in the course of history commit the doctor to certain duties in his relations with his patients and therefore imply a recognition of patients' rights. This recognition preceded that of human rights. For example, through the Hippocratic Oath, the doctor undertakes to respect life. "To please no one will I prescribe a deadly drug, nor give advice which may cause his death. Nor will I give a woman a pessary to procure abortion"; "In every house where I come I will enter only for the good of my patients, keeping myself far from all intentional ill-doing and especially from the pleasures of love with women or with men, be they free or slaves. All that may come to my knowledge in the exercise of my profession or outside of my profession or in daily commerce with men, which ought not to be spread abroad, I will keep secret and will never reveal."

In the Chinese tradition, Confucius affirms that the ideal relationship between rational beings is finally one of compassion and benevolence.

But the Confucian, Taoist and Buddhist schools, refusing to admit the conceptual and ontological separation between the human being and the universe, do not make the subject of human rights a specific and independent problem, because for them inter-human relations are simply a step towards a higher goal, that of the harmony of the universe.

In the five commandments (1617) of the Chinese doctor Chen Shih-Kung medical secrecy is imposed on the doctor and it is written: "Prostitutes should be treated as if they were of good family, free services being given to those who are poor."

In the Middle Ages the Christian, Jewish and Arab traditions demanded that the doctor treat his patients like brothers, all being sons of God and created in His image, without difference ("And God said, 'Let us make man in our image, after our likeness'", Genesis, 1, v. 26).

In the recommendation to a doctor (tenth century) by the Persian doctor Haly Abbas (Ahwazi) we read: "Do not prescribe or use harmful or abortive drugs"; "Respect the confidences and protect the secrets of the patients"; "Give yourself

---

1. E.D. Pellegrino and D.C. Thomas, *A philosophical basis of medical practice*, Oxford University Press, 1981.

untiringly to the treatment of patients, especially of the poor. Never expect remuneration from the poor."

Even more evolved is the expression of respect of the human being and of the equality of all patients before the doctor, in the prayer of Moses Maimonides (twelfth century), where we read: "May the love for my art actuate me at all times; may neither avarice nor miserliness, nor thirst for glory, or for a great reputation engage my mind"; "Support the strength of my heart, that it may always be ready to serve the poor man and the rich, the friend and the enemy, the good and the bad. Let me see in them only the man who suffers"; "Let my patients have confidence in me and my art"; "Give me, O Lord, indulgence and patience in the face of stubborn and rude patients."

For Christianity, the relationship with patients is the fundamental expression of charity which according to St Thomas Aquinas, for example, represents the direct consequence of the love of man for God and the formal correlation of the love of God for man.

The exercise of medicine has always imposed on doctors the respect of deontological duties towards their patients for reasons connected not only with the religious and cultural traditions of each country and each epoch, but also through the requirements of the doctor-patient relationship regarding the confidence, collaboration and consent of the patient, essential for the efficacy of the diagnostic, therapeutic, and didactic processes and of the spiritual relief, when there can be no other, of medicine.

In discussing the emergence of patients' rights as they are understood today, it is also necessary to take account of the historic development of the recognition of human rights and of the characteristics of the medical developments which have made necessary the legal protection of patients' rights on top of the voluntarily accepted obligation to act in conformity with these rights.

The sources of human rights are to be found in the Bible as well as in philosophy (Protagoras, Aristotle, Plato, the Stoics), Roman Law and the English Magna Charta of 1215, continuing through the burgeoning of humanism in the Renaissance, where men proclaimed their will and their right to become the masters of nature and their responsibility for organising themselves socially in freedom of spirit.

The Declaration of the Rights of Man and the Citizen of 1789 had the merit of having universal vocation, as Volney pointed out in his address to the constituent Assembly: "Until now we have deliberated about France and for France; today you are going to deliberate for the universe and in the universe."[1]

---

1. J.-F. Raymond, *Les enjeux des droits de l'homme*, Larousse, Paris, 1988.

But it was still necessary that humanity should suffer and become aware of the horrors of the second world war – Jewish genocide, concentration camps, racial laws, crimes committed under the pretext of eugenics or medical experimentation – for human rights to be considered the legitimate foundation for a universal community and, secondly, for an international medical deontology to develop.

Thus the San Francisco Conference opened in April 1945 and closed on 26 June with the signature of the United Nations Charter, which established the basis for an international order oriented towards the safeguard of fundamental rights.[1]

On 10 December 1948, the United Nations General Assembly adopted the Universal Declaration of Human Rights.

On 4 November 1950, in the context of the Council of Europe, the European Convention on Human Rights was signed by all the member states of the Council of Europe.

The European Convention has a human rights protection mechanism consisting of the European Commission of Human Rights and the European Court of Human Rights, with the task of protecting the interests, in the name of common values higher than those of states, of individuals living under the authority of member states.[2]

As for medicine and human rights, in the aftermath of the second world war, the allied judges enshrined in the Nuremberg Code the basic ethical rules for experimentation human subjects, and in 1947 the World Medical Association was created, which proclaimed the Geneva Oath, updating the Hippocratic Oath, in 1948, and the International Code of Medical Ethics in 1949.

Following the philosophy of the Universal Declaration of Human Rights, the Constitution of the World Health Organisation states that health is a fundamental right of all humans, and explains that it is "a state of complete physical, mental and social well-being and does not consist only of an absence of disease or infirmity".

As a specialised agency of the United Nations, the WHO promotes the respect of human rights in all its work, and notably in that concerned with the humanisation of medicine, new technologies, problems of equality of access to health services, health care for children and women, etc. We may cite as examples: the UNAIDS programme, formerly the Global Programme on Aids, which aims at combating this disease in the respect of human rights; the recommendations on the ethical requirements of organ transplants; and the inclusion of Target 38, Health and Ethics, in the WHO European Policy for health for all.

The Council of the Europe has for its part done a great deal for the protection of

---

1. J.M. Becet, D. Colard, *Les droits de l'homme*, Economica, Paris, 1982.
2. F. Sudre, *La Convention européenne des droits de l'homme*, PUF, Paris, 1990.

patients' rights, from different points of view: protection of confidentiality, samples, grafts and transplants of human substances and organs, the protection of persons suffering from mental disorder placed as involuntary patients, artificial human fertilisation, etc., and, specifically on medicine and human rights, it has worked on the legal obligations of doctors *vis-à-vis* their patients and on medicine and human rights.[1]

In addition to the horrors of the second world war and the reflection they triggered on the importance of safeguarding medical ethics, many other factors have stimulated the development of the recognition of patients' rights, among them:

– the growing technicality of medicine, which gives rise to enormous ethical dilemmas;

– the practice of medicine in teams;

– society's belief that medicine is extremely effective and that failures are the fault of the doctors;

– the changes that have come about in the contractual relationship between doctor and patient in both private practice and social protection schemes;

– growing awareness of their own rights on the part of citizens;

– the evolution of the jurisprudence on professional liability in all the developed countries;

– the fact that doctors are increasingly taking out insurance to cover themselves against having to compensate patients;

– changes in the doctor-patient relationship due to the doctor's role in the attribution of social, economic or other rights which depend on the state of health;

– the influence that the evolution of medicine and of the recognition of patients' rights in the United States has had in Europe, from the standpoint of professional liability.

All this has created a need for analysis and normative clarification of the respective rights, duties and responsibilities in the therapeutic relationship, going beyond deontological self-discipline, for the protection of both patients and health professionals, through clarifying the general and specific norms for many particular cases, all this in a debate which, in so far as it concerns fundamental human rights, is necessarily international.

The WHO Regional Office for Europe carried out a study in 1988/89 on patients' rights in Europe. Published in 1993,[2] it clearly demonstrated the need to formulate patients' rights taking account of the international human rights instruments and the conditions of and outlook for the practice of medicine. This problem was discussed at a European Consultation in Amsterdam from 28 to 30 March

---

1. Council of Europe, *Le médecin face aux droits de l'homme*, CEDAM, Padua, 1990 (available in French only).

2. H.J.J. Leenen, J.K.M Gevers., G. Pinet, *The rights of patients in Europe*, Kluwer, Deventer, 1993.

1994, which resulted in "A declaration on the promotion of patients' rights in Europe", the text of which is reproduced below.

Declaration on the promotion of patients' rights in Europe
European consultation on the rights of patients, Amsterdam, 28 to 30 March 1994, World Health Organization, Regional Office for Europe.

1. *Human rights and values in health care*
The instruments cited in the introduction should be understood as applying also specifically in the health care setting, and it should therefore be noted that the human values expressed in these instruments shall be reflected in the health care system. It should also be noted that where exceptional limitations are imposed on the rights of patients, these must be in accordance with human rights instruments and have a legal base in the law of the country. It may be further observed that the rights specified below carry a matching responsibility to act with due concern for the health of others and for their same rights.

1.1. Everyone has the right to respect of his or her person as a human being.

1.2. Everyone has the right to self-determination.

1.3. Everyone has the right to physical and mental integrity and to the security of his or her person.

1.4. Everyone has the right to respect for his of her privacy.

1.5. Everyone has the right to have his or her moral and cultural values and religious and philosophical convictions respected.

1.6. Everyone has the right to such protection of health as is afforded by appropriate measures for disease prevention and health care, and to the opportunity to pursue his or her own highest attainable level of health.

2. *Information*
2.1. Information about health services and how best to use them is to be made available to the public in order to benefit all those concerned.

2.2. Patients have the right to be fully informed about their health status, including the medical facts about their condition; about the proposed medical procedures, together with the potential risks and benefits of each procedure; about alternatives to the proposed procedures, including the effect of non-treatment; and about the diagnosis, prognosis and progress of treatment.

2.3. Information may only be withheld from patients exceptionally when there is good reason to believe that this information would without any exception of obvious positive effects cause them serious harm.

2.4. Information must be communicated to the patient in a way appropriate to the latter's capacity for understanding, minimising the use of unfamiliar technical terminology. If the patient does not speak the common language, some form of interpreting should be available.

2.5. Patients have the right not to be informed, at their explicit request.

2.6. Patients have the right to choose who, if any one, should be informed on their behalf.

2.7. Patients should have the possibility of obtaining a second opinion.

2.8. When admitted to a health care establishment, patients should be informed of the identity and professional status of the health care providers taking care of them and of any rules and routines which would bear on their stay and care.

2.9. Patients should be able to request and be given a written summary of their diagnosis, treatment and care on discharge from a health care establishment.

3. *Consent*

3.1. The informed consent of the patient is a prerequisite for any medical intervention.

3.2. A patient has the right to refuse or to halt a medical intervention. The implications of refusing or halting such an intervention must be carefully explained to the patient.

3.3. When a patient is unable to express his or her will and a medical intervention is urgently needed, the consent of the patient may be presumed, unless it is obvious from a previous declared expression of will that consent would be refused in the situation.

3.4. When the consent of a legal representative is required and the proposed intervention is urgently needed, that intervention may be made if it is not possible to obtain, in time, the representative's consent.

3.5. When the consent of a legal representative is required, patients (whether minor or adult) must nevertheless be involved in the decision-making process to the fullest extent which their capacity allows.

3.6. If a legal representative refuses to give consent and the physician or other provider is of the opinion that the intervention is in the interest of the patient, then the decision must be referred to a court or some form of arbitration.

3.7. In all other situations where the patient is unable to give informed consent and where there is no legal representative or representative designated by the patient for this purpose, appropriate measures should be taken to provide for a substitute decision-making process, taking into account what is known and, to the greatest extent possible, what may be presumed about the wishes of the patient.

3.8. The consent of the patient is required for the preservation and the use of all substances of the human body. Consent may be presumed when the substances are to be used in the current course of diagnosis, treatment and care of that patient.

3.9. The informed consent of the patient is needed for participation in clinical teaching.

3.10. The informed consent of the patient is a prerequisite for participation in scientific research. All protocols must be submitted to proper ethical review procedures. Such research should not be carried out on those who are unable to express their will, unless the consent of a legal representative has been obtained and the research would likely be in the interest of the patient.

As an exception to the requirement of involvement being in the interest of the patient, an incapacitated person may be involved in observational research which is not of direct benefit to his or her health provided that that person offers no objection, that the risk and/or burden is minimal, that the research is of significant value and that no alternative methods and other research subjects are available.

4. *Confidentiality and privacy*

4.1. All information about a patient's health status, medical condition, diagnosis, prognosis and treatment and all other information of a personal kind must be kept confidential, even after death.

4.2. Confidential information can only be disclosed if the patient gives explicit consent or if the law expressly provides for this. Consent may be presumed where disclosure is to other health care providers involved in that patient's treatment.

4.3. All identifiable patient data must be protected. The protection of the data must be appropriate to the manner of their storage. Human substances from which identifiable data can be derived must be likewise protected.

4.4. Patients have the right to access to their medical files and technical records and to any other files and records pertaining to their diagnosis, treatment and care and to receive a copy of their own files and records or parts thereof. Such access excludes data concerning third parties.

4.5. Patients have the right to require the correction, completion, deletion, clarification and/or updating of personal and medical data concerning them which are inaccurate, incomplete, ambiguous or outdated, or which are not relevant to the purposes of diagnosis, treatment and care.

4.6. There can be no intrusion into a patient's private and family life unless and only if, in addition to the patient consenting to it, it can be justified as necessary to the patient's diagnosis, treatment and care.

4.7. Medical interventions may only be carried out when there is proper respect shown for the privacy of the individual. This means that a given intervention may be carried out only in the presence of those persons who are necessary for the intervention unless the patient consents or requests otherwise.

4.8. Patients admitted to health care establishments have the right to expect physical facilities which ensure privacy, particularly when health care providers are offering them personal care or carrying out examinations and treatment.

5. *Care and treatment*

5.1. Everyone has the right to receive such health care as is appropriate to his or her health needs, including preventive care and activities aimed at health promotion. Services should be continuously available and accessible to all equitably, without discrimination and according to the financial, human and material resources which can be made available in a given society.

5.2. Patients have a collective right to some form of representation at each level of the health care system in matters pertaining to the planning and evaluation of services, including the range, quality and functioning of the care provided.

5.3. Patients have the right to a quality of care which is marked both by high technical standards and by a humane relationship between the patient and health care providers.

5.4. Patients have the right to continuity of care, including co-operation between all health providers and/or establishments which may be involved in their diagnosis, treatment and care.

5.5. In circumstances where a choice must be made by providers between potential patients for a particular treatment which is in limited supply, all such patients are entitled to a fair selection procedure for that treatment. That choice must be based on medical criteria and made without discrimination.

5.6. Patients have the right to choose and change their own physician or other health care provider and health care establishment, provided that it is compatible with the functioning of the health care system.

5.7. Patients for whom there are no longer medical grounds for continued stay in a health care establishment are entitled to a full explanation before they can be transferred to another establishment or sent home. Transfer can only take place after another health care establishment has agreed to accept the patient. Where the patient is discharged to home and when his or her condition so requires, community and domiciliary services should be available.

5.8. Patients have the right to be treated with dignity in relation to their diagnosis, treatment and care, which should be rendered with respect for their culture and values.

5.9. Patients have the right to enjoy support from family, relatives and friends during the course of care and treatment and to receive spiritual support and guidance at all times.

5.10. Patients have the right to relief of their suffering according to the current state of knowledge.

5.11. Patients have the right to humane terminal care and to die in dignity.

6. *Application*

6.1. The exercise of the rights set forth in this document implies that appropriate means are established for this purpose.

6.2. The enjoyment of these rights shall be secured without discrimination.

6.3. In the exercise of these rights, patients shall be subjected only to such limitations as are compatible with human rights instruments and in accordance with a procedure prescribed by law.

6.4. If patients cannot avail themselves of the rights set forth in this document, these rights should be exercised by their legal representative or by a person designated by the patient for that purpose; where neither a legal representative nor a personal surrogate has been appointed, other measures for representation of those patients should be taken.

6.5. Patients must have access to such information and advice as will enable them to exercise the rights set forth in this document. Where patients feel that their rights have not been respected they should be enabled to lodge a complaint. In addition to recourse to the courts, there should be independent mechanisms at institutional and other levels to facilitate the processes of lodging, mediating and adjudicating complaints. These mechanisms would, *inter alia*, ensure that information relating to complaints procedures was available to patients and that an independent person was available and accessible to them for consultation regarding the most appropriate course of action to take. These mechanisms should further ensure that, where necessary, assistance and advocacy on behalf of the patient would be made available. Patients have the right to have their complaints examined and dealt with in a thorough, just, effective and prompt way and to be informed about their outcome.

Fertilisation by donor

A married couple, the wife able to bear children and the husband suffering from azoospermia, requests donor insemination.

a. The right to practise
b. Informed consent of couple
c. Liability of doctor for quality of donor's sperm as regards genetics (possibility of incest) and infection (congenital diseases)
d. Anonymity of donor
e. Use of semen from more than one donor
f. Legal problem in the case of obligation to enter father's name on civil status documents
g. Remuneration of donor
h. Relinquishment of all rights by donor
i. Professional secrecy

1. From the standpoint of international law

In general

At present, international law contains no binding provision on either artificial insemination in the strict sense or implantation of an ovule fertilised by the sperm of the husband or partner in the womb of a "surrogate mother".

Nevertheless, a number of guidelines may be drawn from three recommendations issued by the Parliamentary Assembly of the Council of Europe (Recommendation 934 (1982) on genetic engineering, Recommendation 1046 (1986) of 24 September 1986 on the use of human embryos and foetuses for diagnostic, therapeutic, scientific, industrial and commercial purposes and Recommendation 1100 (1989) of 2 February 1989 on the use of human embryos and foetuses in scientific research), Resolutions 327/88 and 372/88 approved on 16 March 1989 by the European Parliament and a number of European case-law decisions.

These recommendations and resolutions, considering that, "by the technique of *in vitro* fertilisation, man has achieved the means of intervening in and controlling human life in its earliest stages", state in their preambles that "human embryos and foetuses must be treated in all circumstances with the respect due to human dignity" and stress the fundamental importance of the human rights dimension.

Accordingly, paragraph 4 of Resolution 372/88 "recognises the value of life and more especially the human being's right to protection and therefore expresses its concern at the "waste" of embryos which *in vitro* fertilisation can entail" and "hopes that techniques and practices will be employed to eliminate this risk".

Paragraphs 5 and 6 of the same resolution "call therefore for the number of egg cells fertilised by *in vitro* fertilisation to be limited to the number that can be actually implanted" and "considers that embryos should only be frozen to keep them alive where immediate transfer *in utero* is impossible for any reason occurring during fertilisation".

Hence, (paragraph 8) "the storage of frozen embryos should be permitted only if the woman's state of health temporarily prevents her from having the embryo implanted and she has stated that she is willing to have it implanted at a later date. Under no circumstances should a frozen embryo be stored for more than three years. If implantation is out of the question (because of refusal, illness or the death of the woman) the embryo should be taken out of storage and allowed to die. Trading in or experimentation with such embryos should be punishable by law" (see also paragraph 36, Resolution 327/88).

In detail

a. Paragraph 9 of Resolution 372/88 EEC states that "*in vivo* and *in vitro* artificial insemination should be used for therapeutic purposes (to remedy infertility) and should therefore be allowed only on a doctor's recommendation and must be carried out by highly qualified doctors" and paragraph 10 adds that "heterologous *in vivo* or *in vitro* insemination is not desirable" as "it is to the child's advantage to have a common 'biological', 'legal' and 'emotional' bond with both father and mother" (paragraph E of the preamble) and because techniques of artificial *in vivo* and *in vitro* insemination, "while they provide a positive solution to the legitimate desire to have children, also raise serious problems with (...) the legal 'status' of the child conceived in this manner and can also provide the opportunity for dangerous experimentation on and manipulation of the human embryo" (paragraph B of the preamble; see also paragraphs 38, 29 and 40 of Resolution 327/88) and, finally, because the child's "right to its own genetic identity" is one of the "main criteria governing this area" (paragraph D of the preamble).

Nevertheless, paragraph 10 of Resolution 372/88 specifies the conditions which should be met "should this principle not be accepted in a member state".

b. Among these conditions are (paragraph 10.3) "informed consent of the couple" and "confirmation of their suitability, in accordance, by analogy, with the regulations governing adoption". Paragraph 10.4 also provides for a "ban on disavowal of paternity in the case of artificial insemination by a donor", and (10.2) "no possibility of economic gain either for the donor or for the medical staff". Paragraph 10.5 prohibits any allowance, even minimal, for the donor.

The consent of the couple is also required by Articles 5 of Protocol 7 to the ECHR, and 23 (4) of the Covenant on Civil and Political Rights according to which "the spouses shall enjoy equality of rights and responsibilities of a private law character between them (...) during the marriage".

c. Heterologous artificial insemination may be performed only where there is "verified irreversible sterility or certified serious risk of malformation of a naturally conceived child" (ibid.) and it may be carried out "only in authorised centres, with medical and hygiene conditions fully guaranteed (...) and with restrictions on the use of sperm to avoid the risk of incest" (ibid.).

It should be pointed out that in the terms of Article 14 of the bioethics convention (for ease of reference this shall be referred to as BC), "The use of techniques of medically assisted procreation shall not be allowed for the purpose of choosing a future child's sex, except where serious hereditary sex-related disease is to be avoided." It should also be noted that in the terms of Article 26 (2), the application of Article 14 cannot be subject to any restriction, including for the reasons set out in Article 26 (1).

As regards the doctor's liability for the quality of the sperm as regards infections, see the reply to point c of case 2.

In the terms of Article 18 (2), "The creation of human embryos for research purposes is prohibited."

Paragraph 3 of the Appendix to Recommendation 1100 further provides that "the human gametes employed for investigation or experimentation shall not be used to create zygotes or embryos *in vitro* for the purpose of procreation".

d. Accordingly (ibid.), the donor of sperm, ovules or embryos must remain anonymous and there is a ban on "even the smallest demand for maintenance payments from the donor" (paragraph 10, Resolution 372/88).

e. Paragraph iv of Recommendation 1046 forbids the "creation of embryos from the sperm of different individuals".

f. No provision of international law stipulates the rule to be applied regarding the compulsory recording of the father's name in civil-status documents. It follows from paragraph 10, Resolution 372/88 quoted above, however, that the legal father is necessarily identified as the spouse of the inseminated woman, for whom any action to disclaim should be prohibited. It should, nevertheless, be recalled that the Court has several times affirmed (Decision No. 106 of 7.10.1986 in the case of *Rees-Commission* v. *United Kingdom*; Decision No. 184 of 27.9.1990 in the case of *Cossey-Commission* v. *United Kingdom*; Decision No. 232 C of 25.3.1992 in the case of *B.-Commission* v. *France*) that states enjoy a large degree of latitude regarding the legal regime governing civil-status documents, provided that the conditions of Article 8 of the ECHR are satisfied. The same applies with respect to amendments to these instruments.

From the standpoint of Articles 8 and 14 of the ECHR, refer *mutatis mutandis* to the decision of 27.6.1995 of the Commission in the case *X, Y and Z,* v. *the United Kingdom* (Application No. 21830/93).

g. As we have already seen, there may be no possibility of economic gain either for the donor or for the medical staff. Paragraphs 20 and 23 of the Appendix to Recommendation 1100 further specify that "the purchase or sale of embryos (...) or parts thereof by their donor parents or other parties (...) shall also be prohibited". "The donation of organs shall be devoid of any commercial aspect."

The prohibition of any form of profit is also affirmed by Article 11 of the DBC, in the terms of which "the human body and its parts shall not, as such, give rise to financial gain". Paragraphs 88 to 90 of the explanatory report state in this connection that "this article applies the principle of human dignity set forth in the preamble and in Article 1 (...) Under this provision organs and tissues proper, including blood, should not be bought or sold or give rise to financial gain for the person from whom they have been removed or for a third party, whether an individual or a corporate entity such as a hospital. However, technical acts (sampling, testing, storage, culture, transport, etc.), which are performed on the basis of these items may legitimately give rise to reasonable remuneration. For instance, this article does not prohibit the sale of tissue which is part of a medical device since the tissue is not sold as such. Further, this article does not prevent a person from whom an organ or tissue has been taken from receiving compensation which, while not constituting remuneration, compensates that person equitably for expenses incurred or loss of income (for example as a result of hospitalisation). The provision does not refer to such tissues as hair and nails, which are discarded tissues, and the sale of which is not an affront to human dignity.

In the same sense, Articles 21 and 26 of the BC.

h. See points *b* and *d.*

i. There is no explicit reply. An implicit positive reply may be derived from Articles 8 (1) and 10 (2) of the ECHR. See also Article 10 (1) of the BC.

The provisions cited above are applicable by analogy to donations of ovules or embryos.

The following relevant points in European case-law should also be noted:

i.   as a general rule, *mutatis mutandis,* "although the right to found a family is an absolute right (....), it does not mean that a person must at all times be given the actual possibility to procreate" (Commission report on Application Nos. 6564/74,

7114/75, 8166/78 and 17142/90), because "there is nothing to support the conclusion that the capacity to procreate is an essential condition of marriage, or even that procreation is an essential purpose of marriage" (Commission report on Application No. 7654/76);

ii. as for the necessary consent of the husband in the light of Article 8 of the ECHR, see, *a contrario*, Judgment No. 290 (26.5.1994) in the *Keegan* case (*Commission* v. *Ireland*) and the Commission report in Application Nos. 6959/75 and 8416/79;

iii. as for the legal presumption of paternity in the case of the break-up of the marriage, see Judgment No. 297 C (27.10.1994) in the case of *Kroon and others* (*Commission* v. *Netherlands*), as well as the two dissenting opinions appended to it;

iv. as for the legal status of the child born of adultery, see the Commission report on Application No. 11418/85;

v. as for the time period set by national legislations for repudiation of paternity, see Judgment No. 87 (28.11.1984) in the *Rasmussen* case (*Commission* v. *Denmark*);

vi. as for the anonymity of the donor, whose name does not appear in official documents but does appear in a confidential file held by the authorities, if the child asked to consult it and the public authorities should refuse access because of the lack of consent by the donor, possible application of Judgment No. 160 (7.7.1989) in the *Gaskin* case (*Commission* v. *United Kingdom*).

vii. as for the legal problems stemming from the obligatory inclusion of the name of the legal father in official documents, if the donor (biological father) applied to acknowledge the child, possible application of paragraph 40 of Judgment No. 297 C (27.10.1994), in the terms of which "in the Court's opinion, 'respect' for 'family life' [as stipulated by Article 8 of the ECHR] requires that biological and social reality prevail over a legal presumption which, as in the present case, flies in the face of both established fact and the wishes of those concerned without actually benefiting anyone".

2. From the ethical standpoint

The WMA has taken a positive view of medically assisted procreation as a way of helping infertile couples to have children. Where the gamete donor or donors will not be the functional parent(s) of the child, the doctor must obtain assurance that the recipients will accept full responsibility for the unborn child and that the donors will renounce all rights or claims to it, without prejudice to its rights after birth.

In its statement on *in vitro* fertilisation and embryo transplantation, Madrid (1987), the WMA specified that:

a. consent must also apply to the procedure used;

b. the patients are entitled to the same confidentiality and privacy as is required with any medical treatment.

The WMA recommends that physicians refrain from intervening in the reproductive process for the purpose of making a choice as to the foetus' sex, unless it is to avoid the transmission of serious sex-linked disease.

The WMA condemns any commercialisation by which ova, sperm or embryos are offered for purchase or sale.

The European Ethics Guide added in its Article 18 that it is ethical for a doctor to refuse on the grounds of his convictions to intervene in the reproductive process, and to suggest that the people concerned seek the opinions of other doctors.

3. From the standpoint of religious moralities

a. *Catholic*

The points of view of Catholic morality are extracted from official documents of the magisterium of the Church contained in the *Acta Apostolicae Sedis* (AAS) the broadcasts, speeches and messages of His Holiness Pius XII, the documents of the Vatican II Council, the documents of various congregations of the Holy See and *L'Osservatore Romano.*

The different positions of theologians have not been taken into account here.

The judgment of Catholic morality on artificial insemination in general is negative, as it implies a separation in the conjugal act between the procreative meaning and the unitive meaning;[1] still more immoral is heterologous artificial insemination, which "is contrary to the unity of marriage, to the dignity of the spouses, to the vocation proper to the parents, and to the child's right to be conceived and brought into the world in marriage and from marriage".[2]

b. *Protestant*

The starting point of our thinking is always the unborn child and his right to unequivocal filiation. From this point of view, most Protestant Churches, without categorically banning heterologous insemination, do not really advise it.

c. *Jewish*

In the Talmud (Haguiga tractate 15.a), we are taught that a virgin may become pregnant by bathing in water containing sperm. This famous text, drafted some 1700 years ago, was the first to envisage the possibility of artificial fertilisation. For us, it is one of the bases for legal thinking on the problem of artificial insemination.

---

1. Paul VI, *Humanae Vitae*, No. 12.
2. Pius XII, AAS 41 (1949), p. 559 and AAS 45 (1953), pp. 674-675.

According to the great majority of our rabbis, an act of fertilisation using sperm from a donor other than the husband is to be utterly condemned. It is even considered by several rabbis as an abomination.

However, if it is definitively proved that no other treatment is possible and that this technique has every chance of succeeding, in this specific case, as a last resort, insemination using the husband's sperm could be tolerated.[1]

d. *Muslim*

Heterologous insemination is strictly forbidden in Islam. In this case, fertilisation may only be effected by the woman's legal spouse.

e. *Buddhist*

With the couple's informed consent, if the donor's anonymity is preserved and if he does not receive any reward – as his participation may be motivated only by the desire to help others, which also implies that he forego any right to paternity and any possibility of knowing the child's identity at a later stage – this practice is acceptable. It seems, however, that the couple could be guided towards the possibility of adoption.

"A man worries himself saying, I have sons, I have goods. In truth he himself is not his own; whose then are his sons, whose his goods?" (Dhammapada, v. 62)

4. From the standpoint of agnostic morality

French law allows the right to medically assisted procreation, but the couple must give free and informed consent. The doctor has no liability with respect to the quality of the sperm. The anonymity of the donor is an absolute rule. The mixing of spermatic liquid is not permitted, but if the attempt is unsuccessful, sperm may be taken from another "flask". The name of the father is not given on the birth certificate and the legal father is the woman's husband. The donor receives no remuneration except for the reimbursement of modest expenses, for example to cover travel costs, time, etc. The donor donates his sperm, and having done so both he and the spermatic liquid remain anonymous.

---

1. M. Gugenheim, "Contre le bébé éprouvette" ("Against the test-tube baby"), *Information juive*, March 1984.

Restoration of fertility by surgical operation

An unmarried adult couple have been living together for five years and are considering getting married to start a family, but pregnancy is impossible because of tubal obstruction.

    a. Right to practise
    b. Informed consent of couple
       Surgical solution to restore tubal continuity
    c. Civil liability of the doctor.

1. From the standpoint of international law

a. The answer is affirmative in the light of the decisions of the Commission cited at the end of case 1, provided that the risks and drawbacks of the surgical operation requested do not exceed the hoped for advantages and do not jeopardise the patient's health.

In fact, according to the Commission "although the right to found a family is an absolute right (...), it does not mean that a person must at all times be given the actual possibility to procreate, the capacity to procreate [not being] an essential condition of marriage, or even that procreation is an essential purpose of marriage" (Application No. 7654/76).

In the same sense, see Article 4 of the BC, in the terms of which "any intervention in the health field (...) must be carried out in accordance with relevant professional obligations and standards" and points 31 and 32 of the explanatory report: "(…) Doctors and, in general, all professionals who participate in a medical act are subject to legal and ethical imperatives (...). Competence must be determined primarily in relation to the scientific knowledge and clinical experience appropriate to a profession or speciality at a given time. "In this respect it is indicated that the administration of care must be consistent with established scientific methods. Nevertheless, it is accepted that" professional standards do not necessarily prescribe one line of action as being the only one possible: recognised medical practice may, indeed, allow several possible forms of intervention, thus leaving some freedom of choice as to methods or techniques. Further, a particular course of action must be judged in the light of the specific health problem raised by a given patient. In particular, an intervention must meet criteria of relevance and proportionality between the aim pursued and the means used" (32-33). Article 4 concerns doctors and members of the health care professions only, it "does not concern persons other than health care professionals called upon to perform medical acts, for example in an emergency" (28).

b. The need for the patient's informed consent may be implicitly derived from either Article 7 of the Covenant on Civil and Political Rights, which states that "no one shall be subjected without his free consent to medical or scientific experimentation" or the fundamental right of everyone to respect for his or her physical integrity. See also Article 5 (1) of the BC, in the terms of which "an intervention in the health field may only be carried out after the person concerned has given free and informed consent to it. This person shall beforehand be given appropriate information as to the purpose and nature of the intervention as well as on its consequences and risks. The person concerned may freely withdraw consent at any time", and points 34 to 40 of the explanatory report : "this article deals with consent and affirms at the international level an already well-established rule, that is that no one may in principle be forced to undergo an intervention without his or her consent. Human beings must therefore be able freely to give or refuse their informed consent to any intervention involving their person. This rule makes clear patients' autonomy in their relationship with health care professionals and restrains the paternalist approaches which might ignore the wish of the patient. The word 'intervention' is understood in its widest sense, as in Article 3 – that is to say, it covers all medical acts, in particular interventions performed for the purpose of preventive care, diagnosis, treatment, rehabilitation or research. In order for their consent to be valid, the persons in question must have been informed about the relevant facts regarding the intervention being contemplated. This information must include the purpose, nature and consequences of the intervention and the risks involved. Information on the risks involved in the intervention or in alternative courses of action must cover not only the risks inherent in the type of intervention contemplated, but also any risks related to the individual characteristics of each patient, such as age or the existence of other pathologies (...). Moreover, this information must be sufficiently clear and suitably worded for the person who is to undergo the intervention. The patient must be put in a position, through the use of terms he or she can understand, to weigh up the necessity or usefulness of the aim and methods of the intervention against its risks and the discomfort or pain it will cause. Consent may take various forms. It may be express or implied. Express consent may be either verbal or written. Article 5, which is general and covers very different situations, does not require any particular form. The latter will largely depend on the nature of the intervention. It is agreed that express consent would be inappropriate as regards many routine medical acts. The consent is therefore often implicit, as long as the person concerned is sufficiently informed. In some cases, however, for example, invasive diagnostic acts or treatments, express consent may be required. Moreover, the patient's express, specific consent must be obtained for participation in research or removal of body parts for transplantation purposes (...). Freedom of consent implies that consent may be withdrawn at any time and that the patient's decision shall be respected once he or she has been fully informed of the consequences. Furthermore,

Article 26 of the convention, as well as Article 6 concerning protection of persons not able to consent, Article 7 concerning protection of persons who have mental disorders and Article 8 concerning emergency situations, define the instances in which the exercise of the rights contained in the convention and hence the need for consent may be limited."

As regards the consent of the partner, no international text requires it in this case, even though according to the established case-law of the Court, Article 8 of the ECHR guarantees the respect of family life, in the case both of a family based on marriage and a *de facto* family. But it would be the same if, in the present case, the couple were married, notwithstanding the wording of Article 5 of Protocol 7 to the ECHR, which stipulates that "spouses shall enjoy equality of rights of a private law character during marriage and in the event of its dissolution". A possible disagreement between the man/husband and the women on the subject of procreation of a child would in fact be at a subsequent stage to the surgical intervention intended to restore the patient's tubular continuity. Attention should also be drawn to the Commission's decision in Application No. 8416/79, in the terms of which "it is first of all necessary to take account of the wife's right to private and family life, for she is the one most concerned by pregnancy".

c. See Article 24 of the BC, in the terms of which "the person who has suffered undue damage resulting from an intervention is entitled to fair compensation according to the conditions and procedures prescribed by law". Points 143 to 146 of the explanatory report explain in this connection that "this article sets forth the principle that any person who has suffered undue damage resulting from an intervention is entitled to fair compensation. The convention uses the expression 'undue damage' because in medicine some damage, such as amputation, is inherent in the therapeutic intervention itself. The due or undue nature of the damage will have to be determined in the light of the circumstances of each case. The cause of the damage must be an intervention in the widest sense, taking the form of either an act or an omission. The intervention may or may not constitute an offence. In order to give entitlement to compensation, the damage must result from the intervention. Compensation conditions and procedures are prescribed by national law. In many cases, this establishes a system of individual liability based either on fault or on the notion of risk or strict liability. In other cases, the law may provide for a collective system of compensation irrespective of individual liability. On the subject of fair compensation, reference can be made to Article 50 of the ECHR, which allows the Court to afford just satisfaction to the injured party".

As regards European case-law, see, *mutatis mutandis*, the Decision of 22.5.1995 of the Commission on the admissibility of Application No. 20948/92 (*Isiltan* v. *Turkey*).

It should be noted in passing that as regards a child born within a "consensual union", "the Court discerns no objective and reasonable justification for the differences of treatment between an 'illegitimate' and a 'legitimate' child" with regard, *inter alia*, to rights of inheritance (Judgment in the *Marckx* case, 13.6.1979 and Decision No. 214 C of 29.11.1991 in the *Vermeire* case, *Commission v. Belgium*).

See also Judgment Nos. 112 (18.12.1986) in the *Johnston and others* case (*Commission v. Ireland*); 138 (21.6.1988) in the *Berrehab* case (*Commission v. Netherlands*); 290 (26.5.1994) in the *Keegan* case (*Commission v. Ireland*) and 307 B (24.2.1995) the *McMichael* case (*Commission v. United Kingdom*), as well as the Commission reports on Application Nos. 10961/84, 10978/84 and 16106/90.

2. From the ethical standpoint

The doctor must obtain the subject's freely given, informed consent, preferably in writing (Helsinki I, *i*),[1] after explaining the aims, methods, anticipated benefits and potential hazards of the intervention and any discomfort it may entail.

Neither the Declaration of Helsinki nor that of Brussels[2] raises the question of the spouse's consent. However, in the WMA Declaration of Brussels (1985), reference is made to information to be given to patients and to the couple (which implies both parties concerned).

3. From the standpoint of religious moralities

a. *Catholic*

A surgical operation to eliminate a real pathology does not pose problems for Catholic morality, as this operation is anterior to any situation involving the act of procreation.[3]

b. *Protestant*

The act in itself does not pose any specific ethical question. The decision must, as far as possible, be taken by the couple on the basis of informed consideration.

c. Jewish

Surgical intervention is authorised provided that it does not endanger the mother's life.

---

1. Declaration of Helsinki, WMA, Helsinki, Finland, June 1964, paragraph i.
2. Provisional declaration on the ethical aspects of *in vitro* fertilisation, WMA Brussels, Belgium, October 1985.
3. Therapeutic or totality principle: Pius XII, AAS 45 (1953), pp. 674-675, AAS 48 (1956), pp. 461-462.

d. Muslim

Extramarital sexual relations are strictly prohibited. However, if a stable couple made up of adults who have reached the age of majority is envisaging marriage to start a family and pregnancy is rendered impossible by tubal obstruction, the couple could have recourse to a surgical operation or to artificial procreation, namely *in vitro* fertilisation, on condition that both ovum and sperm originate with the couple, and subject to the freely given, informed consent of both spouses.

e. *Buddhist*

Whether or not the couple is married, if the risks of an operation and the subsequent complications are not too severe, this practice is acceptable.

4. From the standpoint of agnostic morality

The right to perform an operation to remedy a tubal obstruction is admitted in France. The consent of the couple is necessary to permit this surgical solution. There is no civil liability for the doctor.

A married woman still has the right without the consent of her husband, and a single woman also has this right.

Surrogate motherhood

A couple has recently married. After a haemorrhage, probably post abortum, the wife undergoes a hysterectomy at the age of 25.
The couple rejects adoption and opts for implantation of an ovule from the wife fertilised by the husband's sperm in the womb of a "surrogate mother".

    a. Right to practise
    b. Informed consent of couple
    c. Consent of donor
    d. Anonymity of donor
    e. Professional secrecy
    f. Liability of doctor (quality of ovule)
    g. Remuneration of the surrogate mother.

1. From the standpoint of international law

a. Paragraph 11 of European Parliament Resolution No. 372/88 states that "in general, any form of surrogate motherhood should be rejected", in particular when adoption would be possible. Accordingly, see the Commission reports in the cases of *X.* v. *United Kingdom* (Application No. 6564/74) and *Van Oosterwijck* v. *Belgium* (Application No. 7654/76): "apart from the fact that a family can always be founded by adopting children, it should be noted that while impotence is sometimes considered to be a cause for annulling a marriage, this is not generally the case with sterility".

b. In the case where the implantation of an ovule of a woman fertilised by the sperm of the husband in the matrix of a surrogate mother is not prohibited by national law, the necessity for the prior informed consent of the woman's husband stems from Article 5 of Protocol 7 to the ECHR, and Article 23 (4) of the Covenant on Civil and Political Rights.

As regards the informed consent of the couple of which the surrogate mother forms part, according to paragraph 22 of Council of Europe Recommendation 1100, "the donation and use of human embryological material shall be conditional on the freely given written consent of the donor parents", and the same conclusion stems from Article 5 of Protocol 7 cited above. There is no reply in the case where the surrogate mother should refuse to hand over the child born from this pregnancy to the infertile woman, and this even though the majority of the national laws of the Council of Europe member states have moved towards the maxim *mater semper certa est*. No reply either as regards a repudiation action by the husband of the surrogate mother.

c. No explicit reply, but the need for this may be derived from the rules and principles referred to above. See Article 5 of the BC. It should also be noted that in the terms of Article 19 (1) of the BC, "Removal of organs or tissue from a living person for transplantation purposes may be carried out solely for the therapeutic benefit of the recipient and where there is no suitable organ or tissue available from a deceased person and no other alternative therapeutic method of comparable effectiveness." According to Article 19 (2) of the BC, "The necessary consent as provided for under Article 5 must have been given expressly and specifically either in written form or before an official body." In the terms of Article 26 (2) of the BC, no exception is permitted to the application of Article 19, including in the circumstances set out in Article 26 (1) of the BC.

d. An affirmative reply: application by analogy of paragraph 10 of European Parliament Resolution 372/88. We may also recall in this connection that "the Court cannot but be struck by the fact that domestic law of the great majority of the member states of the Council of Europe has evolved and is continuing to evolve, in company with the relevant international instruments, towards full juridical recognition of the maxim *mater semper certa est* (*Marckx* Judgment – 13.6.1979). According to this rule the surrogate mother would be the legal mother of the child conceived for others. See, however, Judgment No. 160 (7.7.1989) in the *Gaskin* case (*Commission* v. *United Kingdom*), but also Judgment No. 297 C (27.10.1994) in the *Kroon and others* case (*Commission* v. *Netherlands*) and the two dissenting opinions appended to it.

e. There is no explicit reply. An implicit affirmative reply may be derived from Article 10 (2) of the ECHR. See also Article 10 (1) of the BC and point 63 of the explanatory report.

f. See Articles 4 and 24 of the BC. As regards the conservation of ovules, possible reference to Article 22 of the BC.

g. Paragraph 11 of European Parliament Resolution 372/88 states that "the procuring of surrogate mothers for gain should be punishable by law". It further states that "undertakings carrying on such activities should be banned and trade in embryos and gametes should be prohibited". See Articles 21 and 26 of the BC.

2. From the ethical standpoint

The WMA has taken a positive view of medically assisted procreation as a means of helping infertile couples to have children. In its Declaration of Brussels (1985), the WMA notes that *in vitro* fertilisation, a new medical technique for treating sterility, is being increasingly practised throughout the world, and urges physicians to act ethically and with appropriate respect for the health of the prospective mother and for the embryo from the beginning of life.

As regards remuneration of the surrogate mother, there is no absolute prohibition, but surrogate motherhood for commercial ends is indeed condemned.

In its statement on *in vitro* fertilisation and embryo transplantation, Madrid (1987), the WMA specified that:

a. consent must also apply to the procedure used;

b. the patients are entitled to the same confidentiality and privacy as is required with any other medical treatment.

The WMA recommends that physicians refrain from intervening in the reproductive process for the purpose of making a choice as to the foetus' sex, unless it is to avoid the transmission of serious gender-related disease.

The WMA condemns any commercialisation by which ova, sperm or embryos are offered for purchase or sale.

The European Ethics Guide added in its Article 18 that it is ethical for a doctor to refuse on the grounds of his convictions to intervene in the reproductive process, and to suggest that the people concerned seek the opinions of other doctors.

3. From the standpoint of religious moralities

a. *Catholic*

This is a case of homologous *in vitro* fertilisation, which is illicit for Catholic morality because it separates in the conjugal act the dimension of union from that of procreation[1] and does not allow the life of the human embryo to be safeguarded.[2] Furthermore, from the point of view of Catholic morality, "surrogate motherhood" cannot be accepted as it infringes human dignity by intentionally breaking the only possible context for procreation and gestation, which is within the married couple.[3]

b. *Protestant*

The proposed solution is unacceptable because it seriously calls into question the child's right to guaranteed filiation and reduces the body of a human being to the status of merchandise.

---

1. Paul VI, *Humanae Vitae*, No. 1.
2. Congregation for the doctrine of the faith, *Donum Vitae*, Part I, No. 1, and Part II, No. 5; *Quaestio de abortu*, Nos. 12 and 13, AAS 66 (1974), p. 738ff.
3. *Donum Vitae*, Part II, No. 3.

c. *Jewish*

We may affirm that any arrangement whereby a woman "lends her womb" to a sterile wife as a surrogate mother is utterly prohibited. We must always remember the importance of the relationship between the mother and the foetus, which is indissoluble, as pregnancy is not merely a mechanical act of carrying; during pregnancy, strong bonds are formed between the foetus and the mother who bears it. In the case of surrogate mothers, the child is treated as a means, and not an end. The child becomes a good subject to the laws of supply and demand, and in current economic conditions, the child is in danger of being subjected to growing violence.

d. *Muslim*

Recourse to a surrogate mother is authorised only where this mother is the husband's second wife, as this is possible in Muslim countries, where polygamy is not forbidden.

e. *Buddhist*

Biology shows that an embryo results from the fusion of spermatozoid and ovule, but buddhism postulates that in addition to these two elements a third one is necessary for life: the continuum of consciousness. When the genetic conditions are realised in a favourable context, the mental continuum penetrates and supports the embryo. The texts reports the words of the Buddha on this:

"O monks, where the three elements are found in combination, a seed of life is planted. Thus, if the father and mother unite but the time is not right for the mother and the being to be reborn (*gadhabba*) is absent, no seed of life will be planted. Monks, if the father and mother unite and it is the time for the mother, but the being to be reborn is absent, here too no seed of life will be planted. And if the mother and father unite and the time is right for the mother and the being to be reborn, then by conjunction of these three elements, a seed of life will be planted" (*Sutta-pitaka, Majjhima-nikaya, I, 265-266, Pali Cannon*).

The principle of a surrogate mother may be acceptable if the motives are altruistic and with the informed consent of all the persons concerned.

4. From the standpoint of agnostic morality

The principle of surrogate motherhood does not appear to be permitted by the law, even with the consent of the donor of the ovocytes, and despite anonymity and medical secrecy.

The doctor has no liability regarding the quality of the ovocyte, but has a penal liability for having practised the implantation.

The surrogate mother can obviously never have the right to any kind of remuneration.

Artificial insemination for a female homosexual couple

A young adult woman, living in a stable homosexual relationship with another adult woman, requests donor insemination.

a. Right to practise
b. Informed consent: moral validity, legal validity
c. Liability of doctor (quality of sperm)
d. Anonymity of donor
e. Professional secrecy.

1. From the standpoint of international law

a. Paragraph 14.A.iv of Council of Europe Recommendation 1046 (1986) forbids the creation of children from people of the same sex. Paragraph D of the preamble to Resolution 372/88 states in turn that the main criteria governing artificial insemination *in vivo* and *in vitro* are not only "the mother's right to self-determination" but also "the respect of the rights and interests of the child, namely the right to life and physical, psychological and existential integrity, the right to a family, the right to be looked after by its parents and to grow up in a suitable family environment and the right to its own genetic identity".

b. If the member states of the Council of Europe, invited by the Committee of Ministers to forbid "anything that could be considered as undesirable use or deviations" as regards artificial insemination, prohibit the creation of children from people of the same sex, there is no occasion to speak of consent, be it legally valid or not.

c. See case 2, point c. As regards the conservation of ovules, possible reference to Article 22 of the BC.

d. Possible application by analogy of paragraph 10 (sub-paragraph 3, *in fine*) Resolution 372/88.
As regards European case-law on homosexual relations, see Judgment Nos. 45 (22.10.1981) in the *Dudgeon* case (*Commission* v. *United Kingdom*); 142 (26.10.1988) in the *Norris* case (*Commission* v. *Ireland*) and 259 (22.4.1993) in the *Modinos* case (*Commission* v. *Cyprus*), as well as the Commission reports in Application Nos. 16106/90 and 17279/90.

As regards the inclusion of the name of the biological father in official documents, possible application of paragraph 40 of Judgment No. 297 C (27.10.1994), cited in the reply to case 1 *in fine.*

e. An implicit affirmative reply may be derived from Articles 8 (1) and 10 (2) of the ECHR, as well as Article 10 (1) BC, the latter being specifically concerned with health information.

2. From the ethical standpoint

This issue has not been considered. The Declaration of Brussels regards the technique as legitimate because it enables couples who cannot procreate to have children.

The WMA has taken a positive view of medically assisted procreation as a means of enabling infertile couples to have children. It has set up rules on this practice and bans the use for research purposes of fertilised eggs which are not reimplanted (Brussels 1985).[1] It may be noted that most sperm banks only supply stable couples where the partners are of different sexes.

3. From the standpoint of religious moralities

a. Catholic

This is a case of artificial insemination by a donor outside marriage which "must be purely and simply condemned as immoral".[2] Further, for the Catholic Church, the existence of a stable homosexual couple is absolutely immoral.[3]

b. Protestant

The only issue of importance is that of the child's right to a father and a mother.

c. Jewish

According to the great majority of our rabbi, any fertilisation using sperm from a donor other than the husband is to be utterly condemned. This prohibition is aggravated by the fact that the couple is, in this case, a homosexual one.[4]

---

1. Interim declaration on the ethical aspects of *in vitro* fertilisation, WMA, Brussels, 1985.
2. Pius XII, AAS 41 (1949), p. 559 and Congregation for the doctrine of the faith, *Donum Vitae*, Part II, No. 2.
3. Congregation for the doctrine of the faith: Declaration *Persona Humana*, No. 8, 1975; letter *Homosexualitatis Problema*, AAS 79 (1987), p. 543.
4. Leviticus, 18, v. 22; 20, v. 13.

d. Muslim

Artificial fertilisation *in vitro* is authorised only for legally married couples. Islam regards the existence of a homosexual couple as utterly immoral and forbidden.

e. Buddhist

In this case, there seems to be an absence of the family unit, which threatens to create psychological problems for the child.

In a different context relating to the same problem, his Holiness the Dalai Lama, who is one of the great contemporary spiritual authorities for Buddhists of all denominations, said:

"Psychological problems arise in children whose families are broken or divided because of adultery, children who do not know their father and who never see his face. Without a father, the child will lack the natural paternal warmth and will feel confused or melancholic. This lack will leave a life-long impression" (*Selected works of the Dalai Lama II*, commentary by the present Dalai Lama, p. 117).

4. From the standpoint of agnostic morality

This situation should not be permitted by the law, in particular to protect the future of the child to be born (fatherless). It is, nevertheless, permitted in certain European Union countries, but is practised above all outside the European Union.

Voluntary female sterilisation

A married woman with children requests tubal ligation.

    a. Right to practise (age of patient)
    b. Informed consent of patient, informed consent of couple
    c. Medical liability: ligation or permanent resection
    d. Medical secrecy *vis-à-vis* the husband.

1. From the standpoint of international law

a. At the present stage of its development, international positive law provides no rules or principles referring specifically to voluntary sterilisation. The fundamental texts (for instance the Universal Declaration of Human Rights) effectively prohibit any state, group or person from engaging in any activity or performing any act "aimed at the destruction of rights and freedoms" which are recognised (these include the right to procreate), but the question as to whether the right to procreate freely and consciously also includes the right to refrain from (or to stop) procreating remains open, especially when this aim would be achieved by elimination (currently irreversible) of the object on which legal possession of this right is based. Nor do the standards and principles of international law at present in force resolve the question of whether, and to what extent, individuals can legitimately renounce not only to exercise of but also to the entitlement to (as would be the case here) one or other of the fundamental rights.

See also Article 1 of the BC, in the terms of which "Parties to this convention shall protect the dignity and identity of all human beings and guarantee everyone, without discrimination, respect for their integrity and other rights and fundamental freedoms with regard to the application of biology and medicine", and point 17 of the explanatory report: "the aim of the convention is to guarantee everyone's rights and fundamental freedoms and, in particular, their integrity and to secure the dignity and identity of human beings in this sphere".

See also Articles 4 and 24 of the BC.

The question would, of course, be an entirely different one if voluntary sterilisation carried a risk to the patient's health, for instance in view of the patient's age, or if, on the contrary, the patient was unable to use contraceptive products for health reasons and any further pregnancy or abortion would constitute a danger to her health. Then the absolute obligation to protect health would apply.

b. While the need for the patient's prior informed consent goes without saying, it should be pointed out that Articles 5 of Protocol 7 to the ECHR and 23 (4) of the Covenant on Civil and Political Rights provide for "equality of rights and responsibilities of spouses" in relation to marriage. As a result, and although the Commission (Application No. 8416/76, *X* v. *United Kingdom*) did not find "that the husband's and potential father's right to respect for his private and family life can be interpreted so widely as to embrace such procedural rights as (...) a right to be consulted (...) about an abortion which his wife intends to have performed on her", the husband's consent to surgical sterilisation should be requested, particularly if sterilisation by irreversible tubal resection is envisaged. In addition, attention is drawn to the provisions of the ECHR and the Covenant on Civil and Political Rights (Articles 8 and 17) and which stipulate the right to the respect of private life, also stipulate the respect of family life. See, nevertheless, Article 10 (1) of the BC. In the same sense, possible application, *mutatis mutandis*, of Judgment No. 290 (26.5.1994) in the *Keegan* case (*Commission* v. *Ireland*).

c. There can be no reply *in abstracto*. The choice between ligation and irreversible tubal resection depends on the patient's state of health, the foreseeable risks and disadvantages and physical and psychological side-effects. At all events, the doctor has a duty to preserve the patient's health. In the same sense, see Articles 4, 24 and 1 of the BC.

d. The reply depends on points *a* and *b* and the provisions mentioned therein. See Article 10 (1) and Article 26 (1) of the BC.

2. From the ethical standpoint

There is no specific international ethical text here.

The European Ethics Guide (1986) says only that the doctor shall provide the patient on request with any useful information on reproduction and contraception.

The Declaration of Rancho Mirage of 1986 on physicians' independence refers clinical and ethical decisions on treatment to the doctor's professional judgment and discretion. However, the Declaration of Vienna of 1988 adds that this must be in the best interest of patients and always following informed consent (Declaration of Lisbon of 1981 and European Ethics Guide 1986, Article 4), but the doctor may not allow his own conception of quality of life to prevail over the patient's.

3. From the standpoint of religious moralities

a. *Catholic*

According to the doctrine of the Catholic Church, sterilisation for contraceptive purposes is absolutely forbidden, even where the subjective intention is a proper one.[1]

---

1. Congregation for the doctrine of the faith: AAS 68 (1976), pp. 738-740.

b. *Protestant*

This issue is the sole responsibility of the couple or the mother; this is a responsibility which may require to be informed and be guided by particular counselling.

c. *Jewish*

To marry and have children is one of the first commandments that God gave to man. The aim is not only to continue the divine work but also to permit the renewal of the generations. Hence, anything which can limit procreation goes against the spirit of the law.

Tubal ligature or permanent resection could, nevertheless, be performed if the life or health of the mother were in danger.

d. *Muslim*

Provided there is consent by both spouses, tubal ligation is licit provided that the operation does not lead to irreversible sterility and is expected to benefit the couple psychologically.

e. *Buddhist*

Problems arise here with the irreversibility of the methods. It may, nevertheless, be accepted when there are major obstacles to the use of other methods and where pregnancy would endanger the life of the mother. In any event it is a decision for the couple. Professional secrecy *vis-à-vis* the spouse may be envisaged if it is necessary for the wife's survival. The acceptability of the act depends upon the motives of the applicant and the circumstances of the case.

4. From the standpoint of agnostic morality

Consulted on this problem, the French National Consultative Ethics Committee decided to refuse tubal ligation as a method of contraception. On the other hand, it is permissible in the case of therapeutic necessity, in which case the doctor is bound to medical secrecy *vis-à-vis* the husband.

Under certain conditions, however – depending on such things as the woman's age, number of children, financial difficulties – after the mother has been informed and has given her free and informed consent, voluntary female sterilisation should be accepted as a form of contraception.

Voluntary male sterilisation

An unmarried adult man requests ligation of the vas deferens (deferent duct)
to allow him a freer sex life.
He often has relations with casual partners.

    a. Right to practice (age of patient)
    b. Informed consent of patient (disadvantage)
    c. Accuracy of patient's statement
    d. Medical liability.

1. From the standpoint of international law

a. Reference should be made to point *a* of case 5. The reply would obviously be different if the operation endangered the patient's health. In this case, protection of the individual's health would be the primary obligation of the doctor, whose duty is to treat or alleviate suffering and certainly not to harm his patient (Article 4 of the BC). In the case of a minor, however, reference should now also be made to Article 6 (1) of the BC.

b. The need for patients' informed consent and prior provision of any information which may help him to understand precisely the advantages and disadvantages of any therapy or medical act, goes without saying (Articles 7 of the Covenant on Civil and Political Rights, and 4 and 24 of the BC.

c. No reply.

d. See Articles 4 and 24 of the BC.

2. From the ethical standpoint

There is no specific international ethical text here.

The European Ethics Guide (1986) says only that the doctor shall provide the patient on request with any useful information on reproduction and contraception.

The Declaration of Rancho Mirage of 1986 on physicians' independence refers clinical and ethical decisions on treatment to the doctor's professional judgment and discretion. However, the Declaration of Vienna of 1988 adds that this must be in the best interest of patients and always following informed consent (Declaration of Lisbon of 1981 and European Ethics Guide, 1986, Article 4), but the doctor may not allow his own conception of quality of life to prevail over the patient's.

3. From the standpoint of religious moralities

a. *Catholic*

Voluntary sterilisation is not acceptable from the Catholic point of view unless for therapeutic reasons, as it is contrary to the principle of the "non-disposability" of the body.[1]

b. *Protestant*

This is a case for the individual responsibility of both patient and doctor. The question is: "what constitutes a responsible course of action?". The motives mentioned seem, to say the least, irresponsible and highly debatable. By listening attentively to the person in question, it would doubtless be possible to help him to understood better what he is truly seeking and to act accordingly.

c. *Jewish*

The obligation to procreate is essentially incumbent upon men; it is therefore forbidden for a man to take any measure with a view to putting an end to his ability to procreate.[2]

d. *Muslim*

Ligature of the vas deferens ducts in an unmarried man is unacceptable; it is immoral and reprehensible as it is being requested by this man as a means of allowing him a freer sexual life.

e. *Buddhist*

The acceptability of the act depends upon the motives of the applicant and the circumstances of the case. If the reason for the request is to have a "freer sex life", it is not acceptable to the Buddhist. It would be if the man endangered his partner or himself (virus, etc.). Debauchery being a source of sufferings for the self and for others, it is not recommended by Buddhist ethics.

4. From the standpoint of agnostic morality

Same situation as with a woman requesting tubal ligature. Ligation of the vas deferens is virtually irreversible. The doctor would then be liable, unless the operation was for therapeutic purposes.

---

1. Paul VI, *Humanae Vitae*, 17, Pius XII, AAS 50 (1958), pp. 734-735.
2. The Torah condemns and abhors the act of Onan (Genesis, 38, v. 9) defined as one of the most serious transgressions of the Law as it destroys life at its very source.

Sterilisation of an imprisoned offender

In the case of a serious sexual offender with multiple convictions, permanent castration is proposed in exchange for a reduced sentence.

  a. Right to practise
  b. Absence of consent
  c. Judicial decision in contravention of the WMA Declaration of Tokyo
  d. Medical liability.

1. From the standpoint of international law

a. In the light of all fundamental texts on human rights, the respect of the integrity of the human being and other rights and fundamental freedoms with respect to the application of medicine is guaranteed to everyone (Article 1 of the BC), and the answer in this case is no. In fact "the interests and welfare of the human being shall prevail over the sole interest of society or science" (Article 2 of the BC), the only exceptions possible being "such as are prescribed by law and are necessary in a democratic society in the interest of public safety, for the prevention of crime, for the protection of public health or for the protection of the rights and freedoms of others" (Article 26 (1) of the BC). It should be pointed out that according to points 159 and 160 of the explanatory report "the reasons mentioned in Article 26.1 should not be regarded as justifying an absolute exception to the rights secured by the convention. To be admissible, restrictions must be prescribed by law and be necessary in a democratic society for the protection of the collective interest in question or for the protection of individual interests, that is the rights and freedom of others. These conditions must be interpreted in the light of the criteria established with regard to the same concepts by the case-law of the European Court of Human Rights. In particular, the restrictions must meet the criteria of necessity, proportionality and subsidiarity, taking into account the social and cultural conditions proper to each state. The term "prescribed by law" should be interpreted in accordance with the meaning usually given to them by the European Court of Human Rights, that is a formal law is not required and each state may adopt the form of domestic law it considers most appropriate".

Even serious sexual offenders may not be deprived of their right to procreate, however high the risk of recidivism.

The same goes for offenders of unsound mind, people suffering from mental disorder placed as involuntary patients, the mentally retarded and the disabled (see Rules 31, 32, 70 and 82.2 of Resolution (73) 5 adopted by the Committee of Ministers of the Council of Europe on 19 January 1973 containing standard minimum rules for the treatment of prisoners; Articles 5 (1) and 10 of Recommendation No. R (83) 2 adopted by the Committee of Ministers of the Council of Europe on 22 February 1983 concerning the legal protection of persons suffering from mental disorder placed as involuntary patients; Articles 1, 2 and 6 of the Declaration on the rights of mentally retarded persons (United Nations) and Article 3 of the Declaration on the rights of disabled persons (United Nations). See also Resolution DH (82) 2 concerning the Court's judgments of 24.10.1979 in the *Winterwerp* case and 23.2.1984 in the *Luberti* case as well as, more recently, Decision No. 185 A of 27.9.1990 in the *Wassink* case (*Commission* v. *Netherlands*).

Moreover, point 7.iii.c of Recommendation 1235 (1994) adopted on 12 April 1994 by the Parliamentary Assembly of the Council of Europe stipulates with respect to imprisoned or detained persons that "there must be no permanent infringement of individuals' rights to procreate".

As regards specifically the treatment of insane prisoners, see the decisions of the Court Nos. 185 B of 25.10.1990 in the *Koendjbiharie* case (*Commission* v. *Netherlands*); 185 C of 25.10.1990 in the *Keus* case (*Commission* v. *Netherlands*); 237 A of 12.5.1992 in the *Megyeri* case (*Commission* v. *Germany*); 244 of 24.9.1992 in the *Herczegfalvy* case (*Commission* v. *Austria*) and 268 B of 14.9.1993 in the *Kremzov* case (*Commission* v. *Austria*), as well as the Decision of 4.7.1995 of the Commission in the case *Bizzotto* v. *Greece* (Application No. 22126/93) and the Decision of 18.5.1995 of the Commission on the admissibility of Application No. 22520/93 (*Johnson* v. *United Kingdom*), notably as regards the relations between Articles 5 (1) a and 5 (1) e.

See also Resolutions DH (94) 57 of 21.9.1994 and (94) 70 of 19.10.1994 of the Committee of Ministers of the Council of Europe in the cases *Clarke* v. *United Kingdom*; *Oldham* v. *United Kingdom* and *PJB* v. *Netherlands* (Application Nos. 15767/89, 17143/90 and 15672/89).

The reply is all the plainer since the "freely given" consent of an offender who is being offered a reduced sentence is open to serious doubt.

We may add that, according to Resolution 37/194 of the United Nations General Assembly of 18 December 1982 containing principles of medical ethics (see principles 2 and 6), "it is a gross contravention of medical ethics, as well as an offence under applicable international instruments, for health personnel, particularly physicians, to engage, actively or passively, in acts which constitute participation in, complicity in, incitement to, or attempt to commit torture or other cruel, inhuman or degrading treatment or punishment".

b. The reply is, *a fortiori*, negative, all the more so as in the terms of Article 6 (3) of the BC, even "where, according to the law, an adult does not have the capacity to consent to an intervention" (in the meaning of Article 4 of the BC and point 29 of the explanatory report) "because of a mental disability (...), the individual concerned

137

shall be as far as possible take part in the authorisation procedure". See also points 43 and 46 of the explanatory report.

It should also be pointed out that according to Article 6 (1) of the BC "an intervention may only be carried out on a person who does not have the capacity to consent, for his or her direct benefit", and that, according to Article 7 of the BC, "a person who has a mental disorder of a serious nature may be subjected, without his or her consent, to an intervention aimed at treating his or her mental disorder only where, without such treatment, serious harm is likely to result to his or her health". Point 52 of the explanatory report adds to this that in case of intervention not aiming to treat specifically a mental disorder, "the practitioner must (...) seek the consent of the patient, insofar as this is possible, and the assent or refusal of the patient must be followed."

Lastly, it should be noted that point 151 of the explanatory report, appended to the BC, states as following: "No restrictions shall be placed on the exercise of the rights and protective provisions contained in this convention other than such as are prescribed by law and are necessary in a democratic society (...) for the prevention of crime (...) or for the protection of rights and freedoms of others"; "A person who may, due to his or her mental disorder, be a possible source of serious harm to others may, according to the law, be subjected to a measure of confinement or treatment without his or her consent. Here, in addition to the cases contemplated in Article 7, the restriction may be applicable in order to protect other people's rights and freedom".

c. The doctor, even though he may be a prison official, must refrain from carrying out the castration.

d. Refer to United Nations Resolution 37/194 quoted above, as well as Articles 23, 24 and 25 of the BC and the relevant points of the explanatory report, (139 to 147).

2. From the ethical standpoint

Here, sterilisation is conceived of as a crime prevention measure. According to the Declaration of Tokyo of 1975, the doctor shall not countenance the practice of degrading procedures, whatever the offence of which the victim of such procedures is suspected, accused or guilty. A doctor must have complete clinical independence in deciding upon the care of a person for whom he or she is medically responsible. The doctor's fundamental role is to alleviate the distress of his or her fellow men.

According to the Declaration of Lisbon of 1981, the patient has the right to accept or to refuse treatment.

According to the Declaration of the International Council of Prison Medical Services (Athens, 1978), health professionals working in prisons undertake:
– to base their diagnoses only on the needs of the patients, whose state of health overrides any other considerations;
– to provide imprisoned persons with the best possible care without offending against their professional ethics.
The European Ethics Guide, 1986, Article 22, takes a similar position.

3. From the standpoint of religious moralities

a. *Catholic*
Catholic morality absolutely rejects any action seeking to damage a person's physical integrity, regardless of his consent, and any cruel punishment inflicted by public authorities for crimes committed or to prevent future crimes.[1]

b. *Protestant*
It is of primary importance to implement, in conscience, only those procedures and practices which fully respect the dignity of the individual. Who is behind this act? And why?

c. *Jewish*
According to most rabbinical leaders, the prohibition on castration is a rule of universal law,[2] valid for all human beings. Anyone who destroys man's reproductive organ is acting as if he held the Creator's work in contempt and is making himself guilty of its destruction. Judaism therefore forbids the doctor to use medical art to such ends, whatever reasons may be given.

d. *Muslim*
Definitive castration is not acceptable to Islam as it leads to definitive sterility. It is all the more immoral since it is proposed in exchange for a favour, namely a reduced sentence for the serious sexual offender. Moreover, the integrity of the human body must be respected in Islam save for a therapeutic purpose.

e. *Buddhist*
If the offender asks for help, it is possible to use chemotherapeutic methods which may be used just for a while.

---

1. Pius XI, *Casti Connubii*, AAS 22 (1930), pp. 564-565.
2. *Le livre des commandements*, translated by Robert Samuel, CLKH, Paris, 1974, p. 311.

"Even if he has committed awful crimes, man effaces them if he resorts to the thought of Bodhi or the Awakened Spirit" (*Bodhisattvacharya-Vatara*, 33, No. 13).

4. From the standpoint of agnostic morality

The sterilisation of an imprisoned offender should be prohibited.

However, a serious sex offender may be given hormonal treatment administered by a doctor from outside the prison establishment and at the same time receive psychiatric help.

Non-treatment of a disabled and mentally impaired new-born child

A child is born with an imperforate anus and mongolism (Down's Syndrome).
An immediate surgical operation would mean the survival of a person who may never exceed a mental age of 4 for a probable span of some twenty years.
The parents refuse permission to operate, preferring to let the child die a natural death.

    a. Withholding of care (passive euthanasia)
    b. Medical liability.

1. From the standpoint of international law

a. The definition of passive euthanasia depends on the interpretation given to the content of the right to life ("right to live" – "right to quality of life"). Although positive international law does not specify the meaning of the adverb "arbitrarily" used by Article 6 (1) of the Covenant on Civil and Political Rights ("no one shall be arbitrarily deprived of his life") and Article 4 (1) of the American Convention on Human Rights ("no one shall be arbitrarily deprived of his life"), the wording of Article 2 (1) of the ECHR ("No one shall be deprived of his life intentionally") and the United Nations Declarations on the Rights of Disabled and Mentally Retarded Persons (Resolution 2856 (XXVI) and Resolution 3447 (XXX)) stipulate that these persons enjoy the same rights as others and therefore, *a fortiori*, the right to live.

The parental authority over a minor provided for by all international instruments on human rights (see Article 8 of the ECHR, Article 17 and 23 (1) of the Covenant on Civil and Political Rights and Article 17 (1) of the American Convention on Human Rights) would not only be in conflict with the child's fundamental right to life (Article 8 (2) of the ECHR), but would eliminate this right if the surgical operation did not take place.

The parents' refusal to consent to the preservation of the child's right to life, even a life subject to all the limitations of congenital disease, thus amounts to suppression of the child's life.

We would also mention the *obiter dictum* of the Court in Judgment No. 255 (23.6.93) in the *Hoffmann* case (*Commission* v. *Austria*) (in the same sense, see Articles 1 and 2 (1) of the BC and the relative points of the explanatory report, points 17, 21 and 22), concerning the health of the children of Jehovah's Witnesses, notably with regard to the problem of blood transfusions and the reference made there to Article 5 of Protocol 7 to the ECHR (on the other hand, concerning the right of Jehovah's Witnesses to proselytise, see Court Decision No. 260 of 25.5.1993 in the *Kokkinakis* case (*Commission* v. *Greece*)).

See also, *mutatis mutandis*, Judgment No. 307 B of 24.2.1995 in the *McMichael* case (*Commission* v. *United Kingdom*).

b. The doctor's right/duty being to cure or treat as far as possible, particularly in emergencies, the family's refusal to consent cannot constitute a circumstance justifying the withholding of care. Article 8 of the BC stipulates in fact that "when because of an emergency situation the appropriate consent cannot be obtained, any medically necessary intervention may be carried out immediately for the benefit of the health of the individual concerned". Points 56 to 59 of the explanatory report state in this connection that "in emergencies, doctors are faced with a conflict between their duty to provide care and their duty to seek the patient's consent. This article allows the practitioner to act immediately in such situations without waiting until the consent of the patient or the authorisation of the legal representative where appropriate can be given. As it departs from the general rule laid down in Articles 5 and 6 it is accompanied by conditions. First, this possibility is restricted to emergencies which prevent the practitioner from obtaining the appropriate consent. The article applies both to persons who are capable and to persons who are unable either *de jure* or *de facto* to give consent. An example that might be put forward is that of a patient in a coma who is thus unable to give his consent, or that of a doctor who is unable to contact an incapacitated person's legal representative who would normally have to consent to an urgent intervention. Even in emergency situations, however, health care professionals must make every reasonable effort to determine what the patient would want. Next, the possibility is limited solely to medically necessary interventions which cannot be delayed. Interventions for which a delay is acceptable are excluded. However, this possibility is not reserved for life-saving interventions. Lastly, the article specifies that the intervention must be carried out for the immediate benefit of the individual concerned. "See also Article 24 of the BC and point 144 of the explanatory report: "the cause of the damage must be an intervention in the widest sense, taking the form of either an act or an omission". Lastly, see the Commission reports in Application Nos. 16593/90 and 16734/90, according to which: "the principle established by Article 2 of the ECHR, "everyone's right to life shall be protected by law", obliges states not only to abstain from inflicting any kind of death intentionally, but also to take the measures necessary for the protection of life. Article 2 imposes positive obligations on states.

See also Article 6 (1) of the BC, stipulating that "an intervention may only be carried out on a person who does not have the capacity to consent, for his or her direct benefit", as well as Article 6 (2) idem, in the terms of which "Where, according to law, a minor does not have the capacity to consent to an intervention", for his or her direct benefit, "the intervention may only be carried out with the authorisation of his or her representative or an authority or a person or body provided for by law". According to Article 6 (4) of the BC, "The representative, the authority, the person or the body mentioned in paragraphs 2 and 3 above shall be given, under the same conditions, the information referred to in Article 5." Said authorisation "may be withdrawn at any time in the best interests of the person concerned" (Article 6 (5) of the BC).

As regards the case of a major surgical intervention decided on and performed on a minor instead of a less invasive therapy, without informing nor seeking the consent of the parents, see the Decision of 22.2.1995 of the Commission on admissibility of Application No. 20948/92 (*Isiltan* v. *Turkey*) with respect to Article 2 of the ECHR.

2. From the ethical standpoint

In New York in 1950, the WMA condemned euthanasia in any circumstances. The Declaration of Venice of 1983, which takes a more differentiated view of passive euthanasia, states that "the duty of the physician is to heal and, where possible, relieve suffering and act to protect the best interests of his patients. There may be no exception to this principle, even in the case of incurable disease or malformation".

3. From the standpoint of religious moralities

a. *Catholic*
The corrective surgical operation falls within commensurate therapeutic resources and is right and just, even when it is certain that full health will not be achieved. For Catholic morality, it is not acceptable to omit therapy.[1] Even in this case, "neonatal euthanasia" is placed on a par with infanticide.

b. *Protestant*
It would seem difficult to impose a solution which does not take the greatest possible account of the opinion of the parents, who will have to live with the child and with whom the child will have to live. In protestantism, there are doubtless differing positions in this connection. However, none of them should support those who think and act with a view to avoiding personal investment, involvement and assistance.

---

1. Congregation for the doctrine of the faith, AAS 72 (1980), pp. 542-552.

c. *Jewish*

A physically or mentally abnormal child has the same right to life as a normal child, the more so since there may be a chance for the child to become normal. Science has not yet exhausted its resources; discoveries are made every day. The unhappy destiny is made to be put right.

d. *Muslim*

In Islam, no one is authorised to put an end to the life of another or his own. Even in a case where the child will never exceed a mental age of 4, the doctor whose mission is to heal and save human lives must persuade the parents to accept the surgical operation even if the new-born child's probable life expectancy is no more than twenty years.

Consequently, this new-born child with Down's Syndrome must be operated upon provided that the operation will not endanger its life.

e. *Buddhist*

Even though he is trisomic, this baby is a human being. The proposed operation is surgically simple, and not performing it raises the question of the difficult choice between failure to assist a person in danger and relentless prolongation of life. The principle of benevolence and non-aggression will enable the problem to be solved.

A human life, even imperfect and handicapped, must be preserved and respected. If there is a life to be saved, it must be saved.

4. From the standpoint of agnostic morality

Failure to treat a handicapped and mentally impaired new-born baby places us in an exceptional moral context. We can agree that once a reasoned opinion has been given by a college of paediatricians the parents should be authorised to request that no treatment should be given and that the child be allowed to die.

It seems that we should be against relentless prolongation of life when it leads to mere survival for a being deprived of what makes a truly human life.

Mother's refusal to abort a foetus at risk

A young woman with a stable partnership is pregnant for the first time. Examination of the amniotic fluid reveals a 60% chance of spina bifida. The woman refuses an abortion.

   a. Right to practice.
   b. Absence of mother's consent.

1. From the standpoint of international law

   a.b. No medical act may be performed without the patient's freely given and informed consent, particularly where the act is not urgent and not indispensable to save the patient's life. See also the Commission's decision in *X* v. *United Kingdom* (Application No. 8416/79); the pregnant woman being the person primarily concerned with the pregnancy and its continuation or termination, it is for her to decide. See also Article 5 of the BC and points 34 to 40 of the explanatory report.

   Regarding the contrary view, see the reports of the Commission in Application Nos. 6959/75 and 8416/76 and, more recently, the Court decision in the *Door and Dublin Well Woman* case (*Commission* v. *Ireland*, No. 246 of 29.10.1992).

2. From the ethical standpoint

   The doctor may in no case perform an abortion without the mother's consent, even if he considers it to be in the interests of the mother and of the seriously abnormal unborn child (WMA: Lisbon 1981).

   Where consent is forthcoming, the legitimacy or otherwise of abortion on grounds of abnormality has not been determined by the WMA, which leaves the matter to the law and the convictions of the individual.

3. From the standpoint of religious moralities

a. *Catholic*
In principle, for Catholic morality, abortion on eugenic grounds cannot be countenanced.[1] In this case, moreover, the spina bifida malformation can be treated surgically during the neonatal period. Deliberate abortion in this situation would

---

1. Pius XII: *Broadcast speeches and messages*, Vol. X, 1948-49, pp. 98-99.

145

therefore be all the more unjustified, and the refusal to abort is therefore morally right.

b. *Protestant*
The informed and considered decision of the mother – and of the couple if possible – must be absolutely respected.

c. *Jewish*
In Judaism, abortion is considered as a fundamental absurdity, and to refuse to have children or to abort is to fly in the face of history. The only condition to be taken into account is the mother's life or health.

In this particular case the mother refuses abortion. What right do we have to impose on her an act which she refuses? Furthermore, her refusal is morally justified and existing or future therapies may be able to treat the malformation.

Is the aim of medicine not to provide care?

d. *Muslim*
As we have seen in the introduction, the embryo becomes really human on the hundredth day of gestation. Deliberate termination of pregnancy is possible where the foetus shows an anomaly. In the present case, the examination of the amniotic fluid reveals probable spina bifida.

A deliberate termination of pregnancy is licit in this case provided that the spouses have both freely given their informed consent. Furthermore, present biological progress allows the anomaly in question to be detected at an earlier stage and hence reduces the risks to the mother's life.

e. *Buddhist*
From the Buddhist standpoint, killing is the most serious negative action (an action is positive or negative depending on whether or not it generates suffering, in the short or long term, for the performer of the act or for the other persons involved). In the present case, it is not at all fitting that action should be taken against the mother's will or without her consent. The mother can draw on the Buddhist point of view, acting in full responsibility.

4. From the standpoint of agnostic morality

The mother's refusal to abort a foetus at risk is justifiable if the refusal is licit, free and informed. The refusal to have an abortion is a right.

146

Transplantation of organs (a cornea from a corpse)

The body is that of a woman of 40 who has been killed in an accident.
Must authorisation be requested from her next of kin before the cornea is removed
for grafting purposes?

1. From the standpoint of international law

Article 10 of Resolution (78) 29 adopted by the Committee of Ministers of the Council of Europe on 11 May 1978 and entitled "harmonisation of legislations of member states relating to removal, grafting and transplantation of human substances" reads as follows: "1. No removal must take place when there is an open or presumed objection on the part of the deceased, in particular, taking into account his religious and philosophical convictions; 2. In the absence of the explicit or implicit wish of the deceased the removal may be effected. However, a state may decide that removal must not be effected if, after such reasonable inquiry as may be practicable has been made into the views of the family of the deceased (...), an objection is apparent (...)".

Points 35-37 of the explanatory report appended to this resolution explain in detail the meaning of Article 10. In particular, where it has not been possible to learn of the deceased's wishes, "it has been considered that a presumed consent exists since in most states, where everybody knows that removals can take place, those who are strongly against any possible removal ought to have made it known. In adopting such a solution, which is the one adopted by the most recent legislations in Europe, the majority of experts was essentially inspired by the invaluable importance of substances for transplantation, the shortage of substances available and the interests of sick persons. The experts were aware that such a rule of presumed consent is for the moment and for some states a far-reaching one, since legislations or practices require an enquiry into the views of the family of the deceased person or his legal representative, if the deceased is legally incapacitated. Therefore Article 10 must be considered as a long-term aim, states which are not yet ready to accept it having the possibility of providing for the inquiry in question."

It should be noted in passing that while, in the terms of Article 9 of the BC, "the previously expressed wishes relating to a medical intervention by a patient who is not, at the time of the intervention, in a state to express his wishes shall be taken into account", points 60 to 62 of the explanatory report seem to limit the application of this rule to "situations where individuals have foreseen that they might be unable to give their valid consent, for example in the event of a progressive disease such as senile dementia". In fact, point 62 states that "the article lays down that when persons have previously expressed their wishes, these shall be taken into account. Nevertheless, taking previously expressed wishes into account does not mean that they should necessarily be followed. For example, when the wishes were expressed a long time before the intervention and science has since progressed, there may be grounds for not heeding the patient's opinion. The practitioner should thus, as far as possible, be satisfied that the wishes of the patient apply to the present situation and are still valid, taking account in particular of technical progress in medicine."

Reference should also be made to Recommendation 1159 (1991), adopted on 28 June 1991 by the Parliamentary Assembly of the Council of Europe on the harmonisation of autopsy rules.

It should also be pointed out that in the contrary case of a part of the human body removed in the course of an intervention, Article 22 of the BC stipulates that "it may be stored and used for a purpose other than that for which it was removed, only if this is done in conformity with appropriate information and consent procedures". Points 135 to 137 of the explanatory report state in this connection that "parts of the human body are often removed in the course of interventions, for example surgery. The aim of this article is to ensure the protection of individuals with regard to parts of their body which are thus removed and then stored or used for a purpose different from that for which they have been removed. Such a provision is necessary in particular, because much information on the individual may be derived from any part of his body, however small (for example blood, hair, bone, skin, organ). Even when the sample is anonymous the analysis may yield information about identity. This provision thus establishes a rule consistent with the general principle in Article 5 on consent, that parts of the body which have been removed during an intervention for a specified purpose must not be stored or used for a different purpose unless the relevant conditions governing information and consent have been observed. The information and consent arrangements may vary according to the circumstances, thus allowing for flexibility since the express consent of an individual to the use of parts of his body is not systematically needed. Thus, sometimes, it will not be possible, or very difficult, to find the persons concerned again in order to ask for their consent. In some cases, it will be sufficient for a patient or his or her representative, who have been duly informed (for instance, by means of leaflets handed to the persons concerned at the hospital), not to express their opposition. In other cases, depending on the nature of the use to which the removed parts are to be put, express and specific consent will be necessary, in particular where sensitive information is collected about identifiable individuals."

To this we would add the provisions of the BC concerning organ and tissue removal from living donors for transplantation purposes, and in particular the general rule set out in Article 19 (1) and (2), according to which "Removal of organs or tissue from a living person for transplantation purposes may be carried out solely for the therapeutic benefit of the recipient and where there is no suitable organ or tissue available from a deceased person and no other alternative therapeutic method of comparable effectiveness. The necessary consent as provided for under Article 5 must have been given expressly and specifically either in written form or before an official body."

Reference should also be made to Article 20 (1) and (2) of the BC, on the protection of persons not able to consent to organ removal. In the terms of this provision, "No organ or tissue removal may be carried out on a person who does not have the capacity to consent under Article 5. Exceptionally and under the protective conditions prescribed by law, the removal of regenerative tissue from a person who does not have the capacity to consent may be authorised provided the following conditions are met: i. there is no compatible donor available who has the capacity to consent; ii. the recipient is a brother or sister of the donor; iii. the donation must have the potential to be life-saving for the recipient; iv. the authorisation provided for under paragraphs 2 and 3 of Article 6 has been given specifically and in writing, in accordance with the law and with the approval of the competent body; v. the potential donor concerned does not object."

Lastly, reference should be made to Articles 13 and 22 of the BC.

2. From the ethical standpoint

The WMA refers to legislation on consent in the various countries. Accordingly, the Declaration of Sydney (point 5) states as follows: "determination of the point of death of the person makes it ethically permissible to cease attempts at resuscitation and in countries where the law permits, to remove organs from the cadaver provided that prevailing legal requirements of consent have been fulfilled."

According to the Declaration of Madrid (1987) on human organ transplantation, "the fullest possible discussion of the proposed procedure with the donor and the recipient or their respective responsible relatives or legal representatives is mandatory."

3. From the standpoint of religious moralities

a. *Catholic*

Removal of organs from a cadaver for grafting purposes is licit in itself but, for Catholic morality, it must be done with respect for the rights and feelings of those with whom care of the cadaver lies, that is primarily the family.[1]

---

1. Pius XII, AAS 48 (1956), p. 462ff.

149

b. *Protestant*

The feeling behind the Catholic position is shared. No commercial interest is acceptable.

c. *Jewish*

Removal of organs from the body of a dead man for the purposes of a graft contravenes three prohibitions:
– one may not take profit from a dead body;
– a dead body may not be mutilated in any way;
– the body must be buried.

However, autopsies may be authorised in the following cases:
– where the purpose is to save a human life and this human life to be saved is a real and immediate case;
– it may only be performed if the deceased has given his agreement before death;
– if it is otherwise impossible to determine the cause of death, on condition that the facts are established by three specialist doctors;
– if there is a legal necessity;
– if the purpose is to save other beings;
– if the purpose is to determine the presence of genital disease with a view to preserving the health of close relations or children still alive.

It is obvious that, despite all the foregoing, an autopsy can only be carried out on the express condition that the doctors who operate do so in a dignified and honourable fashion, which shows respect for the dead (no smoking, no trivial conversations, the presence of a rabbi during the operation if the family so wishes, etc.), and that, after the operation, they hand over the body and the parts of the body to the undertaker for burial.[1]

In the case which concerns us here, everything should be done to persuade the family to authorise the removal of the cornea so that they can be grafted, for the donation of organs is a great *mitswah* (merit) if all the conditions necessary for the respect of life and the dead person are complied with.

d. *Muslim*

Transplantation of organs – in this case the cornea – from a dead person is licit under certain conditions:
1. establishment of death by a committee of three doctors including a neurologist (the surgeon who is to perform the transplant must not be a member of this committee);

---

1. E. Gugenheim, *Les portes de la Loi*, Albin Michel, 1982, pp. 257-265.

150

2. the dead person must not have expressed an objection to organ removal while he lived. Otherwise, the consent of the next of kin may be sufficient;

3. the transplantation must be carried out in centres approved by the Ministry of Health of the country concerned.

e. *Buddhist*

If the person gave his prior agreement, there is no problem in removing the cornea after death. The donation of an organ may be able to help another person, which is in conformity with the Buddhist concept of compassion. It appears that in the case of minors it is necessary to have the agreement of the close relatives and would-be donors are advised to carry a card clearly indicating their wishes in the case of death.

For Buddhists, death comes when the spirit leaves the body. This is generally at least three days after clinical death. Thus anybody removing an organ to save another life takes a positive responsibility but also a negative one.

4. From the standpoint of agnostic morality

The transplantation of an organ – here a cornea taken from a corpse – brings into play the law on bioethics, for example the Caillavet Act in France.

In the case of a woman who dies in an accident, if she has not clearly expressed her opposition to organ removal, then it is legally permissible.

Objection to autopsy on religious grounds

The deceased is a 60-year-old man of Muslim faith.
The family objects to an autopsy for religious reasons.

1. From the standpoint of international law

The family's objection must be respected as an expression of the freedom of religion recognised by all the relevant international instruments (see Article 18 of the Universal Declaration of Human Rights, Article 9 (1) of the ECHR, and Article 18 of the Covenant on Civil and Political Rights) if it is accepted that the corpse is the object of a right of succession *erga omnes* pertaining to the family.

Conversely, Articles 11 (1) and 12 (3) of Resolution (78) 29 referred to above state that "death having occurred (...) and having been established by a doctor who does not belong to the team which will effect the removal, grafting or transplantation (...) a removal may be effected". However, we should also bear in mind Article 10 (2) of the same resolution and the relevant points in the explanatory report as quoted in case 10.

If the autopsy is ordered by the judicial powers in an inquiry on a suspect death, neither the family's objection nor use of the corpse for removal of organs can take precedence: Article 11 (2) of Resolution (78) 29 provides that "a removal can be effected if it does not interfere with a forensic examination or autopsy as required by law. A state may, when such requirement exists, decide that a removal can only be effected with the approval of a competent authority". Paragraph 39 of the explanatory report appended to the resolution reads as follows: "Sometimes the law requires a forensic examination or autopsy on the body of the deceased donor. The general rule is that even in the instances where the law requires a forensic examination or autopsy, a removal of substance may be effected if this does not interfere with the results of those examinations or autopsy (...). This being the general rule, the experts also noted that in a number of member states, to effect a removal, an authorisation of a competent authority (other than the doctor or the removal team) was necessary when a forensic examination or autopsy is required by law (in some member states the law requires an autopsy not only for crime investigation but also in other cases, for example to enquire into the causes of an industrial accident) (...). In order for those member states to maintain their law and practice, the experts added a second sentence which allows the state to require an authorisation of a competent authority".

Regarding the harmonisation of autopsy rules, see Recommendation 1159 (1991) of the Parliamentary Assembly of the Council of Europe .

See also Article 9 of the BC, bearing in mind autopsy does not seem to be able to be classified as "an intervention in the health field".

2. From the ethical standpoint

There are no WMA rules on autopsy. The International Conference of Medical Councils (CIO, 1983, Paris) enjoins respect for the family's religious convictions and any objections they may have.

3. From the standpoint of religious moralities

a. *Catholic*
For Catholic morality, respect of the family's rights and religious convictions in relation to the body is right. However, it is licit from the moral point of view for the authorities to go against the family's wishes for serious reasons concerning the common good, for example it is suspected that the death could be due to a crime or where there are risks to public health.[1]

b. *Protestant*
This problem is governed only by the national legislation of the country concerned and in this particular case Islam's position on the matter.

c. *Jewish*
In this case, there should be no autopsy as the family is opposed to it for religious reasons. However, this opposition should be waived in the case of an autopsy imposed for legal reasons in an investigation into a suspect death or if there is possible danger to public health.

In this case it seems to me to be important to apply to the competent religious authority for an opinion.

d. *Muslim*
Autopsy poses a thorny problem for Islam as it damages the physical integrity of the human body, which is a divine creation and must be respected. However, it is licit when it may be of scientific interest (correlation of lesions and symptoms of a disease). It is also authorised when it can serve to establish the truth in a case of criminal justice.

In some Muslim countries, it must be authorised by a committee of two doctors in addition to the attending physician.

e. *Buddhist*
The Buddhist position is in line with the standpoint of international law, while respecting the view expressed by the family, provided that the latter is not in

---

1. Pius XII, AAS 48 (1956), p. 462ff.

contradiction with the legislation in force in the country concerned. It is also necessary to take account of the reasons for the autopsy and the value to medicine of any research.

4. From the standpoint of agnostic morality

Unless there are legal proceedings involved and/or the person of the Muslim faith has consciously requested it, the autopsy can be refused by a member of the family, which represents the deceased person.

Participation in genocide by a physician

The Declaration of Tokyo prohibits any participation by doctors in genocide.

1. From the standpoint of international law

The Convention on the Prevention and Punishment of the Crime of Genocide (United Nations, 9.12.1948-12.1.1951), the four Geneva Conventions of 1948 on the Law of Warfare and the two additional protocols (12.8.1977), the International Convention on the Elimination of all Forms of Racial Discrimination (21.12.1965-4.1.1969), the International Convention on the Suppression and Punishment of the Crime of Apartheid (30.11.1973-18.7.1976) and the New York Convention against the Use of Especially Inhumane Conventional Weapons (10.10.1980) forbid all forms of participation by a physician in genocide (that is actual or attempted collective putting to death) and any incitement to, or complicity in, genocide, whether the doctor is an official or acting as a private individual.

It should be recalled that the *ad hoc* convention also considers the following as genocide (Article II): causing serious bodily or mental harm to members of a (national, ethical, racial, or religious) group; forcibly transferring children of the group to another group; imposing measures intended to prevent births within the group and deliberately inflicting on the group conditions of life calculated to bring about its physical destruction in whole or in part.

Reference should also be made to the Council of Europe's Framework Convention for the Protection of National Minorities, signed in Strasbourg on 1 February 1995.

2. From the ethical standpoint

a. The International Code of Medical Ethics requires the doctor to respect life, and hence humanity.

b. The preamble to the Declaration of Tokyo (1975) states that: "It is the privilege of the medical doctor to practise medicine in the service of humanity, to preserve and restore bodily and mental health without distinction as to persons, to comfort and to ease the suffering of his or her patients.

The utmost respect for human life is to be maintained even under threat, and no use made of any medical knowledge contrary to the laws of humanity."

c. The Lisbon Resolution of 1981 states that "It is unethical for physicians to participate in capital punishment".

d. The Regulations in Time of Armed Conflict (Havana 1956, amended in Venice in 1983) lay upon doctors the obligation to preserve health and save life and to give the required care impartially and without consideration of sex, race, nationality, religion, political affiliation or any other similar criteria (points 2 and 4).

The WMA forbids participation by any physician in genocide (Havana, 1956; Tokyo, 1975; Geneva, 1947).

3. From the standpoint of religious moralities

a. *Catholic*

Genocide, like all that is against life and offends human dignity, is condemned by the Catholic Church.[1] This is why participation by a physician in an act which is in itself intrinsically illicit remains strictly prohibited.

b. *Protestant*

To dare to ask the question is problematic in itself. Who could think that anyone, be he doctor or ordinary mortal, is authorised to take part in a genocide?

c. *Jewish*

Genocide literally means the destruction of all genes, that is any possibility of a people's reproduction through the total massacre of its members. A typical example is Hitler's genocide, which was an attempt to totally exterminate the Jewish people through the use of the most sophisticated criminal methods.

Unfortunately, German doctors who could have constituted an obstacle to this moral downfall largely contributed to the extermination of innocent people through slow death and in the gas chambers.

Nazi doctors transformed the prisoners, men, women and children, into guinea-pigs for brutal pseudo-scientific experiments.

We must oppose any genocide with all our strength, through reinforcing and reaffirming the doctor's professional ethic. It is not enough to train doctors who have a thorough knowledge of their profession; we need to educate people of integrity who have a conscience and are imbued with a love of their neighbour.

A thorough study of medical ethics should be an integral part of university medical courses. It is impossible to put doctors on the market without giving them the resources necessary to be able to respond appropriately to the moral and ethical problems of our societies.

Medical science can exist only if it is based on professional ethics; we must banish and combat science when it is applied without conscience and act in accordance with God's Commandment "Thou shalt love thy neighbour as thyself".

---

1. Vatican Council II, *Gaudium et Spes*, Nos. 27 and 79, AAA 58, (1966), pp. 1025-1120.

Our neighbour is not only the Jew, it is the Christian, the Muslim, the non-believer as well as the believer; it is not only the white man, but the coloured man too; it is not only the European, but all men from all continents.

d. *Muslim*

Islam through the voice of the Koran is very explicit on this matter. The Koran asserts (Sura V, verse 32): "he who slayeth anyone (...) shall be as though he had slain all mankind; but he who saveth a life shall be as though he had saved all mankind alive". The verses of the Koran are therefore still more explicit than the Declaration of Tokyo, which forbids participation by any physician in genocide.

e. *Buddhist*

The doctor is obliged by his deontology to respect and promote human life in all its expressions without discrimination, an approach in conformity with Buddhist ethics.

4. From the standpoint of agnostic morality

Regarding a doctor's participation in genocide, it should simply be recalled that opposition to genocide is a universal imperative and must be scrupulously observed. It concerns human dignity, and thus *a fortiori* that of the doctor.

Passive euthanasia

A man aged 50 suffering from obstructive arterial disease has already undergone several arterial grafts and amputation of both lower limbs.
He is suffering from bronchopneumonia and cardiac decompensation.
Treatment is possible only in an intensive care unit.
Does administration of symptomatic treatment only amount to passive euthanasia?

1. From the standpoint of international law

Several provisions of international positive law state that no one may be arbitrarily deprived of life (Article 3 of the Universal Declaration of Human Rights, Article 6 (1) of the Covenant on Civil and Political Rights and Article 4 (1) of the American Convention on Human Rights), setting aside the problem of the legitimacy of capital punishment (however, see in this connection Protocol 7 to the ECHR), everyone's right to life being protected by the law (Article 2 (1) of the ECHR).

So-called "active" euthanasia is therefore clearly and absolutely forbidden by international human rights law, even if death is inflicted at the request of a patient experiencing acute suffering and pain (see case 14).

However, the case put forward here raises the problem of the definition of and limits to so-called "passive euthanasia" and the definition of and limits to "relentless prolongation of life", as well as the problem of the frontier between the two.

If treatment in intensive care is the only form of treatment capable of ensuring the patient's survival, the doctor has a duty to implement it (see Article 4 of the BC).

The facilities of an intensive care unit should be used for an elderly patient whose situation seems to be irreversible, even to the detriment of a younger person. The content of international provisions concerning the right to life seems to rule out any choice on the part of the doctor (or anyone else) between two patients as to which one should benefit from the available technical resources (which we assume to be limited) which alone can ensure survival, on pain of violating the fundamental principle of non-discrimination (see Article 14 of the ECHR, Article 2 of the Covenant on Civil and Political Rights and Article 1 of the American Convention on Human Rights). However, international human rights law has not so far codified the distinction between ordinary and extraordinary means of assistance, nor has it established the relevant definitions.

See also Article 3 of the BC, in the terms of which "Parties, taking into account health needs and available resources, shall take appropriate measures with a view to providing, within their jurisdiction, equitable access to health care of appropriate quality", and points 23 to 26 of the explanatory report: "this article defines an aim and imposes an obligation on states to use their best endeavours to reach it.

The aim is to ensure equitable access to health care in accordance with the person's medical needs. 'Health care' means the services offering diagnostic, preventive, therapeutic and rehabilitative interventions designed to maintain or improve a person's state of health or alleviate a person's suffering. Access to health care must be equitable. In this context, 'equitable' means first and foremost the absence of unjustified discrimination. Although not synonymous with absolute equality, equitable access implies effectively obtaining a satisfactory degree of care. The Parties to the Convention are required to take appropriate steps to achieve this aim as far as the available resources permit. The purpose of this provision is not to create an individual right on which each person may rely in legal proceedings against the state, but rather to prompt the latter to adopt the requisite measures as part of its social policy in order to ensure equitable access to health care."

See also the Commission decisions in Application Nos. 16593/90 and 16743/90.

The question as to whether the use of intensive care facilities for a patient whose situation appears to be irreversible may be considered as "relentless prolongation of life" remains unanswered in international law. See, however, also Article 4 of the BC.

2. From the ethical standpoint

The WMA first tackled the problem of euthanasia in New York in 1950. It condemned it "in all circumstances".

More recently in Lisbon (2 October 1981) in the Declaration on the Rights of the Patient, the WMA acknowledged the right to die in dignity (e). The patient has the right to refuse treatment (c).

In Venice (1983), a declaration of principle was issued on terminal illness and withholding of treatment.

According to the Declaration of Venice,[1] the duty of the physician is to heal and, where possible, relieve suffering and act to protect the best interests of his patient. There may be no exception to this principle, even in the case of incurable disease or malformation.

3. From the standpoint of religious moralities

a. *Catholic*

Catholic morality, which is against euthanasia including the passive form, acknowledges the right to die in all serenity with human, Christian dignity. That is why it considers it licit to interrupt the application of resources available to the most advanced forms of medicine, when the results disappoint all hopes placed in them.

---

1. WMA Declaration on the terminal phase of illness, Venice, Italy, October 1983.

159

Nevertheless, all routine care (feeding in any form possible, administration of water, hygiene, help with breathing)[1] remains obligatory.

b. *Protestant*

As a general rule, respect for life and respect for the dignity of an individual go hand-in-hand. Where this no longer seems to be true, we must seek, meticulously and with humility, the least unsatisfactory solution. The right to die in dignity is undoubtedly a genuine right.

c. *Jewish*

Helping a patient to survive is an obligation. Everything must be done to preserve life. It is not admissible to economise when it is a matter of saving a human life. However, maintaining an artificial vegetable existence in the case of a terminal patient is by no means a humanitarian act.

The Shulhan Arukh (Code of Jewish Law) states: "if there is any cause which prevents the dying man from expiring, it is permitted to remove this cause. If there is some outside element, an external noise which retains the attention of the patient, it is permitted to remove this obstacle which attaches him to life, provided that he is not touched directly, and none of his members are moved" (*Yoré Déah* 339, 1 *Haga*).

Judaism thus demands the right for the human being to die in dignity, calm and peace, without the sterile relentless use of sophisticated medical technology.

Despite the imminence of death, doctors must maintain parenteral and nasogastric feeding because the suppression of all feeding condemns the patient to certain death.

d. *Muslim*

The Muslim religion does not allow anyone to put an end to his life or anyone else's, even if the person is suffering from a serious or apparently incurable disease. The practice of euthanasia, even in its passive form, is prohibited in Islam.

e. *Buddhist*

The dividing line between passive euthanasia and non-assistance to a person in danger is sometimes difficult to define. The problem does not lend itself to any general solution, but has to be resolved case by case.

However, according to Buddhist thought, the decision could be taken on the basis of the following criteria:
– never intervene directly to end a life;

---

1. Declaration of the Congregation for the doctrine of the faith on euthanasia, No. 2, AAS 72 (1980), p. 542ff.

– relieve suffering;
– avoid relentless prolongation of life;
– if there is no longer anything that can be done, help the person to die in the best conditions.

4. From the standpoint of agnostic morality

The distinction between passive and active euthanasia is a question of semantics; it is in fact purely academic.

If the conscious and informed patient requests the cessation of care and goes on repeating this request, then he has a right to refuse care, regardless of where this leads.

The patient is in fact the sole judge of his quality of life, and may prefer to die in dignity and without any more suffering.

161

Active euthanasia

A man aged 45, suffering from amyotrophic lateral sclerosis, at the stage of phonation and deglutition disorders, requests active euthanasia.
The results of a psychological examination are normal.

1. From the standpoint of international law

Several provisions of positive international law already quoted state that no one may be arbitrarily deprived of life (see Article 6 of the Covenant on Civil and Political Rights and Article 4 (1) of the American Convention on Human Rights).[1] As regards active euthanasia at the patient's request, it is highly doubtful, firstly, whether it is possible to waive the fundamental right to life by means of an intervention by another person with rights and duties under the law, and, secondly, whether the latter can legitimately give his assistance when he is perfectly conscious of the consequences of his act. It should be noted that in some systems of domestic law, destruction of life at the request of the person concerned is not defined as euthanasia, but as murder by consent.

It is, moreover, very debatable whether the patient's request can be considered as legally valid, in particular because acute and prolonged suffering can very well weaken the human consciousness and the human mind.

In the case postulated here, the results of the psychological examination are normal; however, this does not make any difference to the fact that the doctor's specific duty is to treat, cure or alleviate suffering. This is clear from Article 4 of the BC, which refers to "professional standards". In this connection, point 31 of the explanatory report states in its turn that "doctors and, in general, all professionals participating in a medical act are subject to legal and ethical imperatives. They must act with care and competence, and pay careful attention to the needs of each patient", and although the same point admits that "if professional standards are not identical in all countries", Article 1 of the BC stipulates that "Parties to this Convention shall protect the dignity and identity of all human beings and guarantee everyone, without discrimination, respect for their integrity and other rights and fundamental freedoms with regard to the application of biology and medicine". The duty to protect human life, as stated in Article 2 of the ECHR, not only admits no exceptions, but imposes the positive obligation on member states to enact any law necessary to guarantee *de facto* such protection.

---

1. As regards recourse to force in police and military actions and operations aimed at capturing suspected terrorists, resulting in the death of these suspects (namely prevention of terrorism and Article 2 of the ECHR), see Decision No. 324 of 27.9.1995 in the case of *McCann and others* (*Commission* v. *United Kingdom*).

As regards European case-law, see the summary of the facts in report 17.5.1995 of the Commission concerning the decision on the admissibility of Application No. 25949/94 (*Sampedro Camean* v. *Spain*).

2. From the ethical standpoint

The WMA first tackled the subject of euthanasia in New York in 1950. It condemned it "in all circumstances".

More recently in Lisbon (2 October 1981) in the Declaration on the Rights of the Patient, the WMA acknowledged the right to die in dignity. The patient has the right to refuse treatment.

In Venice (1983), a declaration of principle was issued on terminal illness and withholding of treatment.

According to the Declaration of Venice[1] (WMA Declaration on terminal illness of October 1983), the duty of the physician is to heal and, where possible, relieve suffering and act to protect the best interests of his patient. There may be no exception to this principle, even in the case of incurable disease or malformation.

In its Marbella Declaration (1992) on medically assisted suicide, the WMA declared that medically assisted suicide is like euthanasia, contrary to ethics and should be condemned by the medical profession. The doctor who, intentionally and deliberately, helps an individual to put an end to their life acts contrary to ethics.

3. From the standpoint of religious moralities

a. *Catholic*

For Catholic morality, it is wrong to request, for oneself or others, interventions which lead directly to the murder of a human being, though he may be incurably ill or dying.[2] A request for active euthanasia is neither acceptable nor lawful, whatever the patient's situation.

b. *Protestant*

The utmost must be done to enable this man to be himself to a maximum until the end. Over and above the technical act, there arises the equally complex and much more intricate question of the identity of a person and the best way to help him to preserve this identity at various times in his life and up to the end.

---

1. Declaration on terminal illness, Venice, Italy, October 1983, WMA.
2. Declaration of the Congregation for the doctrine of the faith on euthanasia, No. 2.

c. *Jewish*

For Judaism the respect of human life is absolute, sacred, inviolable. Human life has infinite value because it is a gift of God.

Rabbi Yossef Caro in his Shulhan Arukh writes: "it is forbidden to do anything whatever which will hasten death".

To legalise euthanasia is to leave the door open to all abuses, to all excesses. The doctor does not have the right to base his attitude on the notions of curability or incurability.

If the patient's life is in danger, it is the doctor's duty to do everything possible to convince the patient or his family of the need for treatment and thus to obtain their consent. Everything must be done to save the patient's life. The doctor's vocation is to combat disease and death. This is the very essence of medicine.

Thus active euthanasia is categorically prohibited by Judaism. However, the doctor also has the duty to alleviate the physical and mental suffering of his patient by all medical, psychological and social means; it is forbidden to let any living creature suffer. Judaism, an invitation to action and solidarity when another is suffering, cannot be the pretext for inaction disguised as pity.

d. *Muslim*

In Islam, no one is authorised to put an end to his life or anyone else's, even if the person is suffering from an incurable disease. Furthermore, experience has proved that the prognosis can never be completely certain. Finally, the psychological state of the person requesting euthanasia cannot be taken into consideration given his or her physically weakened state.

e. *Buddhist*

Suicide is discouraged in all cases, and this can be well understood if we accept that death is not the final end of a person's mental continuum. But suicide does not have the same causal weight as voluntary murder of a third person out of hatred, for example; it is necessary to bring into play here the concept of intention with all its nuances.

However, in the case of active euthanasia, the doctor or medical team takes the responsibility for an act whose consequences will be considered from the standpoint of the motivation, which is generally to put an end to the patient's suffering.

4. From the standpoint of agnostic morality

Under certain legal conditions, a conscious request for active euthanasia is accepted in the Netherlands. The same is true in certain states in Australia and the United States.

Active euthanasia – an assisted suicide, as it were – is considered by many people to be the last vestige of freedom which remains to a conscious and informed person who rejects the indignity of his final condition.

In France, relentless prolongation of life – as opposed to medical perseverance – is no longer accepted.

In practice, both in hospitals and outside, euthanasia procedures are very often employed.

Relentless prolongation of life

A man aged 60 was operated on five years ago for gastric cancer and three years ago for pulmonary metastasis.
He now has a cerebral metastasis. A surgical operation is being proposed.

1. From the standpoint of international law

As we saw earlier (see commentary on case 13), it is sometimes difficult to draw the border line between passive euthanasia and avoidance of relentless prolongation of life, since no provision (binding or otherwise) of international law defines the concept of relentless prolongation of life, and since the absolute nature of the right to life seems to imply that every means should be employed to safeguard it.

There can therefore be no reply in law.

However, see Article 4 of the BC, in the terms of which "any intervention in the health field, including research, must be carried out in accordance with relevant professional obligations and standards", as well as points 28 to 33 of the explanatory report. In particular, "an intervention must meet criteria of relevance and proportionality between the aim pursued and the means employed" (point 33).

2. From the ethical standpoint

If there is a chance that the patient will benefit from a treatment, however hazardous, its administration does not constitute relentless prolongation of life (WMA, Venice, 1983).

3. From the standpoint of religious moralities

a. *Catholic*

The morality of a possible surgical operation in the case of multiple cancer metastases must be the outcome of thorough consideration on the part of the physician, who must give an assessment on the basis of the criteria of "proportionality of treatment": what will be the benefits for the patient, what risks does he run and what subsequent sacrifices and suffering will result for the patient?[1] In the present case, the decision to operate does not seem to have been taken on ethical grounds.

---

1. Pius XII, AAS 48 (1956), p. 568ff.

b. *Protestant*

The utmost must be done to enable this man to be himself to a maximum until the end. Over and above the technical act, there arises the equally complex and much more intricate question of the identity of a person and the best way to help him to preserve this identity at various times in his life and up to the end.

c. *Jewish*

The doctors (a minimum of three), must look into all possibilities, in agreement with the family. If there is one single chance to save this man's life, the operation should be attempted. If the outcome of the operation is likely to be fatal and will only cause the patient unnecessary suffering and pain, the operation should not be attempted. Nevertheless, in all cases, normal treatment required by the disease must be continued.

d. *Muslim*

In Islam, no one is authorised to put an end to his life or to anyone else's. The doctor, whose mission is to save human lives and not to abbreviate them, is the only person capable of assessing the patient's prognosis and deciding whether a surgical operation is possible without endangering the patient's life.

e. *Buddhist*

As we have already seen, in the Buddhist approach, all relentless prolongation of life, which is a form of aggression upon the body, must be avoided. Here again, it is preferable to help the patient die in the best conditions.

4. From the standpoint of agnostic morality

No harm must be done to the body. In this particular case, the operation is a matter for the doctor's conscience and the family's wishes.

Here again, a distinction has to be made between relentless prolongation of life and medical perseverance.

If the operation is not going to improve the patient's condition substantially and for a reasonable time, then love of one's neighbour and respect for human dignity suggest that comfort care only should be given, and this to the greatest possible extent.

Relentless prolongation of life

A 3-year-old girl suffering from hydrocephalus has been operated on three times for draining of the cerebro-spinal fluid (csf).
She has since developed myelocytic leukaemia.
There are two problems: starting treatment for leukaemia and continuing csf drainage.

1. From the standpoint of international law

The case illustrates the need for a precise as possible legal definition of relentless prolongation of life, a definition which does not yet exist in international law on human rights, despite the text of Article 4 of the BC.

The only possible reply is that treatment for leukaemia cannot be withheld, nor treatment for hydrocephalus broken off, at the request of the parents, and that parental protest may not call into question or override the child's fundamental rights, particularly her right to life (on this point, see Articles 8 (2) and 9 (2) of the ECHR and Articles 18 (3) and (4) of the Covenant on Civil and Political Rights).

In fact, even in cases other than emergencies (Article 8 of the BC), Article 6 (1) and (2) and Article 26 (1) of the BC seem to imply that the physician cannot be satisfied with the refusal of the child's parents or legal representative to give authorisation, since the authorisation of an authority, person or body provided for by law is also necessary (see also Article 6 (4) of the BC).

2. From the ethical standpoint

The interests of the patient and the benefit he can expect will determine the decision (WMA, Venice 1983),[1] but the physician shall refrain from employing any extraordinary means which would prove of no benefit for the patient and where the sole purpose is to keep alive organs intended for grafts.

3. From the standpoint of religious moralities

a. *Catholic*

The judgment of Catholic morality must take the risk-benefit ratio into account. However, as the two treatments envisaged (drainage and leukaemia therapy) constitute "ordinary treatment", for the condition, they are compulsory.[2]

---

1. WMA Declaration on the terminal phase of illness, Venice, Italy, October 1983.
2. Declaration of the Congregation for the doctrine of the faith on euthanasia, No. 4.

b. *Protestant*

The question cannot be resolved without reference to the people close to the child, that is primarily its parents or those who care for it on a day-to-day basis.

c. *Jewish*

We are not told the state of the child as a result of the hydrocephalus. If the patient's life is acceptable, the doctors must use every means open to them.

In any event, it is necessary to continue the normal treatment required by the disease and administer all the treatment which can reduce the suffering.

d. *Muslim*

The doctor's duty is to save lives, not to abbreviate them. The criteria determining the incurability of a disease are sometimes difficult to define. Where there is some doubt concerning pursuit of a treatment or performance of a surgical operation, the attending physician may be assisted by other colleagues, but he may under no circumstances break off treatment of this child.

e. *Buddhist*

This child should be helped by commencing the treatment, taking care to avoid causing her any suffering disproportionate to the benefit obtained.

4. From the standpoint of agnostic morality

We can but be sorry for this little girl. If she cannot have a decent life, namely one which is fairly independent both intellectually and physically, the cessation of medical treatment is justified. However, palliative care must be continued for the hydrocephalic child with myelocytic leukaemia.

Torture

A man aged 30 is a witness and subjected to police interrogation.
Presence of a doctor to monitor the level of tolerance to physical or psychological coercion.
Declaration of Tokyo

1. From the standpoint of international law

All international instruments concerning human rights ban torture and participation in torture (see Article 5 of the Universal Declaration, Article 3 of the ECHR, Article 7 of the Covenant on Civil and Political Rights, and Article 5 (2) of the American Convention). The same is true, *a fortiori*, of the international instruments specifically concerned with the prevention and repression of torture and cruel, inhuman or degrading punishments, namely the UN *ad hoc* Convention (10.12.1984-27.6.1987) (Articles 1 and 11) and the European convention of the Council of Europe (26.11.1987-1.2.1989). In the terms of Article 11 of the UN Convention, "Each State Party shall keep under systematic review interrogation rules, instructions, methods and practices as well as arrangements for the custody and treatment of persons subjected to any form of arrest, detention or imprisonment in any territory under its jurisdiction, with a view to preventing any cases of torture". In particular, UN General Assembly Resolution 37/194 referred to above (particularly principle 4.*a* and *b*) states that "it is a contravention of medical ethics for health personnel to apply their knowledge and skills in order to assist in the interrogation of prisoners and detainees in a manner that may adversely affect the physical or mental health or condition of such prisoners or detainees" and "to certify, or to participate in the certification of, the fitness of prisoners or detainees for any form of treatment or punishment that may adversely affect their physical or mental health and which is not in accordance with the relevant international instruments, or to participate in any way in the infliction of any such treatment or punishment which is not in accordance with the relevant international instruments". In the same sense, see the judgment of the Court in the *Greek* case, as well as the decisions cited in cases 18 and 19 and, more recently, the statement of the facts of the *Hurtado* case (Decision No. 280 A of 28.1.1994, *Commission* v. *Switzerland*).

See also Recommendation No. 1235 (1994) adopted on 12 April 1994 by the Parliamentary Assembly of the Council of Europe on psychiatry and human rights. In the terms of point 7.ii.*b*, even "electroconvulsive therapy may not be performed unless informed written consent has been given by the patient or a person, counsellor or guardian, chosen by the patient as his or her representative and unless the decision has been confirmed by a select committee not composed exclusively of psychiatric experts".

Lastly, see the many observations of the UN Human Rights Committee establishing patent violations of Article 7 of the Covenant on Civil and Political Rights.

2. From the ethical standpoint

Declarations were issued by the WMA in Tokyo in 1975 and the ICPMS in Athens in 1979 prohibiting any participation by a physician in torture.

International ethical declarations condemn participation by physicians in any form of torture.

a. WMA, Tokyo, October 1975

The doctor shall not be present during any procedure during which torture is used, he may not provide any premises, instruments, substances or knowledge to facilitate the practice of torture, nor may he diminish the ability of the victim to resist such treatment.

b. ICPMS, Athens, 11 September 1979

Prison doctors undertake to condemn any participation in any form of torture whatsoever.

In its Declaration of Marbella (1992) on hunger strikers, the WMA gives several ethical guidelines for doctors for the treatment of hunger strikers, notably the informed agreement of the patient, his protection against acts of coercion and the measures to take in the case of a loss of lucidity.

3. From the standpoint of religious moralities

a. *Catholic*

For Catholic morality, participation in torture by a physician is unacceptable as the aim of his conduct must always be to help and heal, not to damage the integrity of the person.[1]

b. *Protestant*

It is surprising to see such a question included in a manual on human rights. Article 5 of the Universal Declaration on Human Rights radically condemns torture together with "cruel, inhuman or degrading punishment". Protestantism cannot claim to say more.

c. *Jewish*

Torture must be condemned and stigmatised in such terms that it is inconceivable that doctors might be willing or able to be involved in it.

---

1. Pius XII, AAS 45 (1953), pp. 744-754.

d. *Muslim*

For Muslim morality, torture or damage to physical or mental integrity are strictly forbidden. *A fortiori*, this applies to the doctor whose mission is to care for human lives.

e. *Buddhist*

Torture is to be condemned and is unacceptable under any circumstances, all the more so when it is a case of making it even more effective through medical intervention.

4. From the standpoint of agnostic morality

No physical coercion is acceptable, and no psychological coercion either. The doctor called in can but declare whether the witness' condition authorises the continuation of the interrogation.

This doctor must also ensure that the interrogation is clearly humane, that is without violence of any sort, all the more so because under French law confession is not proof.

Inhuman and degrading treatment

A man aged 40 is serving a prison sentence.
Intervention of a doctor during application of corporal punishment (solitary
confinement, restricted diet or continuous wearing of handcuffs).

1. From the standpoint of international law

See commentary on case 17. Under all the international instruments (see also Articles 25, 31, 32 (1) and 33 of Resolution (73) 5 adopted by the Committee of Ministers of the Council of Europe on 19 January 1973 containing the standard minimum rules for the treatment of prisoners and Principle 1 of UN General Assembly Resolution 3452 (XXX) of 9 December 1975 containing the Declaration on the protection of all persons from being subjected to torture and other cruel, inhuman or degrading treatment or punishment), the intervention of a doctor is required solely to protect the individual against all abuses banned as torture and cruel, inhuman or degrading treatment.

Participation by a physician in restraining a prisoner or detainee is prohibited under Principle 5 of UN General Assembly Resolution 3452 (XXX) of 9 December 1975 unless it is "determined in accordance with purely medical criteria as being necessary for the protection of the physical or mental health or the safety of the prisoner or detainee himself, of his fellow prisoners or detainees, or of his guardians, and to present no hazard to his physical or mental health".

In the same sense, see Recommendation 1235 (1994) on psychiatry and human rights adopted by the Parliamentary Assembly of the Council of Europe on 12 April 1994. In the terms of point 7.iv.c, this recommendation applies not only to handicapped and mentally ill patients involuntarily committed, but also imprisoned or detained persons. Point 7.iii.c states that no mechanical restraint should be used on these persons. As for pharmaceutical means of restraint, these "must be proportionate to the objective sought, and there must be no permanent infringement of individual's rights to procreate". Furthermore, "the use of isolation cells should be strictly limited and accommodation in large dormitories should also be avoided" (7.iii.b).

In the case of detained persons, in the terms of point 7.iii.a of the same recommendation, "the code of ethics must explicitly stipulate that it is forbidden for therapists to make sexual advances to patients" and "a psychiatrist and specially trained staff should be attached to each penal institution" (7.iv.b).

It should also be pointed out that in the terms of point 7.ii.f, "an inspection system similar to that of the European Committee for the Prevention of Torture and Inhuman or Degrading Treatment or Punishment should be set up".

Lastly, it should be noted that the order of a superior or of a public authority cannot be invoked to justify torture (Article 2 (3) of the United Nations Convention).

As regards European case-law, see Judgment No. 25 of 18.1.1978 in *Northern Ireland* v. *United Kingdom* and Judgment No. 26 of 25.4.1978 in *Tyrer* v. *United Kingdom*. See also the statement of the facts of the *Hurtado* case (Decision No. 280 A of 28.1.1994, *Commission* v. *Switzerland*) and the decisions cited in case 19, as well as Judgment No. 201 of 20.3.1991 in the *Cruz Varas* case (*Commission* v. *Sweden*) and Judgment No. 161 of 7.7.1989 in the *Soering* case (*Commission* v. *United Kingdom*).

More recently, see Judgment Nos. 215 of 30.10.1991 in the *Vilvarajah and others* (*Commission* v. *United Kingdom*); 241 A of 27.8.1992 in the *Tomasi* case (*Commission* v. *France*); 224 of 24.9.1993 in the *Herczegfalvy* case (*Commission* v. *Austria*); 269 of 22.9.1993 in the *Klaas* case (*Commission* v. *Germany*) and 336 of 4.12.1995 in the *Ribitsch* case (*Commission* v. *Austria*). Reference should also be made to the observations of the UN Human Rights Commission, notably that of 1.11.1992 on Communication No. 240/1987, that of 31.3.1993 on Communication No. 282/1988; that of 30.7.1993 on Communication No. 470/1991 and the dissenting opinions appended thereto, and the observation of 5.11.1993 on Communication No. 469/1991 and the dissenting opinions appended thereto.

2. From the ethical standpoint

The ICPMS condemns participation in any corporal punishment (Athens, 11 September 1979).

The WMA (Tokyo, October 1975) declares that:

– "the doctor shall not countenance, condone or participate in the practice of (...) forms of cruel (...) treatment, nor shall he provide knowledge to facilitate (...) such treatment;

– the doctor shall not be present during any procedure during which (...) degrading treatment is used or threatened;

– what constitutes degrading punishment is left to the evaluation of the doctor on the basis of the facts, particularly with regard to solitary confinement and the attendant conditions."

See also the Commission's decision in the *Greek* case (3), which states that "there is violation of medical ethics if members of the health staff, in particular doctors, participate in any way whatever in the containment of prisoners or detainees, unless it is determined in accordance with purely medical criteria as being necessary for the protection of the physical or mental health or the safety of the prisoner or detainee himself, of his fellow prisoners or detainees, or of his guardians, and to present no hazard to his physical or mental health".

174

In its Declaration of Marbella (1992) on hunger strikers, the WMA gives several ethical guidelines for doctors for the treatment of hunger strikers, notably the informed agreement of the patient, his protection against acts of coercion and the measures to take in the case of a loss of lucidity.

3. From the standpoint of religious moralities

a. *Catholic*
For the Catholic Church, it is morally unacceptable to make of medical science an instrument to serve aims damaging to the integrity of the person, regardless of the situation he or she is in. The presence and work of a physician in the case referred to can be licit only if their aim is to tend and calm the physical suffering imposed without his consent.[1]

b. *Protestant*
It is surprising to see such a question included in a manual on human rights. Article 5 of the Universal Declaration on Human Rights radically condemns torture together with "cruel, inhuman or degrading punishment". Protestantism cannot claim to say more.

c. *Jewish*
In this connection, the doctor has a huge responsibility. But over and above the responsibility of the doctor involved in physical and mental torture, a broader responsibility lies with the medical profession as a whole. Only a formal position on the part of medical organisations at national and international level will help the doctor to put up resistance to the torturers if he is called to a tortured fellow human being.

d. *Muslim*
In Islam, any damage to a person's physical or mental integrity is prohibited. *A fortiori* when a doctor is called upon to apply corporal punishment.

e. *Buddhist*
See case 17.

4. From the standpoint of agnostic morality

When he undergoes his sentence the prisoner must not be subjected to inhuman or degrading treatment. The limitation of food, for example, is inexcusable, as is the

---

1. Pius XII, AAS 45 (1953), pp. 744-754.

continuous wearing of handcuffs, the deprivation of clothing or the presence of harsh lighting in the cell. All such treatment is inadmissible, and in France the infamous "punishment cell" regime is being revised because it offends the democratic conscience. It will no longer be left solely to the judgment of the prison administration whether the sentence passed by a judge will be made harsher for offences committed in prison.

It is obviously necessary to take account of the danger represented by some prisoners, but the disappearance of the punishment cell and the high security block is to be desired.

However horrible the crime committed, the prisoner always remains a human being.

Abusive practices in psychiatry

An accused man aged 28 is suspected of taking part in a hold-up perpetrated by an organised gang; interrogation is impossible because of the accused's psychological resistance.
Co-operation of a psychiatrist either in the interrogation or in order to prescribe drugs which will change his mental state.

1. From the standpoint of international law

The case postulated here amounts to an example of the abuse of psychiatry, something prohibited not only by all the international instruments referred to in connection with cases 17 and 18, but also by Resolution R (83) 2 adopted by the Committee of Ministers of the Council of Europe on 22 February 1983 concerning the legal protection of persons suffering from mental disorder placed as involuntary patients (Article 5 and points 29 to 32 of the explanatory report).

See also Recommendation 1235 (1994) on psychiatry and human rights adopted by the Parliamentary Assembly of the Council of Europe on 12 April 1994, in particular point 7.ii.c, in the terms of which "there must be an accurate and detailed recording of the treatment given to the patient"; point 7.ii.e, according to which "patients must have access to a 'counsellor' who is independent of the institution; similarly, a 'guardian' should be responsible for looking after the interests of minors" point 7.ii.f, in the terms of which "an inspection system similar to that of the European Committee for the Prevention of Torture and Inhuman or Degrading Treatment or Punishment should be set up".

In the same connection, see also the judgments of the Court in the Winterwerp case (24.10.1979) and, in particular, the case of *X* v. *United Kingdom* (5.11.1981).

In connection with the various aspects of torture and cruel, inhuman or degrading treatment or punishment, see the judgments of the Court in the following cases: *Ireland* v. *United Kingdom* (18.1.1978), *Tyrer* v. *United Kingdom* (25.4.1978), *Silver and others* v. *United Kingdom* (25.3.1983), *Boyle and Rice* v. *United Kingdom* (27.4.1978) and *Schonenberg and Durmaz* v. *Switzerland* (20.6.1988). See also the Commission's Decisions of 18.10.1985 and 31.12.1985 in the cases of *Farrant, Gleaves and others* v. *United Kingdom* and *Byrne, McFadden and others* v. *United Kingdom* respectively, and Resolution DH (87) 7 of 20.3.1987.

More recently, see the Commission decisions on Application Nos. 14289/88; 14178/89; 14610/89; 14718/89; 15271/89; 16832/90; 16848/90; 17232/90 and 19184/91, as well as Resolution DH (91) 6 of the Committee of Ministers (13.2.1991) in *D.* v. *Belgium*. See also Judgment No. 244 of 24.9.1992 in the *Herczegfalvy* case (*Commission* v. *Austria*).

As regards the question of treating corporal punishment inflicted on school-children as inhuman or degrading treatment, see Resolution (87) 9 adopted by the Committee of Ministers of the Council of Europe on 25.6.1987, the judgment of the Court in the case of *Campbell and Cosans* v. *United Kingdom* (25.2.1982) and the Commission's reports of 23.1.1987 and 16.7.1987 on Application Nos. 9119/80, 9014/81 and 10592/83, all against the United Kingdom. See also Decision No. 247 C of 25.3.1993 in the *Castello-Roberts* case (*Commission* v. *United Kingdom*) and the statement of the facts in Decision No. 247 A of 29.10.1992 in the case of *Y* v. *United Kingdom*.

2. From the ethical standpoint

As regards abusive use of psychiatry, the major reference text is the World Psychiatric Association's Declaration of Hawaii 1977, which reiterates that the doctor's role *vis-à-vis* his fellow men is to heal them in respect for their dignity, refusing all influence extraneous to the treatment. In its Declaration of Marbella (1992) on medically assisted suicide, the WMA stated that medically assisted suicide, like euthanasia, is contrary to medical ethics and should be condemned by the medical profession. The doctor who intentionally and deliberately helps an individual to put an end to his own life acts contrary to medical ethics.

3. From the standpoint of religious moralities

a. *Catholic*
Direct or indirect participation by the psychiatrist in actions damaging to a person's psycho-physical integrity and for the purposes of detention and confession is morally unacceptable.[1] In this specific case, as there is no "medical indication" in the form of mental illness, the psychiatrist's co-operation is illicit.

b. *Protestant*
It is surprising to see such a question included in a manual on human rights. Article 5 of the Universal Declaration on Human Rights radically condemns torture together with "cruel, inhuman or degrading punishment". Protestantism cannot claim to say more.

c. *Jewish*
The collaboration of a psychiatrist either in an interrogation or to prescribe drugs to modify a prisoner's mental structure is morally unacceptable. It brings discredit

---

1. Pius XII, *Broadcast speeches and messages*, Vol. XX, 1958, p. 331ff.

on the medical function and constitutes a disgraceful attack on the dignity of man, who should be treated "as an end and not as a means".

d. *Muslim*

Any damage to a person's physical or mental integrity is proscribed by Islam, even in the case of an accused suspected of some crime.

e. *Buddhist*

Anything intended to modify a person's behaviour or consciousness without his consent is contrary to the Buddhist ethic based on compassion and non-aggression.
The medical act must have no other aim than that of relieving suffering.

4. From the standpoint of agnostic morality

The active presence of a psychiatrist during an interrogation should be prohibited.

Application of penalties by doctors

Application by doctors of penalties imposed by civil or ecclesiastical courts. Penal amputation, castration (Denmark): no intervention without the victim's consent.

1. From the standpoint of international law

A sentence imposing on any basis whatsoever, amputation or castration would be contrary to the provisions of international law already referred to in connection with cases 17, 18 and 19. Moreover, Article 10 (1) of the Covenant on Civil and Political Rights states that "all persons deprived of their liberty shall be treated with humanity and with respect for the inherent dignity of the human person". The doctor must therefore refuse to carry out the sentence, *a fortiori* where the condemned person has not been asked for his consent. In the terms of Article 11 of the Covenant on Civil and Political Rights in fact, "nobody may be imprisoned simply because he is unable to fulfil a contractual obligation".

Such an intervention even with the victim's consent would still be contrary to the provisions of international law, which does not take any position as regards renouncing the exercise and possession of fundamental rights. Such a waiver could, at all events, not be exercised through the intermediary of a person whose "institutional" duty is to care and heal, nor to destroy the mental and/or physical integrity of individuals. Article 4 of the BC stresses this, reference being made here to "professional obligations and standards", namely the ethical and legal requirements with which doctors and members of the health care professions must comply. These requirements now certainly include Article 2 (3) of the UN Convention for the Prevention of Torture, according to which the order of a superior or of a public authority cannot be invoked to justify torture, this provision being a *jus cogens* rule in international law.

Where the doctor in question is a prison official, the same applies.

See also the answer to case 7 and point 7.iii.*c* of Recommendation 1235 (1994) of the Parliamentary Assembly of the Council of Europe.

As regards prisoners subjected to scientific research, Article 17 (1) of the DBC (F) states that "scientific research on a person without the capacity to consent as stipulated in Article 5, can be undertaken "only if all the following conditions are met: i. the conditions laid down in Article 16, sub-paragraphs i to iv, are fulfilled; ii. the results of the research have the potential to produce real and direct benefit to his or her health; iii. research of comparable effectiveness cannot be carried out on individuals capable of giving consent; iv. the necessary authorisation provided for under Article 6 has been given specifically and in writing; and v. the person concerned does not object".

Article 17 (2) adds that "Exceptionally and under the protective conditions pre-scribed by law, where the research has not the potential to produce results of direct benefit to the health of the person concerned, such research may be authorised sub-ject to the conditions laid down in paragraph 1, sub-paragraphs i, iii, iv and v above, and to the following additional conditions: i. the research has the aim of contributing, through significant improvement in the scientific understanding of the individual's condition, disease or disorder, to the ultimate attainment of results capable of conferring benefit to the person concerned or to other persons in the same age category or afflicted with the same disease or disorder or having the same condition; and ii. the research entails only minimal risk and minimal burden for the individual concerned.

See also Article 26 (1) and (2) of the BC.

2. From the ethical standpoint

The WMA (Tokyo 1975) forbids absolutely and without restriction any partici-pation in cruel, inhuman and degrading treatment; the subject's consent to castra-tion or amputation is not acceptable.

3. From the standpoint of religious moralities

a. *Catholic*

Regardless of the victim's consent, any participation by a physician in acts, the purpose of which is not to help or heal, but, on the contrary, to damage the integri-ty of the person, is morally unacceptable. A punishment such as that envisaged in this case can have neither a "religious" nor "civil" meaning.[1]

b. *Protestant*

It seems obvious that the roles of doctor and executioner must be carefully dis-tinguished. Is there really any point in mentioning the possibility of a confusion so contrary to common sense and respect for human rights?

c. *Jewish*

The participation of doctors in torture inflicted on a man with or without his consent must be categorically condemned. It is morally and religiously unaccept-able.

It is important to quote here Article 7 of the WMA Declaration of Geneva of 1946: "I will maintain the utmost respect for human life from the time of concep-

---

1. Pius XII, AAS 45 (1953), pp. 744-54.

181

tion; even under threat, I will not use my medical knowledge contrary to the laws of humanity (...). The doctor's position in this connection must be carefully protected and the cornerstone remains traditional medical ethics which has proved itself through the centuries."

d. *Muslim*

In Islam, it is forbidden for anyone to damage a person's physical or mental integrity. This applies *a fortiori* to a physician.

e. *Buddhist*
See case 19.

4. From the standpoint of agnostic morality

No doctor would be able to perform an amputation such as castration, even with the consent of the convicted person.

Even the taking of drugs with a sterilising effect – specific sedatives – is possible only if a lucid request for it is made by the prisoner. This treatment, however, can be started only after the man has left prison, or shortly before his discharge, and must be prescribed by a doctor outside the prison system.

However, chemical hormonal castration is acceptable for a recidivist sex offender.

Organ transplants

One of a pair of heterozygote twin girls aged 3 suffers from polycystic kidneys, hepatomegaly and splenomegaly.
The family consents to removal of a kidney from the healthy sister for transplant, in view of the urgency of the case and the fact that no kidney from a dead donor of suitable age is available.

1. From the standpoint of international law

The case highlights a number of problems: 1. the conflict between the right to life of the sick sister and the right to physical integrity of the healthy one; 2. the conflict between the right to life of the sick sister and the right to future health of the healthy sister; 3. the legitimacy of the parents' consent to the removal of an organ from a minor subject in breach of the latter's fundamental rights. This raises the question of the legitimacy and limits of parental authority.

Today, there is still no explicit answer in positive international law to the questions raised by problems 1 and 2. The right to physical integrity and to future health (of the healthy sister) does, however, seem to imply that she should not be deprived of a kidney, even for the benefit of a sister in a critical situation. Indeed, Article 6 (2) of Resolution (78) 29, referred to in case 10, states that "the removal of substances which cannot regenerate from legally incapacitated persons is forbidden". Paragraph 26 of the explanatory report specifies that "as a general rule, non-regenerative substance removals from legally incapacitated persons are prohibited".

However, the same article allows member states of the Council of Europe the possibility of authorising such removals in very exceptional cases. These removals may only be performed for therapeutic or diagnostic purposes. If a member state wishes to authorise such removals, it must lay down the following conditions: *a.* the donor must have the capacity of understanding; *b.* he must have given his consent; *c.* his legal representative and an appropriate authority must have authorised removal; *d.* the donor and the recipient must be closely genetically related.

Paragraph 27 of the explanatory report explains in this connection that "during the discussions on this article a number of experts expressed an opinion in favour of a total prohibition of the effecting of the removal of non-regenerative substances on legally incapacitated persons, but the majority of experts, while agreeing to the general rule prohibiting removal, preferred to bring an exception to it in limited cases and under the above-mentioned conditions. The main reason behind this position is the invaluable and irreplaceable nature of substances donated from genetically related persons due to much higher chances of success of transplants effected with the substances".

It follows from the above that even where national legislation permits the removal of the organ concerned in this case, parental authority alone does not suffice to dispose of the rights of a minor child incapable of understanding, even for the benefit of a sibling.

As for the BC: the kidney being a substance incapable of regeneration, removal is prohibited. Reference should be made also to Article 26 of the BC, in particular Article 26 (2).

As regards European case-law, see, *mutatis mutandis,* Decision 22.5.1995 of the Commission on the admissibility of Application No. 20948/92 (*Isiltan* v. *Turkey*).

As regards the international sale of organs for transplantation see "Sale of children", report of the UN Human Rights Committee at its 47th Session (28 January 1991) (Doc. E/CN.4/1991/51).

2. From the ethical standpoint

The International Conference of Medical Councils (CIO, 1983) prohibits in principle removal of organs from human beings except in the case of twins who are able to express an opinion, which is not the case here. This opinion must in all cases be confirmed by the opinion of an *ad hoc* commission.

According to the WMA Declaration of Madrid on organ transplants (1987), the doctor must protect the rights of the donor and of the recipient and may not perform a transplant if these rights are not respected.

The procedures envisaged must be discussed as broadly as possible with the donor and the recipient or their next of kin.

3. From the standpoint of religious moralities

a. *Catholic*

For Catholic morality, the consent of parents for removal of a kidney from a healthy child is not acceptable: this consent must be given by an adult and must be expressed freely and spontaneously.[1]

b. *Protestant*

Perhaps we should quote here these words attributed to Jesus: "If thou knowest what thou doest, do it."

---

1. Pius XII, AAS 48 (1956), p. 459.

c. *Jewish*

In the case of a kidney transplant, the question does not arise in terms of authorisation, but in terms of obligation. In a position where I am subject to the requirement to assist a person in danger according to the commandment: "Do not stand idly by when your neighbour's blood is flowing" (Lev., 18, v. 16), am I obliged to offer a patient one of my organs – a replacement which could save the life of a man whose two kidneys are mortally affected?

It is permissible to assist a patient in mortal danger by transplant of an organ taken from the body of a living person, when the removal of this organ does not endanger the donor's life and after obtaining his informed consent.[1]

d. *Muslim*

Islam authorises transplantation of organs removed from a living donor in the case of kidneys, bone marrow or liver tissue. For the conditions imposed, please refer to the introduction.

e. *Buddhist*

Yes, with the parents' consent, if the removal does not endanger the donor's life or entail any consequences for her. But it is a difficult question to the extent that the child can neither give her opinion nor assess the consequences of the act. Respect for the healthy child might be a reason for questioning the parents' right to decide for this child. There is a great risk of abuse here.

4. From the standpoint of agnostic morality

In this situation the transplant can be authorised:

– if a college of medical experts is in favour;

– provided that the consequences of this donation do not represent a potential danger for the donor, while the success of the transplantation will be limited in time.

---

1. See E. Gugenheim, *Les portes de la Loi* ("The gates of the law"), pp. 264-265.

Organ transplants

A 20-year-old with an incurable cranial traumatism is being kept alive artificially to permit removal of various organs for transplant purposes.
Death has been certified by a team independent of the transplant surgeons.
Authorisation is given by some members of the family, while others object.

1. From the standpoint of international law

Under Article 12 (2) and (3) of Resolution (78) 29 quoted in case 10, grafting and transplantation must take place in public or private institutions which possess proper staff and equipment. Death must be established by a doctor who does not belong to the team which will effect the removal, grafting or transplantation (however, this doctor can effect a removal in cases of minor operations when no other suitable doctor is available).

As regards the concept of "death", see Article 11 of Resolution (78) 29 and paragraph 38 of the explanatory report (quoted *in extenso* in the reply to case 23).

As regards the family's consent or objection, see the commentary on case 10 (Article 10 Resolution (78) 29 and points 35 to 37 of the explanatory report appended thereto).

See also Article 9 of the BC, in the terms of which "the previously expressed wishes relating to a medical intervention by a patient who is not, at the time of the intervention, in a state to express his wishes shall be taken into account". In this connection, points 60 to 62 of the explanatory report state that "Whereas Article 8 obviates the need for consent in emergencies, this article is designed to cover cases where persons capable of understanding have previously expressed their consent (that is either assent or refusal) with regard to foreseeable situations where they would not be in a position to express an opinion about the intervention. The article therefore covers not only the emergencies referred to in Article 8 but also situations where individuals have foreseen that they might be unable to give their valid consent, for example in the event of a progressive disease such as senile dementia. The article lays down that when persons have previously expressed their wishes, these shall be taken into account. Nevertheless, taking previously expressed wishes into account does not mean that they should necessarily be followed. For example, when the wishes were expressed a long time before the intervention and science has since progressed, there may be grounds for not heeding the patient's opinion. The practitioner should thus, as far as possible, be satisfied that the wishes of the patient apply to the present situation and are still valid, taking account in particular of technical progress in medicine." It should be noted, however (see the commentary on case 10), that this provision seems to refer to interventions on a living patient, even though incapable of giving his opinion on the intervention. Article 4 of the BC means by intervention all medical acts, whether for the purpose of diagnosis, preventive care, treatment or rehabilitation or in a research context (point 29 of the explanatory report).

Possible reference also to Article 29 of the BC.

2. From the ethical standpoint

The WMA Declaration of Sydney (1986) lays down the conditions for determination of death by doctors not concerned with the performance of a transplantation. See also the Declaration of Venice (1983).

The Declaration of Sydney refers for artificial prolongation of life, organ removal and transplantation to the "prevailing legal requirements of consent", while the Declaration of Venice requires that the doctor act in accordance with the laws of the country or on the basis of the express or tacit presumed consent of the competent person.

The Declaration of the CIO (1983) concerns only an objection on the part of the family. It does not give a view on what is to be done in a case where members of the family of the same degree of kinship hold differing opinions.

3. From the standpoint of religious moralities

a. *Catholic*
For Catholic doctrine, removal of organs from a dead body with the express consent of some members of the family responsible for care of the body is licit; their feelings and rights must be respected.[1]

b. *Protestant*
Transplantation of organs is certainly legitimate, if the "donor" is "respected" at least as much as the recipient – through respect shown to his family. If the family disagrees on what is to be done, this is a genuine obstacle to be overcome. The debate should therefore be pursued until this has been achieved.

c. *Jewish*
The case in question gives rise to the following problems, among others:
– definition of the time of death (see case 23);
– removal and transplantation of organs (see case 10).

---

1. Pius XII, AAS 48 (1956), p. 459.

Furthermore, in the present case, some members of the close family are opposed to the transplant. It is essential to try to continue the dialogue in order to obtain a consensus. If this cannot be achieved, it seems to me difficult to go against the wishes of the family and thus create dissentions between those in favour and those against.

d. *Muslim*

Transplants of organs removed from the body of a dead person are authorised in Islam provided that the following conditions are met:

1. death established by a committee made up of three doctors including a neurologist (the surgeon who is to perform the operation may not be a member of this committee);

2. absence of remuneration;

3. the transplant must be performed in a centre approved by the Ministry of Health of the country concerned;

4. the dead person raised no objection to removal of organs during his life.

In the present case, where one part of the family objects to removal of the organ, the transplant remains possible if the next of kin do not object and, *a fortiori,* if the person gave consent to removal of organs while he was alive.

e. *Buddhist*

If the donor clearly expressed the desire that his organs could be donated after his death, it can but be a beneficial act. If this is not the case then the removal of organs cannot be envisaged.

4. From the standpoint of agnostic morality

On the assumption that the brain-damaged person did not oppose any organ transplants before the accident, there is no need to take any account of the opinion of family members who oppose the removal of organs.

The gift of an organ is a gift of life.

Organ transplants

A man aged 45 in irreversible coma is being kept alive artificially for removal of an organ.
The family consents, but there is a matter of religious conviction (the man is a Muslim).

1. From the standpoint of international law

Under Article 10 (1) of Resolution (78) 29 of the Committee of Ministers of the Council of Europe, "no removal must take place when there is an open or presumed objection on the part of the deceased, in particular, taking into account his religious and philosophical convictions", and paragraph 35 of the explanatory report specifies that "in determining the existence of a presumed objection the religious and philosophical convictions of the deceased person are particularly taken into account".

Article 11 of the same resolution states that "death having occurred, a removal may be effected even if the function of some organ other than the brain may be artificially preserved" and paragraph 38 of the explanatory report specifies that "paragraph 1 of Article 11 states the moment after which a removal can be allowed to be effected on the body of a deceased person. The rules do not intend to give a legal or medical definition of death nor do they give any criteria by which death can be ascertained; these matters are therefore left completely to the rules and established practice existing in the member states. Once a person is considered dead under these rules and practice, a removal may be effected even if the functioning of some of his organs other than the brain is preserved artificially. Therefore a removal is prohibited if the function of the brain has not irrevocably and completely ceased, but states may wish to require additional criteria".

If the person who is in an irreversible coma meets the conditions and any additional criteria which may be required by the domestic legislation, he may be considered dead. Given the fact that he held religious convictions opposed to removal, the removal may not be performed.

As regards previously expressed wishes and Article 9 of the BC, see the replies to cases 10 and 22. As regards the use of a removed part of the human body, reference can be made to Article 22 of the BC.

2. From the ethical standpoint

The CIO (1983) requires the absence of any contra-indication associated with the deceased's religious convictions, regardless of whether or not the family gives its consent.

The deceased will be presumed not to have given his consent as a result of his convictions.

3. From the standpoint of religious moralities

a. *Catholic*
For Catholic morality, it is not right to remove organs from a body if, before the person's death, it became known that he held convictions against such removal, as there is a duty to respect the donor's wishes.[1]

b. *Protestant*
If an individual, for his own reasons, clearly expressed the desire not to have organs removed, it would seem difficult to go against this desire. We might even wonder how a patient would cope with a transplant, knowing that he is carrying the organ of someone who did not wish to give it. Or would one consider hiding the truth? To do so would certainly not auger well for the subsequent course of events.

c. *Jewish*
The problem of removal of organs is linked to the definition of death. The point of view of Jewish law is a very strict one. The definition of death accepted by all contemporary competent authorities is that given by the *Hatam Sofer* (Rabbi Moché Schreiber) (Y.D. 338). According to him, death is to be recognised by absence of movement, heartbeat and respiration. These three conditions must be met before death can be certified.

The same definition was adopted on 18 May 1978 by the General Assembly of the French Rabbinate. The text reads as follows:

The General Assembly of the French Rabbinate, in the presence of various laws and bills concerning, in particular, removal and transplantation of organs, has the duty to recall the following principles of Judaism:

1. the eminently sacred nature of life means that society and individuals must do their utmost to save a human life;

2. for Judaism, death is defined by simultaneous total cessation of respiratory, circulatory, and neurological functions;

3. as long as these three criteria are not met, it is prohibited to perform any of the many actions which habitually follow immediately upon death. Any action performed upon the dying person is considered as having provoked his death.

In recent years there has been a major change. The success rate for operations is over 80%, and over 70% of those operated upon live for at least five years.

---

1. Pius XII, AAS 48 (1956), p. 459.

Thus, because of the technical progress achieved in this field, and taking account of the criteria accepted by medical circles, criteria require the five following conditions:

– exact knowledge of the conditions of the accident;

– definitive cessation of natural breathing;

– existence of detailed clinical proof of the destruction of the brain stem;

– existence of objective proof and scientific and objective BAER examinations proving the destruction of the brain stem;

– certainty that the definitive cessation of respiration and non-functioning of the brain stem are irreversible and this after a waiting period of twelve hours under artificial respiration.

The Chief Rabbinate of Israel is prepared to authorise heart transplants at the Hadassah Medical Centre under the following conditions:

– the existence of all the above conditions establishing the death of the donor;

– participation of a delegate of the Chief Rabbinate as a full member of the committee responsible for establishing the time of death. This delegate shall be designated by the Ministry of Health and be selected from a list proposed by the Chief Rabbinate of Israel once a year;

– the transplant can take place only if the patient or his family have given their prior agreement in writing;

– the creation of a High Committee by the Ministry of Health in collaboration with the Chief Rabbinate of Israel responsible for examining all cases relating to heart transplants in Israel;

– the Ministry of Health should incorporate this regulation in the national legislation.

d. *Muslim*

Transplants of organs removed from the body of a dead person are licit in Islam provided that the following conditions are met:

1. death must be established by a committee of three doctors including a neurologist (the surgeon responsible for the transplant may not belong to this committee);

2. remuneration for the organ is prohibited;

3. the dead person must not have objected to removal of any organ from his body while he lived. The dead person's next of kin must give their consent;

4. the organ transplant must be carried out in a centre approved by the Ministry of Health.

e. *Buddhist*

The same problems arise as in the previous case, namely with respect to keeping someone alive artificially, the three-day period and the consent of the patient

191

while he was alive. In giving its consent or reviewing its position, the family should take into account the points made in case 22.

For an Islamic subject, account should be taken of the positions of this tradition and a solution found regarding removal of organs and artificial prolongation of life.

4. From the standpoint of agnostic morality

The family's agreement does not matter.
The wishes of the person who is about to die must be respected.

Sexual mutilation

The parents of a 9-year-old North African girl ask a doctor to perform a clitoridectomy.

1. From the standpoint of international law

The doctor must refuse to perform the clitoridectomy on the basis of respect for the dignity and psycho-physical integrity of the young girl as well as her right to health (see Article 5 of the Universal Declaration, Article 3 of the ECHR and Article 7 of the Covenant on Civil and Political Rights), as this is a permanent and irreversible lesion which obviously cannot be inflicted at the parents' behest.

In the same sense, see Article 24 (3) of the Convention on the Rights of the Child in the terms of which "States Parties shall take all effective measures to abolish traditional practices prejudicial to the health of children", the child having the right to enjoy the best possible state of health (Article 24 (1)).

The operation requested is, moreover, a discriminatory practice against women, prohibited as such by international law (see Articles 1, 2 and 3 of the Declaration on the elimination of all forms of discrimination against women, Articles 2 and 9 (1) of the Declaration of the rights of the child and Articles 8 (2) and 9 (2) of the ECHR).

In the same sense, see also Recommendation 1229 (1994) adopted on 24 January 1994 by the Parliamentary Assembly of the Council of Europe on the equality of rights between women and men, but also, though indirectly, several provisions of the African Charter on Human and Peoples' Rights (Nairobi, 1981), which came into force on 21 October 1986 between OAU member states. Thus Article 4 stipulates that the human person is inviolable and that every human being has the right to the physical and moral integrity of his person. Nobody may be arbitrarily deprived of this right. Article 5 adds that every individual has the right to the respect of the dignity inherent in the human person (...). All forms of exploitation and debasement, in particular (...) cruel, inhuman or degrading punishment or treatment are prohibited. On the other hand, whereas Articles 17 (3) and 18 (2) refer to the traditional values recognised by the community, Article 18 (3) states that "the state has the duty to ensure the elimination of all discrimination against women and the protection of the rights of women (...) as stipulated in the international declarations and conventions".

With regard, on the other hand, to practices which, while being specific to ethnic, linguistic, religious or other minorities, pose no problem with respect to human rights, reference should be made to Recommendation 1134 (1990) adopted by the Parliamentary Assembly of the Council of Europe on 1 October 1990. In the terms of Article 10.iii, "the special situation of a given minority may justify special measures in its favour". See also the Council of Europe Framework Convention for the Protection of National Minorities signed in Strasbourg on 1 February 1995.

Lastly, as regards sects and new religious movements, reference should be made to Recommendation 1178 (1992) adopted by the Parliamentary Assembly of the Council of Europe on 5 February 1992.

The equality of rights of women and men above and beyond Article 14 of the ECHR was also recently reaffirmed by the Court in Decision No. 263 of 24.6.1993 in the *Schuler-Zgraggen* case (*Commission* v. *Switzerland*) and in Decision No. 280 B of 22.2.1994 in the *Burghartz* case (*Commission* v. *Switzerland*).

See also the prohibition imposed by Article 6 (1) of the BC, the intervention being of no benefit to the patient.

2. From the ethical standpoint

General principles (WMA International Code of Medical Ethics – 1949) require doctors to act only in the interests of their patient and to respect patients' opinions; the Geneva Oath (1948) stipulates that the health of the patient must be the doctor's first consideration and that considerations of religion or race may not intervene.

The Declaration of Tokyo (1975) prohibits the doctor from inflicting suffering or participating in cruel or degrading treatment, whatever the victim's belief or motives. The WMA Declaration of Budapest (1993) on the condemnation of female genital mutilation prohibits doctors from instructing women, men and children in order to prevent the promotion of the practice of genital mutilation while taking account of the psychological rights and cultural identity of the persons concerned. The WMA condemns the practice of female genital mutilation, including the circumcision of women and girls, just as it condemns the participation of doctors in the execution of these practices.

3. From the standpoint of religious moralities

a. *Catholic*

For the Catholic Church, any operation on the body with the aim of destroying or mutilating it or rendering it incapable of exercising its natural functions by any other means is morally unacceptable.[1] Any mutilation devoid of therapeutic intention is morally unacceptable.

b. *Protestant*

Need we point out that excision is not among the characteristic customs of Protestantism?

---

1. Pius XII, AAS 22 (1930), p. 559ff.

c. *Jewish*

To damage one's body or an organ of the human body is absolutely forbidden. Respect for the wholeness of the body is an absolute obligation except when it is a matter of religious imperatives which do not endanger the life of the individual (circumcision, for example, see case 25).

In the case of excision of the clitoris, Judaism cannot give an opinion because this practice does not exist within it. Reference should be made to the competent religious authority which can give an authorised opinion.

d. *Muslim*

Circumcision, namely removal of part of the foreskin on males, is a practice to be found among Jews and Muslims. This practice as a health measure dates back to earliest antiquity. It was common practice among the ancient Egyptians and subsequently among the Syrians and Phoenicians. Among Jews, circumcision had a symbolic significance (consecration to God). Among Muslims, it is practised on very small children. Excision of the clitoris on girls is the removal of the small erectile organ situated at the upper opening of the vulva. This is practised only in certain African countries, independently of religion. The Prophet Mohammed disapproved of it. He said "this is not good for women or for their husbands".

e. *Buddhist*

To cut off the right of pleasure is negative and gives rise to frustrations and suffering which damage the person's mental and physical health. Excision should not be allowed in the case of minors, manipulated and uninformed people and those who are non-consenting.

"Anyone who hurts another or molests others is not a disciple" (*Dhammapada*, 184, *Pali Canon*).

In the case of an Islamic subject it is for this tradition to resolve the problem *vis-à-vis* the laws in force.

4. From the standpoint of agnostic morality

This case concerns the offence of sexual mutilation.

The criminal law protects the human body and human dignity and has primacy over tradition.

In addition, the sexual mutilation of a North African girl of 9 by excision of the clitoris is irreversible. It is therefore reprehensible and constitutes a moral offence against natural rights.

Participation by a doctor in systematic circumcision

Circumcision within a few days of birth is practised routinely as a health measure (United States).
Parental consent.

1. From the standpoint of international law

Article 4 of the BC stipulates that "any intervention in the health field, including research, must be carried out in accordance with relevant professional obligations and standards" and point 33 of the explanatory report states that "a particular course of action must be judged in the light of the specific health problem raised by a given patient. In particular, an intervention must meet criteria of relevance and proportionality between the aim pursued and the means employed".

Since circumcision is not the only health measure which can be practised on new-born babies, it may be disproportionate with the aim pursued.

If the new-born baby is a member of the Jewish community, circumcision is a legitimate health practice under the terms of Article 18 (4) of the Covenant on Civil and Political Rights and Recommendation 1134 (1990) cited in the reply to case 24, as well as the Council of Europe's Framework Convention for the Protection of National Minorities signed in Strasbourg on 1 February 1995.

2. From the ethical standpoint

This question has not been dealt with in the international declarations on medical ethics, but the general principles of health care may justify the doctor's action.

3. From the standpoint of religious moralities

a. *Catholic*

Circumcision as a health measure is morally acceptable to the Catholic Church provided that it is demonstrated by research that it does indeed constitute a measure for the prevention of tumours to which there is no alternative, in accordance with the therapeutic principle.[1]

b. *Protestant*

How can one oppose a health measure? But are we sure that it is indeed a health measure?

---

1. Pius XII, *Broadcast speeches and messages*, Vol. XIV, 1952, pp. 328-329.

c. *Jewish*

Circumcision is a religious act. It is – one might say – the most characteristic act of Judaism because it marks the individual in his flesh and ceaselessly reminds him that he belongs to the Jewish people.

The Torah orders every Jew to circumcise his son (Genesis, 17, v. 10). This circumcision or Brith Milah must be done on the eighth day (Lev., 12, v. 13). However, when the child is not wholly fit, it is forbidden to cause him to run any risk and one must wait as long as is necessary.

d. *Muslim*

The practice of circumcision is approved and encouraged in Islam. It is practised in the United States with the consent of parents as a hygienic measure.

e. *Buddhist*
No reply.

4. From the standpoint of agnostic morality

It appears that apart from the religious sacrificial aspect, circumcision is often a salutary surgical act because it promotes sexual hygiene. Given these circumstances there is no criminal harm done to the body.

Parental consent suffices for the practitioner of this rite, though it must be performed with the greatest attention to safety. If the parents should refuse, however, only an imperative medical reason would authorise overriding this refusal.

Experimentation on humans

A man aged 72 is suffering from cancer of the prostate with osteal and hepatic metastases.
Trial of anti-neoplastic drugs, phase II (first human trial).
The patient's consent is not requested as the measure is considered as therapeutic.
The patient is unaware of his terminal condition.

1. From the standpoint of international law

Therapeutic experimentation without the patient's freely given and informed consent is forbidden in any circumstances by international law. Article 7 of the Covenant on Civil and Political Rights states that "in particular, no one shall be subjected without his free consent to medical or scientific experimentation". This implies of course that the doctor must fully explain the risks involved and any side-effects the drug could have, failing which the consent will be neither freely given nor informed.

In the same sense, reference should be made to Recommendation R (90) 3 concerning medical research on human beings adopted on 6 February 1990 by the Committee of Ministers of the Council of Europe. In the terms of Principle 3: "No medical research may be carried out without the informed, free, express and specific consent of the person undergoing it. Such consent may be freely withdrawn at any phase of the research and the person undergoing the research should be informed, before being included in it, of his right to withdraw his consent. The person who is to undergo medical research should be given information on the purpose of the research and the methodology of the experimentation. He should also be informed of the foreseeable risks and inconveniences to him of the proposed research. This information should be sufficiently clear and suitably adapted to enable consent to be given or refused in full knowledge of the relevant facts."

See also Article 5 of BC and points 34 to 40 of the explanatory report and Articles 15 and 16.v of the BC, in the terms of which "scientific research in the field of biology and medicine shall be carried out freely, subject to the provisions of this convention and other legal provisions ensuring the protection of the human being" and "the necessary consent as provided for under Article 5 has been given expressly, specifically and is documented. Such consent may be freely withdrawn at any time". See also Article 26 of the BC, and in particular Article 26 (2).

The patient may be unaware of his terminal state because the communication of the fatal prognosis may seriously affect his condition or because he himself has asked not to be given information about his health. In fact, Article 10 (3) of the BC permits restrictions on the patient's right to know any information collected about his health, though this is exceptional and must be in the interest of the patient.

National legislation may thus authorise the doctor to sometimes withhold information or in any case to break the news as gently as possible. This is what is commonly known as a "therapeutic necessity (see points 68 and 69 of the explanatory report attached to the BC)". As regards the second case, the second sentence of Article 10 (2) of the BC stipulates a right not to know as well as a right to know. For reasons which concern only him, a patient may wish not to know certain facts about his health. Such a wish must be respected, particularly in the case where knowledge of these facts is not of vital importance for the patient (see point 67 of the explanatory report).

For the contrary case of the patient who is not capable of giving consent, Article 17 (1) of the BC stipulates that "research on a person without the capacity to consent as stipulated in Article 5 may be undertaken only if all the following conditions are met: i. the conditions laid down in Article 16, sub-paragraphs (i) to (iv), are fulfilled; ii. the results of the research have the potential to produce real and direct benefit to his or her health; iii. research of comparable effectiveness cannot be carried out on individuals capable of giving consent; iv. the necessary authorisation provided for under Article 6 has been given specifically and in writing; and v. the person concerned does not object".

It is only exceptionally and under the protective conditions prescribed by law that research may be undertaken where the research has not the potential to produce results of direct benefit to the health of the person. In the terms of Article 17 (2) of the BC), and taking account of the wording of Article 26 (1) and (2) of the BC, it is subject to "the conditions laid down in paragraph 1, sub-paragraphs i, iii, iv and v above, and to the following additional conditions: i. the research has the aim of contributing, through significant improvement in the scientific understanding of the individual's condition, disease or disorder, to the ultimate attainment of results capable of conferring benefit to the person concerned or to other persons in the same age category or afflicted with the same disease or disorder or having the same condition; ii. the research entails only minimal risk and minimal burden for the individual concerned".

2. From the ethical standpoint

Under the terms of the Declaration of Helsinki (WMA, 1964, 1975, 1983), the doctor is always required to obtain the patient's consent; if there are any specific reasons for not doing so, the proposal should be stated in the experimental protocol, even in the case of a therapeutic trial and where the patient is in a terminal state.

The doctor may not combine biomedical research with clinical care with a view to acquiring new medical knowledge unless it can be shown that this research is justified by its potential diagnostic or therapeutic value to the patient.

Moreover, by virtue of the terms of the Declaration of Venice (WMA, 1983), the doctor must refrain from relentless prolongation of life and may only administer drugs necessary for alleviating pain in the terminal phase. The Declaration of Lisbon (WMA, 1981) refers to the right to die in dignity. This makes the obligation to seek consent to the experiment imperative.

3. From the standpoint of religious moralities

a. *Catholic*

According to Catholic morality, administration for therapeutic and experimental purposes of drugs not yet authorised is licit "in desperate cases, where the patient is doomed if nothing is done (...) with the patient's explicit or tacit consent".[1] In this particular case, as there are no other effective remedies "recourse may be had (...) to the resources of the most advanced medical technology, even where they are still at the experimental stage and not entirely free of risk", but the explicit consent of the patient himself is necessary.[2]

b. *Protestant*

Are we sure that the problem cannot be discussed with the patient or those close to him? If this exchange is truly impossible, why prohibit a last attempt to improve the patient's condition, given that the experimental aspect may not become an end in itself, but must be subordinated to the therapeutic action and hence to care and respect for the patient.

c. *Jewish*

In the case of a desperately ill patient, a surgical intervention or to try out a drug is allowed where this attempt is the only remaining chance, because no possibility should be left untried. The same law governs the case of a child in danger of death: the use of a drug as a test is permissible as a last resort if no other treatment exists. In this case it is necessary to explain the implications of the intervention to the patient and obtain his informed consent.

d. *Muslim*

This is a therapeutic trial on a phase II cancer patient. The doctor alone is qualified to assess the advisability of the treatment. Provided there is no toxic effect, such trials may allow the therapeutic value of a drug to be assessed. However, as

---

1. Pius XII, AAS 46 (1954), p. 591.
2. Declaration of the Congregation for the doctrine of the faith on euthanasia, No. 4.

the patient is in a terminal phase, he is not in a position to give his free and informed consent.

e. *Buddhist*

It is essential to ask the patient's opinion. The principle of personal responsibility is essential in Buddhist thought, and it is therefore necessary (imperative) that the patient should be fully informed of his condition.

4. From the standpoint of agnostic morality

Tests of new treatments must be agreed to by the lucid patient. Without informed consent, nothing can be done. If while lucid the patient refuses the experimentation, the doctor must accept this because he has only the rights conferred upon him by the patient.

Experimentation on humans

*A women aged 43 is suffering from cancer of the ovaries with peritoneal
and pleural metastases.*
*The patient consents to injection of substances unrelated to her condition for the
purpose of post-mortem studies.*

1. From the standpoint of international law

Affirmative reply under the terms of Article 7 of the Covenant on Civil and
Political Rights quoted *in extenso* in relation to case 26, provided that the
consent is truly freely given and informed, that is, if the women is aware of her
condition and if her consent has not been obtained under coercion or psychological pressure.

As regards consent to any medical intervention, this expression also covering
research, see in general Article 5 of the BC and points 34 to 40 of the explanatory
report.

More specifically concerning research, see Principles 3 and 13 of Recommendation R (90) 3 cited in case 26: "Potential subjects of medical research should not
be offered any inducement which compromises free consent". As regards the
BC, see Article 16, cited above.

Regarding the conditions for research, Article 15 of the BC sets out the principle
according to which "scientific research in the field of biology and medicine shall be
carried out freely, subject to the provisions of this convention and the other legal
provisions ensuring the protection of the human being", and points 95 and 96 of the
explanatory report add that "freedom of scientific research in the field of biology
and medicine is justified not only by humanity's right to knowledge, but also by the
considerable progress its results may bring in terms of the health and well-being of
patients. Nevertheless, such freedom is not absolute. In medical research it is limited by the fundamental rights of individuals expressed, in particular, by the provisions of the Convention and by other legal provisions which protect the human
being. In this connection, it should be pointed out that the first article of the Convention specifies that its aim is to protect the dignity and identity of human beings
and guarantee to everyone, without discrimination, respect for their integrity as
well as for other rights and fundamental freedoms. Any research will therefore have
to observe these principles".

In the same sense, see Article 1 of the BC, in the terms of which "Parties to this
Convention shall protect the dignity and identity of all human beings and guarantee everyone, without discrimination, respect for their integrity and other rights and
fundamental freedoms with regard to the application of biology and medicine";

and Article 2 of the BC: "The interests and welfare of the human being shall prevail over the sole interest of society or science."

2. From the ethical standpoint

The Declaration of Helsinki (WMA, 1964) permits experiments to be conducted on patients whose condition is unrelated to the study, provided that the general rules concerning the primacy of the patient's interest and the necessity of informed consent are respected.

3. From the standpoint of religious moralities

a. *Catholic*
Use of drugs for a purely experimental purpose with the patient's consent is morally acceptable where there may be some hope for the common good;[1] it must be understood that the drug in question must have been certified inoffensive and have received authorisation for human use.

b. *Protestant*
The greatest care must be taken to ensure that the consent in question has been freely given – on the basis of full information – and not extorted or conceded.

c. *Jewish*
The injection of substances which bear no relation to the illness may be authorised on the following conditions:
– free and informed consent of the patient;
– the injection must have no negative effect upon the patient.

d. *Muslim*
To test on a terminally ill patient a drug which has no therapeutic indication for the illness in question is strictly forbidden in Islam. The patient's freely given and informed consent cannot be taken into consideration, given the patient's mental state at this terminal stage of illness.

e. *Buddhist*
If the patient is in a psychological condition considered such that she can rationally take such a decision, then her decision should be respected and her altruistic motivation will add value to it.

---

1. Pius XII, AAS 44 (1952), p. 784ff.

4. From the standpoint of agnostic morality

If the patient has been informed about the aims of the injection envisaged and if she is conscious and can thus give her informed consent, then the injection is permissible provided that, for example, it is not to cause pain that cannot be controlled and does not unduly hasten the disappearance of life.

Experimentation on humans

A women aged 25 is in hospital for voluntary termination of pregnancy.
Her consent is requested for the injection of products forty-eight hours before the termination in order to study their effect on the organs of the three-and-a-half month foetus post abortum (teratogenic effect of the drugs).

1. From the standpoint of international law

The purpose of the case is obviously to establish whether it is permissible to study the teratogenic effect of a drug on a foetus which the mother intends to abort, in the case where the mother has given her consent and it is assumed that termination of pregnancy with a three-and-a-half month foetus is legitimate under the national legislation.

In the terms of point D.9 of the Appendix to Resolution 1100 (1989) of the Parliamentary Assembly of the Council of Europe "the removal of cells, tissues or embryonic or foetal organs, or of the placenta or membranes, if live, for investigations other than of a diagnostic character and for preventive or therapeutic purposes shall be prohibited". Point 10 goes on to stipulate that "the pregnant woman and her husband or partner must be provided beforehand with as full information as necessary: i. on the technical operations to be performed for the removal of cells, and/or embryonic or foetal tissues, or for the removal of the membranes, the placenta and/or the amniotic fluid; ii. on the intended purposes; and iii. on the risks involved", and point 11 adds that "persons removing embryos or foetuses or parts thereof from the uterus without clinical or legal justification or without the prior consent of the pregnant woman and, where appropriate, of her husband or partner in a stable relationship, and persons using such embryological materials in breach of the relevant legislation or regulations shall be duly penalised".

If the embryo is dead, see points F. 15 and 16.

Paragraph 32 of Resolution 327/88 EEC reads as follows: "As regards research on embryos, the European Parliament calls for the possible applications of research, diagnosis and therapy, particularly at the prenatal stage, to be the subject of legally binding definitions so that procedures involving live human embryos or foetuses or experiments on them are justified only if they are of direct and otherwise unattainable benefit in terms of the welfare of the child concerned and its mother and respect the physical and mental integrity of the woman in question". Paragraph 38 of the same resolution adds that the European Parliament "insists that any commercial or industrial use of embryos or foetuses (...) must be a criminal offence".

The same principle is to be found in a more qualified form in paragraph 14.A.ii of Recommendation 1046 (1986) of the Parliamentary Assembly of the Council of

Europe, which recommends that the Committee of Ministers call on the governments of the member states "to limit the use of human embryos and foetuses and materials and tissues therefrom in an industrial context to purposes which are strictly therapeutic and for which no other means exist, according to the principles set out in the appendix, and to bring their legislation into line with these principles or to enact rules in accordance therewith which should, *inter alia*, specify the conditions in which removal and use may be undertaken for a diagnostic or therapeutic purpose".

The appendix referred to contains the rules to be observed when using and removing tissues from human embryos or foetuses for diagnostic or therapeutic purposes.

Point A.i (intervention for diagnostic purposes) provides that "No intervention for diagnostic purposes, other than those already authorised under national legislation, on the living embryo *in vitro* or *in utero* or on the foetus whether inside or outside the uterus shall be permitted, unless its object is the well-being of the child to be born and the promotion of its development".

Point B, which concerns the rules applicable in cases of intervention for therapeutic purposes, specifies as follows: "i. No intervention on the living embryo (...) *in utero* (...) shall be permitted unless its object is the well-being of the child to be born, that is, to facilitate its development and birth; ii. Therapy on (...) the foetus *in utero* shall not be permitted unless it is for very clear and precisely diagnosed embryonic maladies, with grave or extremely bad prognosis, where no other solution is possible and therapy would offer reasonable guarantees of successful treatment of those illnesses; iii. It shall be forbidden to keep embryos or foetuses alive artificially for the purpose of removing usable material. iv. The use of dead embryos or foetuses must be an exceptional measure, justified in the present state of knowledge by the rare nature of the illness treated, the absence of any equally effective therapy and a manifest advantage (such as survival) for the person receiving treatment; it must comply with the following rules: a. the decision to terminate pregnancy and the conditions of termination (date, technique, etc.) must under no circumstances be influenced by the possible or desired subsequent use of the embryo or foetus; (...) c. total independence between the medical team terminating the pregnancy and the team which might use the embryos or foetuses for therapeutic purposes must be guaranteed; d. embryos and foetuses may not be used without the consent of the parents or gamete donors where the latters' identity is known; e. the use of (...) foetuses or their tissues for profit or remuneration shall not be allowed."

Now see also Articles 15 and 16 of the BC, the problem of the definition of the concepts of "person" and "human being" with respect to the foetus, and in particular a foetus of three-and-a-half months, being unresolved, and not even being considered by the Convention.

2. From the ethical standpoint

In its international directives for biomedical research involving human subjects (Manila 1981), the CIOMS stipulates that no non-therapeutic research may be conducted on a pregnant woman if this represents a potential risk for the foetus, unless the research relates to a problem concerning the pregnancy.

Therapeutic research is permitted only in the interest of the mother's health or for the purposes of improving the foetus' viability.

3. From the standpoint of religious moralities

a. *Catholic*

Catholic morality regards any experimentation on the foetus without therapeutic significance for the foetus itself as absolutely illicit, as the direct personal consent of the subject of the experimentation is absent; this consent cannot even be given by the mother.[1]

b. *Protestant*

To ask a women for permission to test a product – teratogenic into the bargain – on an embryo she is going to part from is irresponsible from every point of view.

c. *Jewish*

Voluntary termination of pregnancy is in itself a prohibited act, especially if this act is undertaken for personal convenience.

In the case concerned, we assume that the foetus is living. In this case, the injection of products in order to study the teratogenic effect of a drug on a foetus which the mother wishes to get rid of seems to me to be morally unacceptable.

If the foetus is dead the door may be left open provided that there is a clearly demonstrated medical value.

d. *Muslim*

To test the effects of a drug which may be teratogenic on a woman hospitalised for a voluntary termination of pregnancy is totally forbidden in Islam even with her consent, as it is impossible to foresee a priori whether the drug will be harmful to her.

e. *Buddhist*

Volunteers must be in a position to give informed consent, according to the Buddhist principle of individual responsibility. Even under the guise of scientific research, it is not acceptable to maltreat the foetus.

---

1. Pius XII, AAS 44 (1952), p. 784ff.

4. From the standpoint of agnostic morality

The free and informed consent of the patient authorises the injection, provided that it does not entail any dangerous effects for her.

Experimentation: ethics committees

During a meeting of an ethics committee,
disagreement arises between doctors and other members
over the informed consent of volunteers.

1. From the standpoint of international law

The need for the individual's prior free and informed consent to any medical or scientific experimentation is asserted in Article 7 of the Covenant on Civil and Political Rights.

In the same sense, see Article 5 of the BC and point 34 of the explanatory report: "This article deals with consent and affirms at the international level an already well-established rule, that is that no one may in principle be forced to undergo an intervention without their consent (...). This rule makes clear patients' autonomy in his or her relationship with health care professionals (...). The word 'intervention' is understood in its widest sense, as in Article 4 – that is to say, it covers all medical acts, in particular interventions performed for the purpose of preventive care, diagnosis treatment, rehabilitation or research."

Reference may also be made to Article 4 of the BC and to points 30 and 31 of the explanatory report, which refer to statutory and professional codes of ethics, medical conduct or any other means of ensuring respect for the rights and interests of patients.

See in addition Articles 15, 16 and 17 of the BC – all of which have already been cited above.

Reference should also be made to Article 12 of the BC: "Tests which are predictive of genetic diseases or which serve either to identify the subject as a carrier of a gene responsible for a disease or to detect a genetic predisposition or susceptibility to a disease may be performed only for health purposes or for scientific research linked to health purposes, and subject to appropriate genetic counselling".

For the rest there is no reply.

2. From the ethical standpoint

The Declaration of Helsinki, I, 9, stipulates the information that must be given (aims, methods, anticipated benefits and potential hazards). Where a trial is conducted on healthy volunteers, this requirement may under no circumstances be waived, as might be justified *vis-à-vis* patients, and the point of view of those who defend this principle must therefore be upheld.

3. From the standpoint of religious moralities

a. *Catholic*

In the case of non-therapeutic experimentation, consent is required by Catholic morality for the sake of the person's dignity and in accordance with the principle of non-disposability of the body;[1] the right to informed consent must be guaranteed either by the medical profession or by non-doctors in the context of ethics committees.

b. *Protestant*

If the members of the commission object, they must have a reason for doing so. These reasons should therefore be looked into and an attempt made to overcome the disagreements. The argument of authority would be hardly likely to help matters, on the contrary.

c. *Jewish*

In general, experimentation is permitted if the volunteer gives his free and informed consent and provided that his life is not endangered. The refusal of the non-medical member of the ethics committee has to be taken into consideration if the reasons are put forward.

d. *Muslim*

If there is disagreement within a committee between a member who is a doctor and one who is not concerning the informed consent of volunteers, Islam would generally authorise the experiments subject to the following conditions:

1. need for the subject's consent;
2. no remuneration for the experiment;
3. a strong probability that the drug will be innocuous not only physically but also psychologically. Scientific progress depends on such trials.
4. It is necessary for such treatment to be related to the subject's pathological condition.

e. *Buddhist*

The question is not clearly formulated and it is therefore impossible to give an opinion.

4. From the standpoint of agnostic morality

It matters little whether one is a doctor or not, or a member of an ethics committee, to express an opinion. Nothing is possible, either legally or morally, without

---

1. Pius XII, AAS 44 (1952), p. 784ff.

the informed consent of volunteers. Experimentation on humans is subject to strict protocols which cannot be transgressed for any reason whatsoever.

Experimentation: ethics committees

A proposal has been put forward for experimentation on prisoners serving long sentences. The volunteers will be remunerated by benefits in kind and improvements in their conditions of detention.
The ethics committee gives a negative opinion.
An appeal is made to the national committee.

1. From the standpoint of international law

Article 7 of the Covenant on Civil and Political Rights asserts that "no one shall be subjected without his free consent to medical or scientific experimentation".

The benefits in kind and the improvement in conditions of detention may constitute means of pressure or psychological coercion, as the individuals to whom they are being offered are in a situation of deprivation of personal freedom which calls into question the very possibility of "free consent" in the true sense of the term.

If (as is possible) the experimentation is of a dangerous nature, there might even be a case of breach of Article 3 of the ECHR. As regards grafts and transplants, see point 19 of the explanatory report to Resolution (78) 29 of the Committee of Ministers of the Council of Europe and Article 3 of the Resolution proper.

It should be noted that, where a long custodial sentence is accompanied, as is frequently the case in western penal systems, by statutory incapacity or the loss of civil and political rights, the prisoner should be considered incapable of expressing a legally valid wish (in this case consent), the more so since it would most probably result in a waiver of the right to life or physical integrity/health. However, see paragraphs 24, 25 and 26 of the explanatory report to Council of Europe Resolution (78) 29, Article 22 of Resolution (73) 5 containing the standard minimum rules for treatment of prisoners and Principles 1 and 4.b of Resolution 37/194 of the UN General Assembly.

While Article 22 of Resolution (75) 5 stipulates that "prisoners may not be submitted to medical or scientific experiments which may result in physical or moral injury to their person", Principle 7 of Recommendation R (90) 3 adopted by the Committee of Ministers of the Council of Europe on 6 February 1990 concerning medical research on human beings stipulates that "persons deprived of liberty may not undergo medical research unless it is expected to produce a direct and significant benefit to their health".

As far as the BC is concerned, neither Article 5 nor Article 6 (3), the latter stipulating the rule of previous and informed consent with specific regard to adults incapable of consenting, range prisoners serving long sentences and legally incapable of expressing valid consent amongst "incapable adults" as such. Moreover, point 43 of the explanatory report assents that "if adults have been declared incapable but at a certain time do not suffer from a reduced mental capacity (...), they must, according to Article 5, themselves consent".

With respect to scientific research in particular, see Articles 17 (1) and (2) of the BC, as well as points 103 to 114 of the explanatory report.

2. From the ethical standpoint

The regulations in time of armed conflict (WMA, 1956) strictly forbid experimentation on all persons deprived of their liberty.

The Declaration of Athens (ICPMS, 1979) takes a less catagoric view, prohibiting all human experimentation on prisoners without their formal consent.

Under the terms of the Declaration of Helsinki (WMA, 1964), doctors should be particularly cautious if the subject may consent under duress. The declaration suggests that the informed consent should be obtained by another independent doctor not engaged in the investigation.

3. From the standpoint of religious moralities

a. *Catholic*

There is no official position on this matter. On the basis of the Catholic Church's doctrine on experimentation, it would seem morally acceptable to experiment on prisoners acting as volunteers, even if they are offered a chance of shortening their sentences; however, it is necessary to safeguard with even more scrupulous attention than usual the objective limits constituted by the protection of the life and physical integrity of the subjects, as well as respect for personal and genuinely freely given consent.

A contrary opinion on the part of the ethics committee must be taken into consideration in relation to the grounds adduced in the opinion itself.

b. *Protestant*

The problem here is that we are only talking about prisoners. Are they perhaps not people like everyone else? Or do they have to make amends twice: by being prisoners, on the one hand, and objects of experimentation, on the other? Admittedly, reference is made to the possibility of a reduced sentence. However, the procedure is too close to blackmail to be truly correct. Furthermore, who is to decide on the reduction in question? It would seem that there would be a need to introduce *ad hoc* legislation here and procedures for its possible implementation. In order to do so, a major public debate would be necessary so as at least to enable the real value of the experiments in question to be assessed.

c. *Jewish*

A prisoner is not in the situation of a free individual who can decide in an informed fashion to participate in an experiment. In this case there is a morally and religiously unacceptable kind of horse-trading.

However, if we are certain that the experimentation presents no danger to the prisoner and that he considers that the benefits in kind and the improvement in his conditions of imprisonment will be of real advantage to him, it may be envisaged.

d. *Muslim*

Islam is wholly opposed to any experimentation on prisoners serving long or short sentences, as these prisoners are in a state of psychological weakness and hence cannot give their consent in a free and informed manner.

e. *Buddhist*

Negative view out of respect for the human being. Moral pressure, whatever form it may take, is unacceptable.

4. From the standpoint of agnostic morality

In France, the National Consultative Ethics Committee had occasion to consider a similar project. It would if necessary confirm the negative opinion of the ethics committee, simply because a prisoner is never a free man.

Agnostic morality is opposed to any such research proposal.

Experimentation : ethics committees

Trial of a new substance on a group of volunteers is proposed.
The ethics committee approves.
The attending physician refuses.

1. From the standpoint of international law

Over and above the disagreement between the ethics committee and the attending physician, the case seems to raise a number of questions which have not yet been dealt with in international law :

a. the question of the consent of the doctor, who is asked to implement the medical trial decided on by others (pharmaceutical products manufacturers) in two cases : where the trials are dangerous for the volunteers and where they are not ;

b. the problem of the consent of healthy individuals who are ignorant of the possible consequences of the experimentation to be performed on them.

As regards the first question, Articles 9 (1) and 10 (1) of the ECHR and Articles 18 (1) and 19 (1) and (2) of the Covenant on Civil and Political Rights confirm the right of the attending physician to object to the treatment, not only if he considers it dangerous for the patients, but also if it is against his convictions.

As regards the second problem, it is obvious that "a medical act" can only be performed with the patient's free and informed consent.

In the same sense, see first of all Council of Europe Recommendation R (90) 3 concerning medical research on human beings adopted by the Committee of Ministers on 6 February 1990, Principle 3 of which stipulates that "1. No medical research may be carried out without the informed, free, express and specific consent of the person undergoing it. Such consent may be freely withdrawn at any phase of the research and the person undergoing the research should be informed, before being included in it, of his right to withdraw his consent; 2. The person who is to undergo medical research should be given information on the purpose of the research and the methodology of the experimentation. He should also be informed of the foreseeable risks and inconveniences to him of the proposed research. This information should be sufficiently clear and suitably adapted to enable consent to be given or refused in full knowledge of the relevant facts".

See also Articles 5 ; 15 ; 16 ; 17 and 26 (1) and (2) of the BC.

2. From the ethical standpoint

The doctor must remain the protector of the volunteer's health and must discontinue or abandon the research if in his/her judgment it may, if continued, be harmful to the individual (Helsinki, 1964, III, 1 and 3), whatever may be the opinion of the ethics committee, which has a purely consultative responsibility.

3. From the standpoint of religious moralities

a. *Catholic*

Catholic morality considers experimentation on volunteers to be licit where the risk does not endanger life or physical and mental integrity.[1] In addition to the subject's explicit consent freely given in person, the opinion of the attending physician must be taken into account, where the latter's opinion is based on the particular conditions of his patient and where the experimentation involves the liability of the attending physician himself.

b. *Protestant*

Let the doctor in question be heard! If he does not convince his discussion partners, let them find a doctor who, without breaking the law, is willing to share their project.

c. *Jewish*

If the ethics committee has given its approval, this means that the substance in question presents no danger.

It is necessary to take account of the individual's doctor, who knows his patient and must certainly have valid reasons for refusing this experimentation.

In any event, the informed consent of the volunteer is essential.

d. *Muslim*

For therapeutic purposes, experimentation with a new substance may be carried out on a group of volunteers provided that the following conditions are fulfilled:
1. free and informed consent of the subject;
2. no remuneration;
3. probability that the drug being tested will be innocuous;
4. experimentation carried out in approved centres;
5. agreement of the ethics committee.

e. *Buddhist*

The informed consent of the person concerned is essential and the final decision will be taken by this person, who may seek several medical opinions.

---

1. Pius XII, AAS 44 (1952), p. 784ff.

4. From the standpoint of agnostic morality

The experimentation must not be dangerous. In any event, the doctor has the right to oppose his conscience clause.

217

Genetic manipulation

An ethics committee is asked to authorise modification of a genome, that is manipulation of a chromosome fragment and creation of a new transmissible characteristic:
   a. *on an animal*
   b. *on man.*

1. From the standpoint of international law

Recommendation 1100 (1989) of the Parliamentary Assembly of the Council of Europe on the use of human embryos and foetuses in scientific research also covers (paragraph 18 of the appendix) scientific research projects on genetic engineering using genetic or recombinatory genetic material.

Such projects "shall be permitted, subject to approval" by "national or regional multidisciplinary bodies" to be set up as a matter of urgency by member states. These bodies are to have the task of "authorising, provided there are appropriate regulations or delegations of authority" (and including the dimension of human rights) "specific projects of scientific investigation or experimentation in these fields" (paragraph 9.B.i) where they are "for purposes of scientific investigation, for studying DNA sequences in the human genome – their location, functions, dynamics, interrelationships and pathology; for studying recombinant DNA within human cells (...); with a view to obtaining a better understanding of the mechanisms of molecular recombination, of expression of the genetic message, of the development of cells and their components and their functional organisation; for studying the ageing process of cells, tissues and organs; and, more particularly, for studying the general or specific mechanisms governing the development of diseases; for any other purpose considered useful and beneficial to the individual and to humanity, and incorporated in projects already approved".

Point G.19 adds that "investigations or acts involving genetic technology shall only be authorised at centres and establishments which have been registered, approved and authorised for such purposes, and which have the requisite specialised personnel and technical resources". Point 9.B.v recommends in this connection that the Committee of Ministers of the Council of Europe invite the governments of member states "to regulate the operations and to draw up national or regional registers of accredited and authorised centres where research or experiments are undertaken on reproductive material (...) and to monitor and evaluate such activities, and to require that the biomedical and scientific teams at such centres are properly qualified and authorised to perform such activities and have the necessary resources". It is further recommended that the Committee of Ministers (see Section D) "establish as a matter of urgency, as a safeguard, an international multidisciplinary body to ensure convergent approaches by the national bodies already operating or to be set up in accordance with paragraph 9.B.i above, and to avoid thereby the creation of 'genetic havens'."

It may be added that under point B.4 of the appendix, investigations of viable embryos ("embryos which are free of biological characteristics likely to prevent their development" – point 25) *in vitro* "shall only be permitted: for applied purposes of a diagnostic nature or for preventive or therapeutic purposes; if their non-pathological genetic heritage is not interfered with".

This recommendation, approved on 2 February 1989 by the Parliamentary Assembly of the Council of Europe, was followed closely by Resolution 327/88 adopted on 16 March 1989 by the European Parliament which concerns the ethical and legal problems of genetic engineering.

In points 7 to 11, the European Parliament "reaffirms the principle of freedom of science and research; regards the restraints imposed on freedom of science and research, arising in particular from the rights of third parties and the society they constitute, as the expression in legal terms of the responsibility assumed by society as a whole for the action of the scientist and for research; recognises that the rights from which these restraints derive are primarily the dignity of the individual and of the sum of all individuals; believes that the legislator has an absolute duty to define these limits; sees the role of ethical committees and professional regulatory bodies solely as translating into practice the rules laid down by legislation". More particularly (paragraph 12), the European Parliament "considers that the absolute preconditions for the use of genetic analysis are that: *a.* genetic analysis and genetic counselling must be designed exclusively for the well-being of those concerned, and be based exclusively on voluntary agreement and the results of an examination must be communicated to those concerned at their request. This also means that a doctor shall not have the right to inform members of the family of those concerned without their consent; *b.* they must on no account be used for the scientifically dubious and politically unacceptable purpose of 'positively improving' the population's gene pool, negatively selecting genetically undesirable characteristics or laying down 'genetic standards'; *c.* the principle of a patient's right of self-determination must have absolute precedence over the economic pressures imposed by health care systems since every individual has an inalienable right to know his genetic make-up or to remain in ignorance; *d.* the establishment of individual gene maps may only be carried out by a doctor; the forwarding, collection, storage and evaluation of genetic data by government or private organisations shall be prohibited; *e.* the development of genetic strategies for the solution of social problems must not be allowed since it would undermine our ability to understand human life as a complex entity which can never be compassed entirely by any scientific approach; *f.* the knowledge acquired by means of genetic analysis must be absolutely reliable and enable unequivocal statements to be made about precisely defined medical facts, knowledge of which may directly benefit the health of the persons affected."

See also the text of Article 13 of the BC, in the terms of which "an intervention seeking to modify the human genome may only be undertaken for preventive, diagnostic or therapeutic purposes and only if its aim is not to introduce any modification in the genome of any descendants", as well as points 89 to 92 of the explanatory report.

Reference should also be made to Article 18 (2) of the BC, which prohibits the creation of human embryos for research purposes, as well as point 116 of the explanatory report.

Lastly, it should be pointed out that research on embryos *in vitro*, where it is allowed by (national) law, "shall ensure adequate protection of the embryo" (Article 18 (1) of the BC and point 115 of the explanatory report).

2. From the ethical standpoint

The WMA adopted in Madrid in 1987 a declaration pointing out that genetic manipulation must take place in the conditions laid down in the Declaration of Helsinki, and envisages such manipulations for the purposes of genetic therapy.

As research in the field of genetic manipulation develops, appropriate standards have to be established by the scientific community, doctors, the professional circles concerned, the government and the public in order to regulate this research.

When the replacement of a gene by a normal DNA becomes a practical reality for the treatment of human troubles, the WMA insists that the following factors should be taken into account:

1. if the manipulation takes place in a research establishment, it will be necessary to take account of the WMA Declaration of Helsinki on biomedical research involving human subjects;

2. if the manipulation does not take place in a research establishment, all the habitual standards relating to medical practice and professional liability, including those of the Declaration of Helsinki, must be respected;

3. the procedure envisaged must be discussed in detail with the patient. The consent of the patient or his legal representative must be informed, free and in writing;

4. there must be no dangerous or undesirable virus in the viral DNA containing the replacement or corrective gene;

5. the DNA inserted must function normally in the receptor cell in order to avoid any metabolic damage which could impair sound tissue and the patient's health;

6. the efficacy of the genetic therapy should be evaluated with the greatest possible precision. This procedure will include the determination of the natural history of the disease and the monitoring of succeeding generations;

7. these procedures should not begin until after a thorough examination of the availability and efficacy of other possible therapies. If there is a simpler and safer remedy, this must be used;

8. these provisions must be reconsidered as necessary in the light of technical progress and scientific information.

In its Declaration of Marbella (1992) on the human genome project, the WMA draws attention in particular to the danger of eugenism in genetic therapy and the use of genes for non-medical purposes.

3. From the standpoint of religious moralities

a. *Catholic*
All attempts to interfere with man's chromosomal or genetic heritage which are not therapeutic "but tend towards the production of human beings selected according to sex or other pre-established qualities" are contrary to the personal dignity of the human being, his integrity and his identity.[1]

Creation of new transmissible characteristics in animals can be ethically acceptable if its purpose is the real good of mankind and on condition that it should not disturb the biological balance of nature.[2]

b. *Protestant*
All the texts referred to in the introduction are categorically opposed to this possibility. By conceiving itself as the object of possible manipulations and experimentations, mankind makes itself an object and loses the very meaning of what gives it human reality. While believing that it can reach some kind of paradise, mankind is in reality only constructing an artificial paradise which, as everyone knows, is but hell.

c. *Jewish*
Genetic research, like all medical research, can be undertaken and pursued if it has a therapeutic purpose and above all if it is aimed at curing transmissible hereditary diseases like haemophilia or Tay-Sachs disease.

---

1. John Paul II, AAS 76 (1984), p. 391.
2. John Paul II, "Message for the world day of peace 1990", 7, *L'Osservatore Romano*, 6 December 1989.

In this case it may be undertaken only after the tacit and informed agreement of the patient or his legal representative and only in the case where no other therapy exists as yet.

The question will arise in other terms when genetic science succeeds in creating and programming monstrous creatures as in present research on drosophilae. In this case are we in the context of research with a view to healing?

In any event, it is essential to set up strict controls as a matter of urgency. Today, we can create races of rats with a particular characteristic. Who will prevent the practitioner from submitting tomorrow to a dictator who might decide to create a race of blond-haired, blue-eyed men? We are not far beyond the age when the world was carried away by the folly of a man who one day decided to impose the Aryan race on humanity.

To perform genetic manipulations to satisfy one's own ego is to fall into the error committed by the men who tried to build the Tower of Babel and reach God. This human pride is in danger of bringing about a new Babel, that is a world in which confusion of values reigns supreme, a world in which man is in danger of being out-stripped by his own inventions.

d. *Muslim*

Genetic manipulation, or rather genetic engineering or genetic recombination, constitutes one of the most prodigious techniques of molecular biology. This technique can be used to modify the sequence of genes contained in the hereditary medium, deoxyribonucleic acid or DNA. To date, a few thousand genes have been identified. For some of them, a correlation can be seen between their structure and the nature of the corresponding hereditary characteristics. By means of genetic engineering, it is possible to add or remove a genetic datum or even to modify an item of genetic information in the case of mutagenesis performed *in vitro*. If we take the case of introduction of a gene into stem cells which reproduce themselves, there are two possibilities:

1. Introduction of the gene into fertilised egg produces germinal cells, this gene will be found in all the cells, since all the cells of the organism come from the egg. This method produces an artificial modification of the human genome which is transmissible to the person's descendants. This modification of the genetic heritage by manipulation of germinal cells is utterly forbidden in Islam, as it leads to the creation of an organism which differs from a divine creation.

2. Introduction of the gene into somatic cells, that is stem cells of an organ deficient in a given substance corresponding to the gene introduced. Examples are the stem cells of the epidermis or those of the haematopoietic series situated in the bone marrow. These somatic cells have the property of rapid self-division. They are first removed and treated *in vitro*, then reinjected or grafted into the organism. This

technique of genetic therapy is still at the experimental stage. Given that the purpose of this technique is essentially therapeutic, it may be tolerated in Islam subject to all the precautions necessary to avoid any aberration.

It should be noted that the first experiments in integration of exogenous genes into the chromosome were performed on animals. These so-called "transgenic" animals serve as an experimental model for fundamental research into disease. This type of trial for purely scientific purposes can be tolerated at a pinch, but research involving transplantation of embryos between humans and animals must be prohibited from the point of view of Muslim morality, as the result is the production of organisms different from divine creations.

e. *Buddhist*

Genetic engineering opens up new therapeutic possibilities and prospects for improving human life, but may also bring uncontrolled abuse which could endanger the future of the human race. The greatest caution is thus called for.

4. From the standpoint of agnostic morality

As things stand, this genetic manipulation would not be prohibited. Authorisation to proceed to the modification of the human genome can be requested under certain conditions, namely:

– modification of the somatic cells;

– modification of the germ cells up to the fifteenth day only;

It can only be carried out for preventive and curative therapeutic purposes, to eradicate certain diseases, with the free and informed consent of the patient or his legal representative.

The transmission of a new characteristic which has become hereditary must not represent any danger or entail any substantial modification.

Genetic manipulation

A marker gene for Huntington's chorea is discovered in an embryo.
Destruction of the embryo is suggested.
The pregnant woman refuses while her partner consents.

1. From the standpoint of international law

As stated in paragraph 4 of the preamble and points D.6, 8 and 10 of Recommendation 1046 (1986) of the Parliamentary Assembly of the Council of Europe, progress in medical science and technology "has made the legal position of the embryo and foetus particularly precarious, and (...) their legal status is at present not defined by law"; hence, "it is urgent to define the extent of (their) legal protection" as "human embryos and foetuses must be treated in all circumstances with the respect due to human dignity".

Accordingly, point B.i of the appendix to this recommendation affirms that "no intervention on the living embryo *in vitro* or *in utero* (...) shall be permitted unless its object is the well-being of the child to be born, that is, to facilitate its development and birth".

In its turn, point 3 of the preamble to Recommendation 1100 (1989) of the Parliamentary Assembly of the Council of Europe on the use of human embryos in research states that "the human embryo and foetus are [to be] treated in conditions appropriate to human dignity", considering that, among other things, "the human embryo, though displaying successive phases in its development which are designated by different terms (zygote, morula, blastula, pre-implantation embryo or pre-embryo, embryo, foetus), displays also a progressive differentiation as an organism and none the less maintains a continuous biological and genetic identity" (point 7).

It stems from this principle (point A.i of the appendix to Council of Europe Recommendation 1046 (1986) of 24.9.1986) that "no intervention for diagnostic purposes, other than those already authorised under national legislation, on the living embryo *in vitro* or *in utero* or on the foetus whether inside or outside the uterus shall be permitted, unless its object is the well-being of the child to be born and the promotion of its development. Concerning interventions for therapeutic purposes, point B.i of the appendix stipulates the same principle as point A.i, while point B.ii adds that therapy on embryos *in vitro* or *in utero* or on the foetus *in utero* shall not be permitted, unless it is for very clear and precisely diagnosed embryonic maladies, with grave or extremely bad prognoses, where no other solution is possible and therapy would offer reasonable guarantees of successful treatment of those illnesses".

We would add that in the terms of point D.11 of the appendix to Recommendation 1100 (1989), "persons removing embryos or foetuses or parts thereof from the uterus without clinical or legal justification or without the prior consent of the pregnant woman and, where appropriate, of her husband or partner (...) shall be duly penalised" and that in the terms of point B.vi.*a* of the appendix to Recommendation 1046 (1986) "the decision to terminate pregnancy and the conditions of termination (date, technique, etc.) must under no circumstances be influenced by the possible or desired subsequent use of the embryo or foetus".

For the rest, there is no reply: neither Article 2 of the ECHR nor Article 1 of the BC, which stipulate respectively everyone's right to life and respect for the dignity and identity of all human beings and respect for their other rights and fundamental freedoms, in fact defines the concept of "human being". Points 18 and 19 of the explanatory report appended to the BC state as following: "The Convention does not define the term "everyone" (in French "toute personne"). These two terms are equivalent and found in the English and French versions of the European Convention on Human Rights, which however does not define them. In the absence of unanimous agreement on the definition of these terms among member states of the Council of Europe, it was decided to allow domestic law to define them for the purposes of the application of the present Convention. The Convention also uses the expression "human being" to state the necessity to protect the dignity and identity of all human beings. It was acknowledged that it was a generally accepted principle that human dignity and the identity of the human being had to be respected as soon as life began".

We would also point out that in Application No. 8416/78, the Commission considered that it was not called upon to decide whether Article 2 does not cover the foetus at all or whether it recognises a "right to life" with implied limitations (such as the necessity to protect the woman's health).

Regarding tests predictive of genetic diseases, attention should also be drawn to Article 12 of the BC, in the terms of which "tests which are predictive of genetic diseases or which serve either to identify the subject as a carrier of a gene responsible for a disease or to detect a genetic predisposition or susceptibility to a disease may be performed only for health purposes or for scientific research linked to health purpose, and subject to appropriate genetic counselling". Reference should also be made to points 78 to 88 of the explanatory report appended to the BC, namely to point 82, in terms of which "because of the particular problems which are related to predictive testing, it is necessary to strictly limit its applicability to health purposes for the individual. Scientific research likewise should be carried out in the context of developing medical treatment".

The wording of this article and the explanations provided by the explanatory report stress that no intervention for diagnostic purposes should be carried out on a living embryo in the case where there is at present no therapy for the disease detected, and hence no aid can be given for the development and well-being of the embryo (or of the child to be born).

225

Lastly, it should be recalled that in the terms of Article 11 of the BC, "Any form of discrimination against a person on grounds of his or her genetic heritage is prohibited". Once again, the concept of "subject" (Article 12 of the BC and points 74 to 77 of the explanatory report) is not defined with respect to the embryo.

2. From the ethical standpoint

The WMA adopted in Madrid in 1987 a declaration pointing out that such manipulations must take place in the conditions laid down in the Declaration of Helsinki and envisages manipulation for the purposes of genetic therapy (see case 32).

3. From the standpoint of religious moralities

a. *Catholic*

A prenatal diagnosis finding the presence of a hereditary disease must not be tantamount to a death sentence.[1] For this reason, destruction of an embryo, which must always be respected as a human being, is a serious wrong.

Furthermore, in the case of Huntington's chorea, it would be destruction of an embryo which will be perfectly healthy for many years: it is known that the disease develops on average around the age of 45.

The patient's partner cannot therefore prevail upon her to destroy the embryo.

b. *Protestant*

The problem is primarily that of the couple. If the couple disagrees on the matter, it will remain essentially – at least for a time – the problem of the mother. The answer is not first and foremost a technical one; the important thing is to support and guide the parents in order to help them to take the least destructive decision for them.

c. *Jewish*

An embryo with a marker gene for Huntington's chorea may be destroyed if:
– the mother's life is in danger;
– or the mother's health so requires.

Economic or social reasons or reasons of personal convenience may never be allowed to prevail.

In the case under consideration, the patient refuses to destroy the embryo. There is therefore no reason to authorise this destruction.

---

1. Congregation for the doctrine of the faith, *Donum Vitae*, Part I, 2, AAS 80 (1988), p. 70ff.

Medicine has not the right to regulate its attitude according to the concept of curability or incurability, as there are no means of unerring diagnosis. For us, science has not come to an end: there are new discoveries every day. The unhappy destiny is made to be remedied. One thing is certain: what we cannot do today in the face of an anomaly, we shall be able to do tomorrow. If it is not we who achieve it, it will be our descendants.

d. *Muslim*

It should be pointed out first of all with regard to Huntington's chorea that a marker gene allows a predictive diagnosis to be established for a disease which, in the majority of cases, allows people to live normally up to the age of 40 or so. It must also be pointed out that this is a chromosomal anomaly, transmitted by the dominant gene. This means that any individual may pass on the disease to half his children who will pass it on to half of theirs. However, if a child has not received the gene for the disease, neither he nor his future descendants will contract it. Hence the importance of prenatal diagnosis, as, in the case of a positive result, a deliberate termination of pregnancy may be carried out. For Islamic religious morality the consent of both spouses must be obtained before the termination may be carried out. If the attending physician cannot persuade the partner to accept the proposal, the patient's decision to keep the child must be respected, the more so since researchers may have discovered effective treatment by the time the disease develops.

e. *Buddhist*

All life must be respected. What is more, although recognisable at birth, this disease does not appear until after the age of 40, and given the rapid progress of medicine and the hope this may bring, the life of this embryo should be preserved.

4. From the standpoint of agnostic morality

The informed woman is entirely free to make her decision. She has the right to refuse the destruction of the defective embryo she is carrying even if this decision is unrealistic.

It does not matter whether the partner agrees or not.

227

Drug dependence

A patient aged 30 regularly injects himself with morphine.
He has made several unsuccessful attempts to end his dependence.
His drug addiction is maintained under the strictest supervision (United Kingdom legislation; in Belgium, this is strictly forbidden
and constitutes a criminal offence under the 1975 Act).

1. From the standpoint of international law

This case seems to raise two questions: firstly that of the existence of an individual legal obligation to health, and secondly that of the legitimacy of legal measures (penal or otherwise) which lead to a limitation of personal freedom, enjoyment of legal personality or respect for privacy.

As regards the first question, it is highly doubtful whether, at the present time, an individual international obligation to look after one's health could be construed (even through *a contrario* interpretation of existing provisions on the right to health).

As regards the second question, the wording of Articles 9 (1) and 17 (1) of the Covenant on Civil and Political Rights and Articles 5.1 and 8.1 of the ECHR proclaims the right to respect for private and family life and the right to liberty of person. However, Articles 5.1.e and 8.2 of the ECHR, nevertheless, refer to the lawful detention of drug addicts and the legitimacy of interference by a public authority in private life when it is necessary for the protection of health (for instance infection by Aids or other contagious diseases affecting drug addicts) respectively.

Measures which restrict personal freedom are therefore legitimate in this case. It should, nevertheless, be recalled that in the terms of the established precedents of the Court, personal freedom being the most important possession of the individual, Article 5 of the ECHR must be interpreted in a restrictive fashion and legal control must be exercised by the competent authorities at regular intervals to ensure that the conditions which determined the privation or limitation of personal freedom still exist. It should be possible for the individual himself or his legal representative or adviser to request a similar control mechanism.

In the same sense and very recently see Article 10 (1) of the BC, in the terms of which "everyone has the right to respect for private life in relation to information about his or her health", but also Article 26 (1), which states that "no restrictions shall be placed on the exercise of the rights and protective provisions contained in this Convention other than such as are prescribed by law and are necessary in a democratic society in the interest of public safety, for the prevention of crime, for the protection of public health or for the protection of the rights and freedoms of others". See also points 63 and 70, as well as points 148 to 156 and point 159 of the explanatory report.

Reference should also be made to Articles 6 (3) and 7 of the BC, "where, according to law, an adult does not have the capacity to consent to an intervention because of a mental disability, a disease or for similar reasons, the intervention may only be carried out with the authorisation of his or her representative or an authority or a person or body provided by the law" and "subject to protective conditions prescribed by law, including supervisory, control and appeal procedures, a person who has a mental disorder of a serious nature may be subjected, without his or her consent, to an intervention aimed at treating his or her mental disorder only where, without such treatment, serious harm is likely to result to his or her health", as well as to points 41 to 44 and 50 to 55 of the explanatory report.

As regards European case-law concerning prisoners and drug addicts, attention should be drawn to the Commission Decision of 4.7.1995 in the case *Bizzotto* v. *Greece* (Application No. 22126/93) which concerns in particular the relationship between Article 5.1.*a* and Article 5.1.*e* of the ECHR.

Lastly, see Article 6 of the Convention for the Protection of Individuals with Regard to Automatic Processing of Personal Data (Council of Europe, 28.9.1981-1.9.1982): "personal data concerning health (...) may not be processed automatically unless domestic law provides appropriate safeguards". This principle is taken up by Article 10 (1) of the BC, as pointed out in point 63 of the explanatory report.

2. From the ethical standpoint

The general principles (patients' interests, choice of treatment and requirement that doctors practise within their competence) laid down by international declarations (WMA, London 1949) apply.

Furthermore, the Declaration of Tokyo on psychotropic drug abuse (WMA, 1975) requires doctors to exercise the greatest caution when prescribing psychotropic drugs and to respect medical indications strictly; they must ensure that prescriptions correspond to a precise diagnosis, are accompanied by appropriate non-pharmacological advice and that drugs are used with caution. The potential dangers of their misuse must always be borne in mind.

3. From the standpoint of religious moralities

a. *Catholic*

In various documents, the magisterium has condemned as illegitimate the false release constituted by recourse to drugs, which leads to physical and mental self-destruction.[1] Referring to the general principles for the purposes of establishing an

---

1. Congregation for Catholic education, "Orientamenti educativi per l'amore umano", 104, *L'Osservatore Romano* of 2 December 1983; Congregation for the doctrine of the faith, *Libertatis conscientia*, No. 14, AAS 79 (1987), pp. 554-599.

effective therapy, it is necessary to consider the human being as a whole, that is not only his physical state but also his psychology, moral and spiritual ideals and social background.[1] Enforced detention must be considered as an *ultima ratio* – on a par with compulsory treatment of mental patients – and applied only where there are no other strictly therapeutic remedies.

b. *Protestant*

People become drug addicts, they are not born that way. Why? If drug addiction is a state into which one can "fall", it is doubtless one from which it is possible to emerge. How? At what cost?

Let anyone who seriously asks himself these questions act in a manner most likely to provide an answer.

c. *Jewish*

In this case, the doctor must avoid at all costs prescribing drugs or amphetamines which can give rise to dependence or mental problems.

Recourse should be had to substitute drugs only in extreme cases for which there is no other treatment available and when the patient's life is in danger. In this case it is permissible to prescribe substitute products which will enable the patient to gradually free himself from the drug and thus become more receptive to the help of psychotherapists or treatment centres.

It goes without saying that in order to be effective such treatment must be monitored by an experienced doctor and involve a multidisciplinary team.

d. *Muslim*

Islam, through the voice of the Koran, considers man as a precious good in his physical and mental wholeness. Aggression against this creature by substances damaging to the human body is forbidden. A detoxification could, however, be applied under medical supervision, provided that it is free of risks.

e. *Buddhist*

As the purpose is to help the patient by sparing him suffering, the solution *per se* seems satisfactory. But the patient must be encouraged to restore his balance and escape his drug dependence through various types of aid, sporting activities, etc.

---

1. Pius XII, *Broadcast of speeches and messages*, Vol. XX (1958), p. 331ff.

4. From the standpoint of agnostic morality

Drug addition raises the problem of individual freedom, just like drinking, smoking, sexual promiscuity, bisexuality or homosexuality. Man has the right to commit suicide, he has the right to destroy himself, even slowly. However, with the addict's consent, it is possible to envisage a substitution policy, that is softer drugs with less harmful effects and leading to a longer life expectancy.

Drug dependence

A patient aged 50 lodges a complaint on grounds of induced drug dependence. He suffers from chronic asthma and was prescribed corticosteroids by his doctor. The patient objects to the side-effects and the impossibility of stopping treatment. The doctor claims that he gave all necessary prior explanations and obtained the patient's consent.

1. From the standpoint of international law

This case would appear to suggest that there is at this time no alternative to corticosteroids for the treatment of chronic asthma, and that the patient's breathing (vital function) can be improved only at the price of the side-effects of long-term cortisone use (*facies lunare*, etc.). This is therefore a problem of individual assessment of the advantages and disadvantages of a treatment, which cannot be resolved *in abstracto*.

In this connection, Article 4 of the BC stipulates that "any intervention in the health field, including research, must be carried out in accordance with relevant professional obligations and standards" and points 28 to 33 of the explanatory report add that "(…) all interventions must be performed in accordance with the law in general, as supplemented and developed by professional rules (…). Doctors and, in general, all professionals who participate in a medical act are subject to legal and ethical imperatives. They must act with care and competence, and pay careful attention to the needs of each patient (…). Competence must be determined primarily in relation to the scientific knowledge and clinical experience appropriate to a profession or speciality at a given time. The current state of the act determines the professional standard and skill to be expected of health care professionals in the performance of their work. In following the progress of medicine, it changes with new developments and eliminates methods which do not reflect the state of the art. Nevertheless, it is accepted that professional standards do not necessarily prescribe one line of action as being the only one possible: recognised medical practice may, indeed, allow several possible forms of intervention, thus leaving some freedom of choice as to methods or techniques. Further, a particular course of action must be judged in the light of the specific health problem raised by a given patient. In particular, an intervention must meet the criteria of relevance and proportionality between the aim pursued and the means employed".

As regards the patient's consent to the treatment in question, there is no provision of international law to the effect that it must be given in writing in such cases or that there must be a written record of the discussion between the doctor and the patient, on the basis of which the breadth and depth of the explanations given (including those given by the patient) can be reconstructed and checked.

Summary table of international instruments concerned with consent:

- General standard and principle:
  - Article 7 of the Convenant on Civil and Political Rights;
  - Convention for the Protection of Human Rights and Dignity of the Human Being with regard to the Application of Biology and Medicine: Convention on Human Rights and Biomedicine (Oviedo, 4.4.1997); Article 5;

- Principle not written, but stemming from:
  - Articles 8 (1); 9 (1) and 10 (1) of the ECHR;
  - Article 5 of Protocol 7 to the ECHR;
  - Articles 17; 18 (1); 19 (1); 23 (4) of the Covenant on Civil and Political Rights;

- Specific standards and principles:
  - Convention for the Protection of Individuals with regard to Automatic Processing of Personal Data (Council of Europe, 28 November 1981-1 January 1982): Article 8;
  - European Convention for the Prevention of Torture and Inhuman or Degrading Treatment or Punishment (Council of Europe, 26 November 1987-1 February 1989): Article 11 (3) = explicit;
  - Convention on the Rights of the Child (UN, 20 November 1989): Article 12;
  - Resolution (78) 29 of the Committee of Ministers of the Council of Europe on harmonisation of the legislation of member States relating to removal, grafting and transplantation of human substances (11 May 1978): Article 2; Article 3 = in writing; Article 6; Article 10;
  - Recommendation R (81) 1 of the Committee of Ministers of the Council of Europe concerning the rules applicable to automatic medical databanks (23 January 1981): Article 5.3.c; Article 5.4 = express and conscious;
  - Recommendation R (83) 2 of the Committee of Ministers of the Council of Europe concerning the legal protection of persons suffering from mental disorder placed as involuntary patients (22 February 1983): Article 5 (2) = express;
  - Recommendation R (83) 10 of the Committee of Ministers of the Council of Europe concerning the protection of personal data used for scientific research and statistical purposes (23 September 1983): Article 3.1;
  - Recommendation R (85) 4 of the Committee of Ministers of the Council of Europe concerning violence in the family (26 March 1985): Principle 15;
  - Recommendation 1046 (1986) of the Parliamentary Assembly of the Council of Europe on the use of human embryos and foetuses for diagnostic, therapeutic, scientific, industrial and commercial purposes (24 September 1986): point B.iv.*d*, appendix;
  - Recommendation R (87) 3 of the Committee of Ministers of the Council of Europe concerning European prison regulations (12 February 1987): Article 27;

– Resolution 327/88 of the European Parliament on the ethical and legal problems of genetic engineering (16 March 1989): point 12.*c*;
– Resolution 372/88 of the European Parliament on artificial fertilisation *in vivo* and *in vitro* (16 March 1989): point G.10.3;
– Recommendation 1100 (1989) of the Parliamentary Assembly of the Council of Europe on the use of human embryos and foetuses in scientific research (2 February 1989): points D.10; D.11; H.22, appendix;
– United Nations General Assembly Resolution 43/173 on the principles for the protection of all persons subjected to any form of detention or imprisonment (9 December 1988): Principle 22;
– Recommendation R (90) 3 of the Committee of Ministers of the Council of Europe concerning medical research on human beings (6 February 1990): Principle 3 = informed, free, express and specific; Principle 4; Principle 5;
– Recommendation R (90) 13 of the Committee of Ministers of the Council of Europe on prenatal genetic screening, prenatal genetic diagnosis and associated genetic counselling (21 June 1990): Principle 6 = free and informed; Principle 7 = free and informed; Principle 8 = fully informed; Principle 13 = free and informed;
– Convention for the Protection of Human Rights and Dignity of the Human Being with regard to the Application of Biology and Medicine: Convention on Human Rights and Biomedicine (Oviedo, 4 April 1997): Article 6; Article 7; Article 8; Article 9; Article 10; Article 12; Article 16.iii; Article 16.v = express, specific and documented; Article 17.1.i; Article 17.1.iv = specific and in writing; Article 17.1.v; Article 17 (2); Article 19 (2) = express, specific, in writing or before an official body; Article 20 (1); Article 20.2.iv = specific and in writing; Article 20.2.v; Article 22; (Article 26).

2. From the ethical standpoint

The general principles (patients' interests, choice of treatment and requirement that doctors practise within their competence) laid down by international declarations (WMA, London 1949) apply.

Furthermore, the Declaration of Tokyo on psychotropic drug abuse (WMA, 1975) requires doctors to exercise the greatest caution when prescribing psychotropic drugs and to respect medical indications strictly; they must ensure that prescriptions correspond to a precise diagnosis, are accompanied by appropriate non-pharmacological advice and that drugs are used with caution. The potential dangers of their misuse must always be borne in mind.

3. From the standpoint of religious moralities

a. *Catholic*
Even in this case, from the moral point of view, the principle of proportionality of treatment and that of evaluation of the risks and benefits of a therapy still holds.

The patient's explicit consent on the basis of proper information is indispensable if harmful side-effects are foreseeable and cannot be eliminated by other means.[1]

b. *Protestant*
The issue must be resolved by proceedings involving both parties before the competent courts.

c. *Jewish*
It seems to me that the doctor is not liable here because in this case:
1. the treatment was justified and there was no other more appropriate treatment available;
2. the doctor states that he gave all the prior explanation necessary and obtained the patient's consent.
I wonder nevertheless whether the consent obtained from the patient was truly informed consent?

d. *Muslim*
The doctor alone is authorised and able to assess the risks associated with the side-effects of a treatment. It is to be hoped that, thanks to research, a new treatment may be found.

e. *Buddhist*
This is not a particular problem of ethics but rather a relational problem between the doctor and his patient, a problem which should be settled by the competent authorities.

4. From the standpoint of agnostic morality

If the doctor can prove that he gave the patient all the necessary prior explanations and obtained his consent, there is no legal foundation for any action brought by the patient.

---

1. Pius XII, AAS 46 (1954), p. 591.

Exercise of the medical profession in conditions of restricted freedom

A doctor is himself in detention (prison camp).
Problem of the neutrality of doctors.
Inadequacies of the Geneva Convention.
Proposal for an international (United Nations) declaration on the protection
of doctors in the case of national or international conflicts.

1. From the standpoint of international law

See Articles 8 (3), (5), (6), (7), (8), (9), (10), (12) and (13); 9; 13; 14; 15; 16; 17; 18 and 21 to 31 of the Additional Protocol to the Geneva Convention relating to the protection of victims of international armed conflicts and Resolution 881 (1987) of the Parliamentary Assembly of the Council of Europe on the activities of the International Committee of the Red Cross (ICRC) (1.7.1987).

As regards the protection of humanitarian medical missions, see Resolution 904 (1988) of the Parliamentary Assembly of the Council of Europe, Article 1 of which states "medical personnel must be protected and respected. They may not be punished or molested for having engaged in medical activity, whoever the beneficiaries of such care may be". As a result, "if a member of a medical staff is, on account of his medical activities, arrested by the authorities of the territory in which he is carrying out his mission or by a party opposed to such authorities, he must be released and repatriated without delay" (Article 4). During his detention, in any event, "no member of a medical staff may be compelled to provide information concerning the persons to whom he has given assistance, with the exception of information concerning contagious diseases" (Article 3).

For their part, medical personnel, who "must be afforded access to all places where medical care is needed" (Article 2), "must scrupulously respect the rules of medical ethics and may not refrain from performing acts required by these rules" (Article 1 *bis*) and "the assistance provided must be based on purely medical criteria of a humanitarian kind" (Article 2 *bis*).

See also the Rules for behaviour in combat published by the ICRC and the *Handbook of rights and duties of health personnel during armed conflicts* published by the ICRC and the League of Red Cross and Red Crescent Societies (1982).

Reference should also be made, by way of example, to Resolution 1989.26 (6.3.1989) of the UN Human Rights Committee on Hostage Taking.

Lastly, see the report of the Secretary General of the UN Security Council to the General Assembly (Doc. S/26358 of 27.8.1993) concerning the security of UN operations and Security Council Resolution S/Resolution/868 (1993) (29.9.1993) on the security of UN operations and of the personnel participating in them.

Now see also Article 4 of the BC.

2. From the ethical standpoint

The Declaration of Havana of 1958, revised in Venice in 1983, states that the doctor as prisoner must be given assistance, freedom of movement and the independence necessary to the exercise of his profession.

3. From the standpoint of religious moralities

a. *Catholic*
Pius XII explicitly refers to the right of doctors to exercise their profession at all times and in all places where their work is required and in a situation of freedom of conscience. Catholic morality also emphasises the need to set up an international law on doctors, sanctioned by the international community.[1]

b. *Protestant*
Why distinguish between a prisoner who is a doctor and a "common" prisoner? The problem concerns the level, causes and conditions of imprisonment. Is it being suggested, for example, that in our "ordinary" prisons, a doctor who has been sentenced under criminal law should enjoy a special status?

c. *Jewish*
In all cases, the doctor must have the possibility of exercising his art without any restraint. The doctor's aim is to help the patient and relieve his suffering; he must therefore enjoy special protection and never be subject to blackmail or any kind of pressure.

d. *Muslim*
Wherever he may be, the doctor must exercise his profession, which means treating the sick and relieving suffering. There appears to be a gap in international law as regards doctors detained in prison camps.

e. *Buddhist*
The doctor, whose status should be seen as a function of the causes and circumstances of his imprisonment, should be allowed to relieve the suffering of others, regardless of any possibility of outside intervention.

---

1. Pius XII, AAS 45 (1959), p. 744ff.

4. From the standpoint of agnostic morality

It all depends on the conditions of imprisonment. In any event the doctor must always endeavour to exercise his art to relieve sickness and suffering to the best of his ability. In the case where disease should strike torturer prison guards suspected of crimes against humanity, the doctor could invoke the conscience clause and take no action.

Women

A girl is brought by her Muslim parents to have her virginity certified.
The girl refuses to undergo the examination.

1. From the standpoint of international law

Neither Article 5 of the Universal Declaration of Human Rights nor Article 7 of the Covenant on Civil and Political Rights nor Article 3 of the ECHR, all of which prohibit inhuman or degrading treatments, draws up any "list" of behaviour considered as inhuman or degrading.

For its part, the Court has affirmed on many occasions that for a behaviour to be degrading and to infringe Article 3, the humiliation or degradation which accompanies it must be of a particular level of seriousness the appreciation of which depends on all the factors involved. The Court, nevertheless, recently affirmed (Decision No. 247 C of 15.3.1993 in the *Costello-Roberts* case, *Commission* v. *United Kingdom*) that the notion of private life as stipulated in Article 8 of the ECHR also encompasses the physical and mental integrity of the person. As a result, the protection afforded by Article 8 to the physical and mental integrity of the person can go beyond that afforded by Article 3 of the ECHR, precisely where a given behaviour is not of sufficient seriousness to fall within Article 3. In particular, certain practices become all the more degrading when they are proscribed virtually everywhere.

Thus Article 4 of the African Charter on Human and Peoples' Rights (Nairobi, 1981), which came into force on 21 October 1986 between OAU member states stipulates that "human beings are inviolable. Every human being shall be entitled to (...) the integrity of his person"; "every individual shall have the right to the respect of the dignity inherent in a human being (...) all forms of exploitation and degradation of man particularly (...) cruel, inhuman or degrading (...) treatment shall be prohibited", and "the state shall ensure the elimination of every discrimination against women".

Article 2 (2) of the Convention on the Rights of the Child stipulates that "States Parties shall take all appropriate measures to ensure that the child is protected against all forms of discrimination or punishment on the basis of the status, activities, expressed opinions, or beliefs of the child's parents, legal guardians, or family members" and in the same sense Articles 2 and 3 of the Declaration on the elimination of discrimination against women enjoins member states to take "all appropriate measures (...) to abolish existing laws, customs, regulations and practices which are discriminatory against women", and "all appropriate measures (...) to educate public opinion and to direct (...) aspirations towards the eradication of prejudice and the abolition of customary and all other practices which are based on the idea of the inferiority of women".

It should also be pointed out that in the terms of Article 12 (1) of the Convention on the Rights of the Child, "States Parties shall assure to the child who is capable of forming his or her own views the right to express those views freely in all matters affecting the child, the views of the child being given due weight", and according to Article 16 "No child shall be subjected to arbitrary or unlawful interference with his or her privacy (...). The child has the right to the protection of the law against such interference".

The concept of intervention as defined in the BC including any kind of intervention in the field of medicine (including diagnosis), Article 6 (2) of the BC is applicable in this case "the opinion of the minor shall be taken into consideration as an increasingly determining factor in proportion to his or her age and degree of maturity". Point 45 of the explanatory report stipulates that "(...) the second and third paragraphs prescribe that when a minor (paragraph 2) or an adult (paragraph 3) is not able of consenting to an intervention, the intervention may be carried out only with the consent of parents who have custody of the minor, his or her legal representative or any person or body provided by the law. However, as far as possible, with a view to the preservation of the autonomy of persons with regard to interventions affecting their health, the second part of paragraph 2 states that the opinion of minors should be regarded as an increasingly determining factor in proportion to their age and capacity of discernment. This means that in certain situations which take account of the nature and seriousness of the intervention as well as the minor's age and ability to understand, the minor's opinion should increasingly carry more weight in the final decision. This could even lead to the conclusion that the consent of a minor should be necessary, or at least sufficient for some interventions. Note that the provisions of the second sub-paragraph of paragraph 2 are consistent with Article 12 of the United Nations Convention on the Rights of the Child, which stipulates that "States Parties shall assure the child, who is capable of forming his or her own views, the right to express those views freely in all matters affecting the child, the views of the child being given due weight in accordance with the age and maturity of the child".

See Article 6 (1) of the BC, in the terms of which "an intervention may only be carried out on a person who does not have the capacity to consent, for his or her direct benefit".

Assuming that the certification of virginity brings a benefit, although indirect and not *stricto sensu* medical for the girl (or rather her parents of the Muslim faith), Article 6 (2) of the BC states that the consent (or even request) of the parents is not sufficient, the authorisation of an authority or a person or body provided for by (domestic) law also being required.

2. From the ethical standpoint

Under the terms of the International Code of Medical Ethics (WMA, London, 1949), doctors are required to practice with due respect for human dignity and the rights of patients and treat all information on patients as strictly confidential.

3. From the standpoint of religious moralities

a. *Catholic*
For Catholic morality, the parents' request is illicit in this case, as it infringes the freedom of the subject and respect for her moral sensibility. Only a court could request such an attestation for reasons of the public good or to establish whether a crime has been committed.[1]

b. *Protestant*
The dignity and freedom of the young girl must be respected first and foremost.

c. *Jewish*
It is essential to obtain the voluntary agreement of the young girl.
As for the doctor, he has to respect absolute secrecy with regard to what he knows about the patient.

d. *Muslim*
Parents have no right to force a young girl to undergo an examination to check her virginity. This is a case of violation of human dignity. Only the judicial authorities may be empowered to order such an examination in a case of rape.

e. *Buddhist*
The girl's wishes should be respected and the examination requested by the parents should be refused for this reason.

4. From the standpoint of agnostic morality

If the girl concerned is a major, she has the right to refuse to submit to an examination concerning her virginity. If she refuses the doctor cannot examine her. Since the lack of virginity in no way endangers the girl's health, there would have to be rape and a criminal action for an examination to be necessary.

---

1. Second Vatican Council, *Gaudium et Spes*, 7, AAS 57, (1966), pp. 1025-1120.

Even if the girl is a minor, she is still a free person who can oppose her parents' wishes. In this case the doctor has no particular right which permits him to examine the girl without her consent.

Old people

A man of 85, in good physical and mental condition, suffers a syncope (Adam-Stokes syndrome); the doctors consider it necessary to implant a pacemaker.
The hospital administration refuses the operation as the patient is insolvent.

1. From the standpoint of international law

There are no international provisions which set out the sickness, invalidity or old age benefits to be covered by national social security, as reference is always made to the "applicable law", that is domestic law. It is therefore on this law that the implantation of a pacemaker will depend.

We would, nevertheless, recall the fundamental principle of non discrimination "for reasons of fortune" stipulated by Articles 14 of the ECHR and 2 of the Covenant on Civil and Political Rights.

See also point 6.v of Recommendation 1153 (1991) on concerted European policies for health adopted by the Parliamentary Assembly of the Council of Europe on 26 April 1991, which affirms "equal access to health care, including new techniques, treatment and products" and Article 3 of the BC, according to which "Parties taking into account health needs and available resources shall take appropriate measures with a view to providing, within their jurisdiction, equitable access to health care, of appropriate quality". Reference should also be made to points 45 to 47 of the explanatory report cited in the reply to case 13.

See also Recommendation 1196 (1992) on severe poverty and social exclusion: towards guaranteed minimum levels of resources, adopted by the Parliamentary Assembly of the Council of Europe on 7 October 1992. This recommendation stems from Article 13 of the European Social Charter, in the terms of which any person without adequate resources should be granted appropriate assistance. (This article has been accepted by almost all member states of the Council of Europe.)

Lastly, see Articles 1 and 2 of the BC: "Parties to this Convention shall protect the dignity and identity of all human beings and guarantee everyone, without discrimination, respect for their integrity and other rights and fundamental freedoms with regard to the application of biology and medicine"; "The interests and welfare of the human being shall prevail over the sole interest of society and science", as well as points 23 to 27 of the explanatory report (namely point 26, in terms of which "the purpose of Article 3 is not to create an individual right on which each person may rely in legal proceedings against the state, but rather to prompt the latter to adopt the requisite measures as part of its social policy in order to ensure equitable access to health care").

2. From the ethical standpoint

According to the WMA Twelve Principles of Social Security of 1963, the doctor must have unrestricted technical and moral independence to decide upon necessary treatment.

Once he has been informed, it is for the patient himself to take the decision, not for his family (WMA, Lisbon, 1981). It is the patient who must judge his material possibilities.

As regards cost coverage, the Standing Committee of Doctors (Nuremberg, 1967) in its statement on the exercise of the profession refers to the obligation of states to take measures to ensure that everyone has access to the necessary medical care.

In Copenhagen (EECSCD, 1979), the standing committee invited governments to bear in mind the quality of life which medicine can give elderly people when judging the necessary restrictions.

The WMA Declaration of Rancho Mirage (1986) states that it is the doctor's duty to defend the patient's interests while being aware of the price of care; the WMA Declaration of Vienna of 1988 states that no one should be refused treatment he or she needs because of insolvency.

3. From the standpoint of religious moralities

a. *Catholic*

A patient's economic circumstances may not constitute an obstacle to the care to which everyone has the right when it is indispensable. A refusal by the hospital administration to apply such treatment is therefore absolutely unacceptable in the view of Catholic morality.[1]

In the case of care dispensed by a private health scheme, the state has always the duty to reimburse the costs of emergency care when the patient is not able to pay (subsidiarity principle).

b. *Protestant*

The social legislation of the country where this problem arises warrants immediate improvement. This also leads us to think of the many countries in which the question does not even arise, for lack of facilities; in such cases, it is the entire country that it is insolvent. What conclusions should we draw from this?

c. *Jewish*

Material reasons may never be an obstacle to provision of medical care. The patient's age, too, should not enter it or be taken into account. As long as a patient

---

1. Second Vatican Council, *Gaudium et Spes*, 29, AAS 58, (1966), pp. 1025-1120.

is alive, the doctor has a duty to do everything to save his life. This right to life should know no barriers or differences due to colour, religion, sex, age or any administrative or customs formalities.

d. *Muslim*

No one can prevent administration of a treatment to a patient. This is a case of failure to help a person in danger. As regards the costs, an appeal may be made to the patient's family. Otherwise, the matter is governed by the legislation of the country concerned.

e. *Buddhist*

Fortunately the question does not arise at present in France, but in any event it would appear impossible not to permit the patient to benefit from existing medical possibilities because of his age and financial problems.

Extending this question, is it possible for us to refuse somebody something that we have which would save his live? And how do we approach this problem as regards the Third World?

4. From the standpoint of agnostic morality

The situation described is unacceptable. This patient could bring an action for failure to assist a person in danger. In the hospital structure, a patient's insolvency is not a valid argument for refusing to implant a pacemaker. Legal action would oblige the hospital administration to comply, and thus accept and treat this patient.

Migrants

A migrant worker, aged 29, suffers from a condition requiring treatment extending beyond the expiry date of his work permit.
The authorities propose deportation.
The doctors propose treatment.

1. From the standpoint of international law

In the terms of Article 1 (1) of Protocol 7 to the ECHR "An alien lawfully resident in the territory of a state shall not be expelled therefrom except in pursuance of a decision reached in accordance with law". Collective expulsion of aliens is prohibited by Article 4 of Protocol 4 to the ECHR.

Article 1 (2) of Protocol 7 to the ECHR states that the alien "shall be allowed: to submit reasons against his expulsion, to have his case reviewed, and to be represented for these purposes before a competent authority or a person or persons designated by that authority".

In this particular case, these "reasons" include Article 19 of the European Convention on the Legal Status of Migrant Workers (Council of Europe, 24.9.1977-1.5.1983); Articles 19 to 26 of the European Convention on Social Security (Council of Europe, 14.12.1972) and Recommendation 1066 (1987) adopted on 7.10.1987 by the Parliamentary Assembly of the Council of Europe, in particular point 11 of the preamble.

If the immigrant worker is a national of a Contracting Party of the European Social Charter and is on the territory of another member state, he has "the right to protection and assistance in the territory of any other Contracting Party" (Principle 19). According to Article 19 (8) of the Social Charter, "such workers (...) are not expelled unless they endanger national security or offend against public interest or morality". Similar provisions are to be found in Article 4 of ILO Convention 111 (1958), Article 1 (1) and (2) of Protocol 7 to the ECHR and Recommendation (86) 5 of the Committee of Ministers of the Council of Europe of 17.2.1986 on making medical care universally available.

European Union Regulations 1612/68 and 1408/71 state that "a worker who is a national of a member state (...) shall enjoy the same social (...) advantages as national workers". "A worker whose condition necessitates immediate benefits during a stay in the territory of another member state" is entitled to "(sickness) benefits provided (...) by the institution of the place of stay or residence in accordance with the legislation which it administers." The length of the period during which benefits are provided shall be governed by the legislation of the competent state."

Migrant workers who are not nationals of a State Party to a specific international agreement, but who are lawfully residing on the territory of a state, should they find themselves in the situation postulated here, cannot be deported either, under the terms of Article 13 of the Covenant on Civil and Political Rights and Article 1 of Protocol 7 to the ECHR, or by virtue of the "minimum standard" rule of general international law.

The established precedents of the Court in fact affirm that the expulsion of the foreigner who is legally on the territory of a Council of Europe member state is likely to infringe Article 8 of the ECHR, that is the right to respect of the private and family life of the individual. On this subject, see, for example, Decision No. 234 A of 26.3.1992 in the *Beldjoudi* case (*Commission* v. *France*) and Decision No. 193 of 18.2.1991 in the *Moustaquim* case (*Commission* v. *France*), but also, *in contrario*, Decision No. 322 B of 13.7.1995 in the *Nasri* case (*Commission* v. *France*).

As regards the contrary case, namely a minor who asks to join his father, holder of a residence authorisation for humanitarian reasons, see the Decision (no number) of 19.2.1996 in the *Gül* case (*Commission* v. *Switzerland*).

Concerning the connection between expulsion and Article 3 of the ECHR, see Decision No. 161 of 7.7.1989 in the *Soering* case (*Commission* v. *United Kingdom*), and also Decision Nos. 201 of 20.3.1991 in the *Cruz Varas* case (*Commission* v. *Sweden*) and 215 of 30.10.1991 in the *Vilvarajah* case (*Commission* v. *United Kingdom*).

See also Recommendation 1236 (1994) on the right of asylum, adopted by the Parliamentary Assembly of the Council of Europe on 12.4.1994 and Recommendation 1237 (1994) of the same date on the situation of asylum-seekers whose asylum applications have been rejected, adopted on the same day.

2. From the ethical standpoint

In the patient's best interest, there must be no restriction on the doctor's right to prescribe necessary drugs or any other treatment (WMA, *Twelve Principles of Social Security*, 1963).

States have a duty to take all measures necessary to ensure that all social classes, without discrimination, have access to all medical care they require.

3. From the standpoint of religious moralities

a. *Catholic*

The migrants' situation may not impinge on the human right to health care.[1] Hence, nations have a moral obligation to safeguard the health of all citizens, regardless of their role as this is one of the conditions of universal peace and general security.[2]

---

1. Pius XII, AAS 45 (1953), p. 744ff.
2. Pius XII, AAS 41 (1949).

247

b. *Protestant*

Somebody once said: "the sabbath was made for man, and man for the sabbath" (St Mark's Gospel, 2, v. 27) and we may add: "if any man have ears to hear, let him hear".

c. *Jewish*

As long as the patient is alive, the doctor has a duty to do everything to save his life. This right must know no barriers nor differences based on colour, religion, sex, age or administrative or customs formalities.

d. *Muslim*

In Islam, the right to health is a fundamental right. The patient's situation (immigrant) may not be an obstacle to this right. The right to health may not be obstructed by any form of discrimination. Here again, we have a problem of failure to assist a person in danger.

e. *Buddhist*

According to Buddhist ethics, all living creatures, and in particular humans, should receive care and attention.

4. From the standpoint of agnostic morality

The administrative authorities' intention to expel the patient is negated by the doctors' proposal to continue the treatment. The concept of danger connected with the possible cessation of treatment outweighs the legal concepts of the French labour code.

Workers

A female worker, aged 35, attends a job interview.
It is stipulated as a condition of employment that she should not have a child during the term of contract.
Prescription of suitable drugs by a doctor or certification of sterility is required.

1. From the standpoint of international law

Article 4.vii of Recommendation 1146 (1991) on equality of opportunity and treatment for women and men on the labour market, adopted by the Parliamentary Assembly of the Council of Europe on 11.3.1991 stipulates that member states should take initiatives "to avoid or to resolve problems arising from unlawful discrimination on grounds of gender or from measures or practices having a discriminatory effect, without prejudice to judicial areas of responsibility". In the same sense, see Recommendation 1229 (1994) on equality of rights between men and women, adopted by the Parliamentary Assembly of the Council of Europe on 24.1.1994.

As regards the (company) doctor to whom the employer wishes to entrust the task of prescribing contraceptive medicaments, respect of the woman's integrity and of her right to the respect of her private life (Articles 8 of the ECHR; 17 of the Covenant on Civil and Political Rights) is imposed by Article 1 of the BC, all the more so since by the very fact of prescribing the drugs he would run the risk of the sanctions provided for by Article 23 of the BC. In the terms of points 130 and 141 of the explanatory report, Article 23 "requires the Parties to make available a judicial procedure to prevent or to stop an infringement of the principles set forth in the Convention. It therefore covers not only infringement which have already begun and are ongoing but also the threat of an infringement (...). The appropriate protective machinery must be capable of operating rapidly as it has to allow an infringement to be prevented or halted at short notice. This requirement can be explained by the fact that, in many cases, the very integrity of an individual has to be protected and an infringement of this right might have irreversible consequences".

See also Decision No. 263 of 24.6.1993 in the *Schuler-Zgraggen* case (*Commission v. Switzerland*).

As regards predictive genetic testing in the context of pre-employment medical examinations, see Article 12 of the BC, which excludes it if it does not serve a health purpose (points 85 and 86 of the explanatory report). "However, national law may allow for the performance of a test predictive of a genetic disease outside the health field for one of the reasons and under the conditions provided for in Article 26.1 of the Convention" (ibid.). It should be noted that "in particular circumstances, when the working environment could have prejudicial consequences on the health of an individual because of a genetic predisposition, predictive genetic testing may be offered without prejudice to the aim of improving working conditions. The text should be clearly used in the interest of the individual's health (second part of point 85 of the explanatory report).

2. From the ethical standpoint

In accordance with its principles, the WMA regards family planning as a right for individuals, affording them greater possibilities and a chance to develop their full potential (WMA, Madrid, 1967), after being adequately informed it is the individual alone who can decide to accept or refuse the "treatment" (WMA, Lisbon, 1981).

3. From the standpoint of religious moralities

a. *Catholic*
An obligation to remain sterile, even temporarily, is illicit. "True promotion of the family requires that work be structured in such a way that it is not required to pay for its advancement by abandoning its own specificity (...)."[1]

b. *Protestant*
To demand this is undoubtedly in contravention of a number of labour laws which should be enforced accordingly; where they do not exist, they should be encouraged. Indeed, one of the fundamental laws of any healthy society is the distinction between life as a citizen and a member of society, on the one hand, and private life, on the other.

c. *Jewish*
This case seems to be immoral. Employers should not be allowed to practice moral blackmail, particularly as we are currently living in a period of crisis and unemployment. A female worker must be able to choose freely when she wishes to have children and how many. No constraint may be tolerated in this area.

d. *Muslim*
In this case, employment of a woman is made conditional upon prescription of contraceptives by a doctor or a certificate of sterility.
This constraint on the woman is totally immoral, as it deprives the woman of her full liberty and the ability to procreate which is a specific characteristic of womanhood.

---

1. John Paul II, *Encyclical Laborem Exercens*, 19, AAS 73 (1981), pp. 577-667.

This form of discrimination towards women is forbidden in Islam.

e. *Buddhist*
This requirement is contrary to the labour legislation of all European countries. Any form of blackmail is illegal and unacceptable.

4. From the standpoint of agnostic morality

The conditions imposed are unconscionable. They are immoral and without foundation. The prescription of such drugs has no legal basis.

Workers

A group of workers in a given department are exposed to substances known to be carcinogens.
The company doctor considers the substances to be harmless.
The private doctor acting as an expert disagrees.

1. From the standpoint of international law

As regards the conflict between the company doctor and the private doctor, there is no reply. However, see ILO Convention 139 of 10.6.1976 concerning Prevention and Control of Occupational Hazards caused by Carcinogenic Substances and Agents.

In the terms of Article 4 of the BC, any intervention in the health field (the term "intervention" being understood here in a broad sense, covering all medical acts, whether for the purpose of diagnosis, preventive care, treatment or rehabilitation or in a research context: point 29 of the explanatory report) must be carried out in accordance with relevant professional obligations and standards. As an intervention is an act performed on a human being, it must be done with care and competence, and pay careful attention to the needs of each patient. Competence must be determined primarily in relation to the scientific knowledge and clinical experience appropriate to a profession or speciality at a given time. The administration of care must be consistent with established scientific facts. A particular course of action must be judged in the light of the specific health problem raised by a given patient. In particular, it is acknowledged that an intervention must meet the criteria of relevance and proportionality between the aim pursued and the means used (points 31, 32 and 33 of the explanatory report). Point 30 makes reference to professional codes of ethics, other codes of medical conduct, health law or any other means of ensuring respect for the rights and interests of patients.

It should also be pointed out that Article 24 of the BC stipulates that a person has a right to fair compensation if he has suffered undue damage resulting from an intervention in the widest sense, taking the form of either an act or an omission. The intervention may or may not constitute an offence (point 144 of the explanatory report).

Reference should also be made, *mutatis mutandis*, to the decision of 6.7.1995 of the Commission on the admissibility of Application No. 14967/89 (the case of *Anna Maria Guerra and thirty-nine other women* v. *Italy*), which concerns the violation of Article 10 of the ECHR through the pollution of an area by local chemical plants.

See also the Community Charter of the fundamental social rights of workers adopted by the European Parliament on 22.11.1989 (Principle 6).

2. From the ethical standpoint

Under the terms of the Code of Ethics (WMA, 1949) and the Declaration of the EU Standing Committee of Doctors on industrial medicine, the doctor must always make his diagnosis in full technical independence and in the patient's interests without concern for financial implications.

3. From the standpoint of religious moralities

a. *Catholic*

According to the doctrine of the Catholic Church,[1] workers have the right to a working environment and production procedures which are not damaging to their physical health. It is therefore necessary for the company doctor to take all measures to check whether or not there is a possibility of carcinogenicity, and for the differences of opinion between him and the private doctor to be resolved through consultation of outside experts, as the company doctor is often responsible not only for protection of the workers' health but also for the smooth running of the company.

b. *Protestant*

This question is primarily a technical, not an ethical one. Who is technically right? Further information and more opinions are required. If, at the end of the investigation, there should remain a doubt, operations likely to be dangerous should be foregone.

c. *Jewish*

In Judaism, respect for human life is not only proclaimed, but expressed in the least acts of daily life. Man is released from the performance of religious obligations to save his life, as divine law seeks above all the protection of man and his life. It is written in the Talmud that "So great is respect for our living creatures that it pushes aside the prohibitions contained in the Torah".

In the present case it is therefore necessary to take all measures required to ensure that the health of the workers cannot be endangered in any way.

Since there is conflict between the company doctor and the private doctor acting as expert, it seems to me important to request an expert opinion from a college of three experts who will produce a report.

d. *Muslim*

Where the company doctor and the private doctor as expert disagree, a further external expert opinion should be sought. The criteria for assessment of the

---

1. John Paul II, *Encyclical Laborem Exercens*, 19.

253

carcinogenicity of a substance are not simple to define. At all events, through the Koran as well the Hadith, respect for the human person is presented as a fundamental and inviolable principle.

e. *Buddhist*

If there is any doubt as to whether the product is innocuous or not, a more thorough investigation is called for. If the doubt persists, the persons exposed to it should be informed. Production should cease if this is possible, otherwise all parties should accept their responsibilities.

4. From the standpoint of agnostic morality

This conflict can be resolved by a submitting the matter for examination by a committee of medical experts.

Right to information

A man aged 38 undergoes surgery (lumbar sympathectomy) for arteritis in the lower limbs without being warned of the risks involved.
He becomes permanently impotent.

1. From the standpoint of international law

As permanent impotence (*generandi*) constitutes an irreversible violation of the right to procreate provided for by all international instruments on human rights (Article 16 of the Universal Declaration, Article 23 (1) and (2) of the Covenant on Civil and Political Rights), the patient must – except in an emergency – give his prior and informed consent to the surgical operation (Article 7 of the Covenant on Civil and Political Rights), which implies that he should be given the opportunity to become well acquainted with the essential data concerning his problem and the consequences of the treatment.

See also Article 5 of the BC, as well as points 34 to 40 of the explanatory report, in particular points 35, 36 and 37, which stipulate that "the patient's consent is considered to be free and informed if it is given on the basis of objective information from the responsible health care professional as to the nature and the potential consequences of the planned intervention or of its alternatives, in the absence of any pressure from anyone. Article 5, paragraph 2, mentions the most important aspects of the information which should precede the intervention but it is not an exhaustive list; informed consent may imply, according to the circumstances, additional elements. In order for their consent to be valid the persons in question must have been informed about the relevant facts regarding the intervention being contemplated. The information must include the purpose, nature and consequences of the intervention and the risks involved. Information on the risks involved in the intervention or in alternative courses of action must cover not only the risks inherent in the type of intervention contemplated, but also any risks related to the individual characteristics of each patient, such as age or the existence of other pathologies. Requests for additional information made by patients must be adequately answered. Moreover, this information must be sufficiently clear and suitably worded for the layman who is to undergo the intervention. The patient must be put in a position, through the use of terms he or she can understand, to weigh up the necessity or usefulness of the aim and methods of the intervention against its risks and the discomfort or pain it will cause. Consent may take various forms. It may be express or implied. Express consent may be either verbal or written. Article 5, which is general and covers very different situations, does not require any particular form. The latter will largely depend on the nature of the intervention. It is agreed that express consent would be inappropriate as regards many routine medical acts. The consent is therefore often implicit, as long as the person concerned is sufficiently informed. In some cases, however, for example invasive diagnostic acts or treatments, express consent may be required."

In the case where the patient does not wish to know information collected about his health, see Article 10 (2) and (3) of the BC and points 67, 68 and 70 of the explanatory report, notably in view of the case where it may be of vital importance for patients to know certain facts about their health, even though they have expressed the wish not to know them.

2. From the ethical standpoint

The doctor must obtain informed consent by providing adequate information under the terms of various declarations: WMA Declarations of Lisbon (1981); Helsinki (1964, revised in 1983) and Venice (1983); WPA/APM Declaration of Hawaii (1983); CIO Declarations on transplantation (1981) and quality of care (1983), CIOMS, Manila (1981), ECHP Declaration on respect for the human individual in hospital treatment (1979), the CISMP Declaration of Athens (1979).

3. From the standpoint of religious moralities

a. *Catholic*

It is morally acceptable to assume consent from the moment the patient entrusts himself to the doctor's care,[1] provided that he is given all information on the implications of the treatment to be administered. There is no single answer to the problem of whether or not to tell the truth to a seriously ill patient. In principle, truth is a criterion of morality and it must be told to the extent and in the proportion that the patient is able to benefit from it. The patient's wishes must be taken into account.

b. *Protestant*

Who is most troubled by this situation: the patient, who wonders what is happening to him, or the doctor, who can no longer remain vague as regards his patient's condition? Here we have two people who will be forced to take the time, finally, to speak about that which concerns them both: the illness and the treatment it requires. The ethical point of view certainly does not consist in avoiding this confrontation, but in helping to ensure the best possible outcome.

---

1. Pius XII, AAS 46 (1954), p. 591.

c. *Jewish*

The patient must be informed of the consequences which may result from the operation. He must be able to evaluate the risks. What right has the doctor to decide without seeking the patient's opinion?

The role of the doctor is to permit the patient to evaluate the risks and be able to decide in full knowledge of the facts, thanks to complete and objective information.

However, if the patient's life is in danger the position may be different, because nobody has the right to put his life in danger. In this case, it is for the doctor to do everything in his power to try to convince the patient or his family of the need for the treatment and to obtain their consent.

d. *Muslim*

The patient must be informed of possible consequences, damaging to his physical and mental integrity, before any surgical operation is performed. However, the doctor alone is in a position to decide whether failure to perform the operation may endanger the patient's life. In any case, the doctor must inform the patient and his family on all these problems. It is the doctor's duty to do all he can to convince them in order to obtain their consent.

e. *Buddhist*

The patient should not have to undergo any operation causing physical or psychological consequences without first being fully informed.

4. From the standpoint of agnostic morality

The failure to inform the patient means that he can justifiably claim damages. The fact is that this patient, if he had been properly informed of his condition and thus able to appreciate the consequences of the surgery, might have refused the operation. He is therefore entitled to fair compensation.

Right to information

A patient is prescribed antineoplastic drugs which cause serious side-effects (hair loss, sterility, diarrhoea) without being informed that he is suffering from cancer.

1. From the standpoint of international law

There is no general provision of international law which obliges the doctor to inform the patient of the nature of the disease from which he is suffering, except where the treatment proposed would entail serious and/or permanent consequences for his fundamental rights and a choice arises between preservation of one fundamental right or that of another. In the case put forward here, the major side-effects are not such as to affect one of the patient's fundamental rights: full prior information on the disease does not therefore seem to be necessarily required, if it is not requested, except for the sterility. On this see the replies to cases 42 and 44.

As regards *ad hoc* international law, the right to information and consent provided for in Article 5 and 10 (2) of the BC also includes the right not to be informed. Article 10 (2) states in fact that "everyone is entitled to know any information collected about his or her health. However, the wishes of individuals not to be so informed shall be observed". Point 67 of the explanatory report states in this connection that "the right to know goes hand in hand with the 'right not to know' which is provided for in the second sentence of the second paragraph. Patients may have their own reasons for not wishing to know about certain aspects of their health. A wish of this kind must be observed. The patient's exercise of the right not to know this or that fact concerning his health is not regarded as an impediment to the validity of his consent to an intervention (...)".

As a result, if the patient did not know he has cancer because he had asked the doctor not to inform him about his health or because he had not asked to know about his condition, he can undergo the antineoplastic treatment provided that he has given consent to the latter.

Article 10 (3) of the BC also stipulates that in exceptional cases, restrictions may be placed by national law on the exercise of the rights contained in the preceding paragraph in the interests of the patient, and point 68 of the explanatory report adds that "in some circumstances the right to know or not to know may be restricted in the patient's own interest". Point 69 states that "for example, the last paragraph of Article 10 sets out that in exceptional cases domestic law may place restrictions on the right to know or not to know in the interests of the patient's health (for example, a prognosis of death immediately might, in certain cases which if passed on to the patient, seriously worsen his or her condition). In these cases, the doctor's duty to provide information which is also covered under Article 4 conflicts with the interests of the patient's health. It is for domestic law, taking account of the social and cultural background, to solve this conflict. Where appropriate under judicial control, domestic law may justify the doctor sometimes withholding part of the information or, at all events, disclosing it with circumspection. ('therapeutic exception').

If knowledge that he has cancer has been withheld from the patient in order not to seriously harm his health, then information stemming from this should be spared him too.

2. From the ethical standpoint

The doctor must obtain informed consent by providing adequate information under the terms of various declarations: WMA Declarations of Lisbon (1981); Helsinki (1964, revised in 1983) and Venice (1983); WPA-APM Declaration of Hawaii (1983); CIO Declarations on transplantation (1981) and quality of care (1983); CIOMS Declaration of Manila (1981); the ECHP on respect for the individual in hospital treatment (1979) and the CISMP Declaration of Athens (1979).

3. From the standpoint of religious moralities

a. *Catholic*

According to Catholic morality, the surgeon has an obligation to explain the purpose of or need for the operation, and to point out remaining uncertainties and all possible consequences. The operation is licit only if there are no valid alternatives and subject to the patient's consent.[1]

b. *Protestant*

No one may dispose of another's health or another's body as simple merchandise.

c. *Jewish*

The doctor must inform the patient of his state and indicate the consequences which the prescribed treatment may have for him. This information must not be given brutally however, but with consideration and solicitude. Above all it must take account of the patient's capacity to accept the truth.

In any event, the doctor must refrain from providing precise information which can plunge the patient into a state of physical or emotional depression. Even if the situation appears hopeless, he must on no account eliminate all hope. His duty is to go on giving advice, reassuring and comforting the patient.

---

1. Pius XII, AAS 40 (1948).

259

d. *Muslim*

The doctor has a duty to warn the patient of side-effects, for instance in the case of cancer therapy. This presupposes that the doctor must tell the truth about the nature and possible seriousness of the disease. The fundamental and essential point is that the doctor must do all in his power to save the patient's life. The informed consent of the patient or his close relatives is, of course, desirable.

e. *Buddhist*

The doctor must warn the patient of the side-effects of any medicines prescribed, but must also respect the attitude adopted by the patient with respect to his disease, respecting his silence or answering his questions.

4. From the standpoint of agnostic morality

The doctor is not morally obliged to tell his patient the truth concerning the fact that he has cancer. On the other hand, he must inform the patient about the secondary effects of the medicines prescribed. The doctor is fully liable and could incur penalties.

Obligation to obtain consent

A patient, aged 60, is suffering from hypertrophy of the prostate.
The doctor intends to carry out a prostatectomy and ligation of the vas deferens.
He does not consider that an operation entailing sterility in a 60-year-old
requires the patient's consent.

1. From the standpoint of international law

Regarding the question of consent in this case, Articles 7 of the Covenant on Civil and Political Rights and 5 of the BC and the need to safeguard the fundamental right to procreate and the physical and mental integrity of the individual imply that the patient should be informed in advance not only of the necessity of the prostatectomy but also of the ligature of the vas deferens and the permanent *impotentia generandi* which will result, and give his consent for the operation, all the more so if he is still sexually active. The ligature of the vas deferens cannot in fact be considered one of the "routine medical acts" for which implicit consent suffices (point 37 of the explanatory report appended to the BC). Being on the contrary an invasive therapeutic intervention, "express consent may be required" (ibid.). Furthermore, even implicit consent assumes that the patient is "sufficiently informed" (ibid.). Deprivation of one of the fundamental rights in fact requires the personal will of the person concerned, even if such deprivation is for health reasons.

As regards the aspect of the case concerned with the choice of therapy, there being several ways of treating hypertrophy of the prostate, reference is made to Article 4 of the BC and to points 32 and 33 of the explanatory report.

2. From the ethical standpoint

The doctor must obtain informed consent by providing adequate information under the terms of various declarations: WMA Declarations of Lisbon (1981); Helsinki (1964, revised in 1983) and Venice (1983); WPA Declaration of Hawaii (1983); CIO Declarations on transplantation (1981) and quality of care (1983); CIOMS Declaration of Manila (1981); the ECHP on respect for the individual in hospital treatment (1979); and the CISMP Declaration of Athens (1979).

3. From the standpoint of religious moralities

a. *Catholic*

In order to obtain the patient's informed consent, the surgeon is obliged to inform him of all the consequences of the surgical operation.[1] In this case, there is no unanimous view that ligation of the vas deferens is a valid preventive treatment for epididymitis; the sterilisation is therefore not therapeutic in the strict sense, because the disease is not present or foreseeable with certainty. At all events, there would remain the obligation to inform the patient in advance – regardless of his age – of possible sterility as a result of the operation,[2] as man can be fertile even after the age of 60.

b. *Protestant*

The doctor simply made a mistake. A human being retains his quality of humanity – and the various functions associated with it – to the end.

c. *Jewish*

Age may never be a valid criterion for allowing any form of abuse. The doctor is bound to inform the patient of the consequences inherent in the treatment administered. However, if this hypertrophy of the prostate can endanger the patient's life, the doctor may, in this case, operate even without the patient's consent. As we have seen throughout this work, defence of life overrides any other considerations. It is obvious that the doctor can act in this way only if it is impossible for him to act otherwise and when there are almost certain guarantees that the operation will be successful.

d. *Muslim*

The doctor is obliged to provide the patient with full information and to point out all the possible consequences of a form of treatment or a surgical operation. The patient's informed consent or that of his family is an important element, but the patient's life is paramount. In this case, it is the doctor and he alone who is able to assess the risks likely to be run in the absence of any treatment or surgical operation.

e. *Buddhist*

The doctor is obliged under all circumstances to request the patient's consent before performing any irreversible act.

4. From the standpoint of agnostic morality

Since the ligature of the vas deferens is virtually irreversible, the patient's consent is a legal requirement.

---

1. Pius XII, AAS 40 (1948).
2. Congregation for the doctrine of the faith, *Qaecumque sterilirati*, 1, AAS 68 (1976), pp. 738-740.

Right to confidentiality

A tram driver aged 40 suffers from epileptic fits.
This is not known to the employer, but it is known to the attending physician.

1. From the standpoint of international law

As far as doctors and health professionals are concerned, the right to confidentiality stems, in general, from the provisions (Article 8 (1) of the ECHR, 17 of the Covenant on Civil and Political Rights) which stipulate the right to the respect of the private life of the patient. More specifically, Article 10 (1) of the BC adds to this that "everyone has the right to respect for private life in relation to information about his or her health". Point 63 of the explanatory report appended to the BC states that Article 10 (1) "establishes the right to privacy of information in the health field, thereby reaffirming the principle introduced in Article 8 of the ECHR and reiterated in the Convention on the Protection of Individuals with regard to Automatic Processing of Personal Data. It should be pointed out that, under Article 6 of the latter convention, personal data concerning health constitute a special category of data and are as such subject to special rules".

Consequently, the right of third parties to receive and communicate information of any kind, provided for in Articles 10 (1) of the ECHR and 19 (2) of the Covenant on Civil and Political Rights, may be subject to restrictions, provided for by law, which are necessary in a democratic society for the respect of the rights of others (Articles 10 (2) of the ECHR and 19 (3) of the Covenant on Civil and Political Rights), including the patient's right to respect of his private life.

However, the protection of health and/or the rights and freedoms of others may justify, in the terms of Article 8 (2) of the ECHR and Article 26 (1) of the BC, interference by a public authority with the right to private life, provided this interference is in accordance with the law.

Point 149 of the explanatory report appended to the BC states that Article 26 (1) of the BC "echoes (…) the provisions of Article 8, paragraph 2, of the European Convention of Human Rights." Nevertheless, "the exceptions made in Article 8, paragraph 2, of the European Convention on Human Rights have not all been considered relevant to this convention. The exceptions defined in the article are aimed at protecting collective interests (…) or the rights or freedoms of others." Consequently, in terms of point 156 of the explanatory report, "defending the economic well-being of the country, public order or morals and national security are not included amongst the general exceptions referred to in the first paragraph of Article 26 (1), unlike Article 8 of the ECHR. It did not appear desirable, in the context of this

263

convention, to make the exercise of fundamental rights chiefly concerned with the protection of a person's rights in the health sphere subject to the economic well-being of the country, to public order, to morals or to national security". Let us also mention in passing that the exercise of the right of the patient to know or not to know any information collected about his or her health (Article 10 (2) of the BC) may, in exceptional cases, be restricted in the patient's own interest (Article 10 (3) of the BC) or else on the basis of Article 26 (1) of the BC, for example, in order to protect the rights of a third party or of society (point 68 of the explanatory report).

As regards European case-law, see Decision No. 160 of 7.7.1989 in the *Gaskin* case (*Commission* v. *United Kingdom*) and the Commission Decision of 2.12.1995 in *Z* v. *Finland*, in which the Commission was of the unanimous opinion that there had been violation of Article 8 on the part of the defendant state in that the doctors of the hospital where the applicant was treated for HIV had been forced, despite their protests, to make statements concerning, among other things, seropositivity of Mrs Z before the Helsinki municipal court during a trial for attempted homicide brought by the prosecutor against the husband of the applicant on the ground that he had knowingly exposed the victims of a series of sexual offences he had committed to the risk of HIV infection.

As regards the contrary case, and in particular the right to information of health service users, refer for example to Decision No. 30 of 26.4.1979 in the *Sunday Times* case (*Commission* v. *United Kingdom*) and Decision No. 165 of 20.11.1989 in the *Markt intern Verlag GmbH and Klaus Beermann* case (*Commission* v. *Germany*).

2. From the ethical standpoint

The attending physician is bound by absolute professional secrecy (WMA, London, 1949; Geneva, 1948; Lisbon 1981, *Twelve principles of social security*, 1963). Even the company doctor appointed by an employer must respect professional secrecy (EEC Standing Committee of Doctors, 1969).

3. From the standpoint of religious moralities

a. *Catholic*
The rules of Catholic ethics explicitly affirm the doctor's obligation to respect professional secrecy. However, professional secrecy does not have an absolute value. It would not be ethically acceptable for secrecy to be placed in the service of crime or fraud.[1] In this particular case, the patient's illness may endanger the physical integrity of other people, and hence the doctor has a duty to inform the

---

1. Pius XII, *Broadcast speeches and messages*, Vol. VI, p. 191ff.

competent authorities if the patient, once informed of his condition, refuses to inform the employer himself.

b. *Protestant*

This is a question of conscience. We may imagine that as a first step, the doctor might try to convince the person that a job other than driving trams might be more appropriate. As a second step, he could warn him that the "secret" is too heavy for him to bear and that he himself is also – at least morally – responsible. As a third step (...), but here we must not try to think too far ahead (...).

c. *Jewish*

Judaism attaches great importance to the respect of professional secrecy. However, and despite the gravity of the violation of professional secrecy, Jewish law recognises that there are exceptions.

Respect for privacy and the inviolability of professional secrecy may not take precedence over protection of human lives and the safety of others. The absolute obligation to protect the lives of others obliges the doctor to take the measures he considers necessary to eliminate all dangers. The doctor must certainly inform the employer that the driver is unfit to drive a tram. Medical secrecy must be maintained with respect to the nature of the disease. The employer must not know what disease his employee suffers from, but must be made aware of the fact that the driver's state of health is incompatible with tram driving.

Non-revelation should be sanctioned, as no one has the right to put others' lives in danger.

d. *Muslim*

There are limits to the doctor's professional secrecy. It may be violated if there is a danger of damage to the physical integrity of another, as this is contrary to Muslim morality. In other words, the person involved must be faced with his responsibilities, which means that the patient must be persuaded to tell his employer of his illness.

e. *Buddhist*

The only possibility open to the patient's doctor is to persuade the patient to inform the company doctor and examine with him the possibility of switching to another job. The company doctor must maintain secrecy *vis-à-vis* the employer while seeking a redeployment solution.

4. From the standpoint of agnostic morality

The doctor must reveal the fact that the patient's disease can have dangerous

265

consequences, in order to avoid endangering innocent lives. However, he should not indicate the nature of the disease. He should help his patient obtain a job which is compatible with his state of health.

Right to confidentiality

A patient with Aids asks the doctor not to inform his or her partner of the diagnosis.

1. From the standpoint of international law

In the terms of Articles 10 (2) of the ECHR and 19 (3) of the Covenant on Civil and Political Rights, the partner's right to receive information of all kinds (stipulated by Articles 10 (1) of the ECHR and 19 (2) of the Covenant on Civil and Political Rights) may be subject to restrictions which, in accordance with the law, constitute necessary measures in a democratic society for the respect of the rights of others, that is the patient. Among these rights there is in particular the patient's right to respect of his private life, affirmed by Articles 8 (1) of the ECHR and 17 of the Covenant on Civil and Political Rights.

On the other hand, since the information concerned is intended to protect the partner's right to health, the patient's right to the respect of his private life is subject to restrictions and limitations provided for by law, which are necessary in a democratic society for the protection of the rights of others (Article 8 (2) of the ECHR).

It is thus for domestic legislation to decide: in such a decision, according to the established case-law of the Court, states have considerable freedom, but the interference with the exercise of the fundamental rights concerned must be necessary and proportionate (see also point 159 of the explanatory report appended to the BC).

As regards the latest developments in international law, reference should be made to the reply to case 45 and in particular to point 70 of the explanatory report appended to the BC, which specifically mentions the case of a disease transmittable to a partner. "In such a case, the possibility for prevention of the risk to the third party might, on the basis of Article 26, warrant his or her right taking precedence over the patient's right to privacy, as laid down in Article 10, paragraph 1, and as a result the right not to know, as laid down in paragraph 2. In any case, the right not to know of the person concerned may be opposed to the interest to be informed of another person and the interests of these two persons should be balanced by internal law".

It should also be pointed out that in the terms of points 2.2.1 and 2.2.3 of Recommendation R (87) 25, adopted by the Committee of Ministers of the Council of Europe on 26.11.1987, concerning a common European public health policy to fight the acquired immune deficiency syndrome (Aids), "screening should be in compliance with the usual strict requirements of informed consent and regulations for the confidentiality of data and individuals should be informed of a confirmed positive result of a blood test; they should be referred to competent medical and counselling services to be informed of precautions to be taken to protect their own health and to avoid spreading the infection to other individuals".

Aids being an infectious disease, Article 5.*e* of the ECHR, which states that no one shall be deprived of his liberty save in accordance with a procedure prescribed by law for the lawful detention of a person to prevent the spreading of infectious diseases might be applied. In the same sense, see Article 26 (1) of the BC and point 150 of the explanatory report, which particularly concerns serious infection diseases. Paragraph 48 of Recommendation R (89) 14 of the Committee of Ministers of the Council of Europe on the ethical issues of HIV infection in the health care and social settings nevertheless invites the authorities of member states to "not resort to restrictive measures such as quarantine and isolation for people infected with HIV or who have developed Aids".

As regards the problem of Aids and prisons, see Recommendation 1080 (1988) adopted by the Parliamentary Assembly of the Council of Europe on 30.6.1988, and in particular principle A.iii, according to which the governments of member states are invited to offer all prisoners the possibility of HIV tests and of counselling, while ensuring that the results of these tests remain secret except for the authorities directly concerned with the health and administration of the prisoners.

As regards European case-law, reference is made to the reply to case 45 and in particular the Commission Decision of 2.2.1995 in *Z* v. *Finland*.

It should also be pointed out that Article 6 of the Convention for the Protection of Individuals with Regard to Automatic Processing of Personal Data (Council of Europe, 28.11.1981-1.9.1982) stipulates that "personal data concerning health or sexual life may not be processed automatically unless domestic law provides appropriate safeguards".

2. From the ethical standpoint

The attending physician is bound by absolute professional secrecy (WMA, London, 1949; Geneva, 1948; Lisbon 1981; *The twelve principles of social security*, 1963). Even the company doctor appointed by an employer must respect professional secrecy (EEC Standing Committee of Doctors, 1969).

The WMA Declaration of Madrid (1987) requires that doctors advise their patients to inform their past and present partners that they may be carriers of the virus. Each confirmed case of Aids must be notified to the responsible authority without disclosure of the patient's identity.

The identity of people affected by Aids or carrying the HIV virus may not be disclosed unless the health of the community may be endangered.

A means must be devised of warning the sexual partners of infected persons while respecting as far as possible the confidential nature of information relating to these persons. This means must guarantee appropriate legal protection for doctors performing their professional duty by warning people who are running a risk.

3. From the standpoint of religious moralities

a. *Catholic*

According to the doctrine of the Catholic Church, professional secrecy does not have an absolute value.[1] In this case, as the issue is a contagious disease, the doctor is obliged to notify the health authority. The doctor must at least demand that the patient inform his or her partner of the diagnosis personally, as only knowledge of the past or future risk would allow him to take all necessary preventive measures. If the patient refuses or acts irresponsibly, the common good requires the doctor to inform the competent authorities, or even the patient's partner, himself.

b. *Protestant*

Why would the patient make this demand? What kind of "partner" can it be when such a "mortal" deception is cooked up? The doctor should provide the patient with an opportunity to explain all these points and to take his own responsibility seriously. Failing that, it is plain that the concern for the health – or even the life – of the partner in question must take precedence over that of respect for a desire which is at the very least questionable.

c. Jewish

Respect of privacy and inviolability of professional secrecy may not take precedence over protection of human lives and the safety of others. The absolute obligation to protect the lives of others obliges the doctor to take the measures he considers necessary to eliminate all dangers. Failure to reveal the truth may be sanctioned, as no one has the right to put others' lives in danger.

However, before revealing the diagnosis to the partner, the doctor must do everything possible to persuade the patient himself to make the revelation, and thus avoid breaking the rule of professional secrecy.

d. *Muslim*

There are limits to professional secrecy. To omit to inform a patient's partner that he or she has been diagnosed seropositive is to expose a human being to a risk of infection and possible damage to his or her integrity.

The alternative would be for the doctor to convince the seropositive individual to inform his or her partner. This is all the more important since, in addition to preventive measures (use of condoms), there are a number of drugs which can inhibit propagation of the virus. Islam prescribes fairness and honesty.

---

1. Pius XII, *Broadcast speeches and messages*, Vol. VI, p. 191ff.

e. *Buddhist*

The doctor must do all within his power to persuade the patient to accept his responsibilities, make him understand the risk to which he is exposing his partner(s) and convince him of the need to protect her, him or them by appropriate means.

4. From the standpoint of agnostic morality

The doctor should be able to reveal to the partner that the patient has Aids, but in the present state of the law he does not have this possibility. There is thus an ethical problem here.

We think that in this case medical secrecy can be violated in order to protect an innocent third party. Not to do so would amount to failure to assist a person in danger. Our decision will be communicated to a magistrate.

To be in accordance with the law we could follow the example of the fight against tuberculosis, where in derogation of medical secrecy the practitioner was obliged to declare all cases of this disease.

The general interest requires the legislator to take action on this point.

Acquired immune deficiency syndrome (Aids)

A surgeon routinely tests patients for HIV without their knowledge and refuses to operate on them if they prove seropositive.

1. From the standpoint of international law

The only text which deals with problems arising from Aids is Recommendation R (87) 25 adopted by the Committee of Ministers of the Council of Europe on 26.11.1987 (following Recommendations R (83) 8 and R (85) 12 concerning the screening of blood donors for Aids markers).

According to the first sub-paragraph of paragraph 2.2.3, "individuals, whether donors or not, should be informed of a confirmed positive result of a blood test". However, the provision takes no position on the legitimacy or otherwise of testing without the patient's knowledge.

Paragraph 2.2.1 of the same recommendation, which deals with screening, provides (in the first and second sub-paragraphs) that "systematic screening programmes should be fully implemented in respect of donations of blood, mother's milk, organs, tissues, cells and, in particular, semen donation in compliance with the usual strict requirements of informed consent and regulations for confidentiality of data; there should be no compulsory screening of the general population nor of particular population groups". In the light of the above provisions and of Articles 5 of the BC and 7 of the Covenant on Civil and Political Rights referred to above, the surgeon must not perform the test for HIV infection without the patient's prior consent.

As regards the second question, paragraph 2.2.3 of Recommendation R (87) 25 states that "if they take appropriate measures, health staff can usually avoid contamination; patients should, therefore, themselves be left to advise health staff of their seropositivity unless the patient has specifically authorised a doctor to pass on this information"; however, it gives no explicit reply to the question raised. See, in the same connection, sub-paragraph 3 of paragraph 2.4 ("staff who may have occupational exposure to infected fluids and secretions should be kept informed of sensible hygienic precautions to be taken both for themselves and for their clients").

As regards the refusal to operate on HIV-positive patients, reference should be made to Article 4 of the BC in connection with professional obligations and standards and Article 8 of the BC in connection with emergency situations (including point 58 of the explanatory report).

See also point 4 of Resolution 1989/11 of the UN Human Rights Committee adopted at the 45th Session on 2.3.1989 entitled "Non-discrimination in the health field", and WHO Resolutions cited in point 4 of the preamble, as Resolution E/CN.4/1994/L.60 adopted at the 50th Session (1994) and entitled "Persons infected with HIV or suffering from Aids". In this resolution the committee, expressing its concern at discriminatory laws and policies and the appearance of new forms of discrimination which prevent persons infected with HIV or suffering from Aids and their family and entourage from enjoying their fundamental rights and freedoms, calls upon states to ensure that their laws, policies and practices, including those adopted to combat HIV and Aids, respect the standards relating to human rights, and to revise their legislation and practices to ensure the respect of the private life and integrity of persons infected with HIV or suffering from Aids and those who are considered likely to risk contamination.

As regards compensation for the prejudice suffered by haemophiliacs infected by the Aids virus by blood transfusions, see among others Decision No. 333 B of 4.12.1995 in the *Bellet* case (*Commission* v. *France*) and Decision No. 317 of 24.5.1992 in the *Marlhens* case (*Commission* v. *France*).

2. From the ethical standpoint

According to the WMA Declaration on the treatment of Aids patients (Vienna, 1988): "Aids sufferers and seropositive persons should receive appropriate medical care; they must not be treated unfairly of suffer arbitrary or irrational discrimination in their daily life. Doctors respect the age-old tradition with consists of treating patients infected with contagious diseases with compassion and courage. This tradition must be continued in the face of this Aids epidemic."

Aids sufferers have the right to receive appropriate medical care given with compassion and respect of their human dignity. A doctor has no moral right to refuse to treat a patient whose malady comes within his field of competence simply because this patient is seropositive. Medical ethics does not authorise discrimination against certain categories of patient solely because they are seropositive. A person suffering from Aids needs to be treated appropriately and with compassion. A doctor who is not able to provide the care and services required by Aids patients should refer them to doctors and services equipped to provide this kind of care. The doctor (man or woman) is duty bound to care for the patient as well as he or she can until the patient is referred elsewhere.

In its Declaration of Marbella (1992) on the problems posed by the HIV epidemic, the WMA adds eleven new recommendations to national medical associations, in particular the study of ways to help improve measures to control HIV infection in hospitals and other medical establishments.

3. From the standpoint of religious moralities

a. *Catholic*

Routine screening for HIV on patients who are to undergo a surgical operation – as is already practised for infectious diseases such as viral hepatitis or syphilis – seems acceptable from the standpoint of Catholic morality because the surgeon and other members of the health staff have the right to take all possible preventive precautions (principle of the common good). The tests may be performed even without the patient's explicit consent, but presuming it, as this test carries no risks for the patient and furthermore is necessary for public health.

However, it is morally unacceptable for the surgeon to refuse to operate on them if they are positive: John Paul II, addressing doctors and all health staff, exhorted: "May your solicitude know no discrimination. Receive, interpret and honour the trust placed in you by your suffering brother."[1]

b. *Protestant*

This surgeon should think of changing jobs. His attitude does not seem to be technically justified and any discrimination *vis-à-vis* patients is unacceptable.

c. *Jewish*

Routine HIV testing without the patient's knowledge seems to me normal. Routine screening is carried out for other diseases and the purpose is to establish the patient's state of health so as to be able to better treat and help him.

However, the position of the doctor who refuses to give treatment seems to me immoral. In this case, as in the case of other contagious diseases, the doctor must take extra precautions to avoid contamination.

What would happen if we were to reach a form of medicine where the practitioner chose his patient?

The unhappy destiny is made to be put right. In all cases, patients must have doctors with them and not against them. The role of the doctor is to relieve pain and combat disease. The doctor's job has never been to execute the sentence, but always to commute the penalty. Such, it seems to me, is the very essence of medicine.

d. *Muslim*

Firstly, the patient who is to undergo surgical operation should not be screened for HIV without his knowledge. The test must be carried out with the patient's agreement, after he has been informed of the consequences and measures to be taken to prevent possible infection, and also in order that general hygiene

---

1. "Address to the participants in the 4th International Conference organised by the Pontifical Council for the Health Services", *L'Osservatore Romano* of 16 November 1989.

precautions may be reinforced to avoid transmission of the HIV infection from a seropositive patient to members of the hospital staff. Indeed, the results of screening should be covered by medical secrecy, but we may wonder whether the requirements of the struggle against an epidemic of particular gravity do not call for, if not derogations from, at least adaptations of the principles of medical secrecy. Moreover, in the present case, the surgeon cannot withdraw from his prime function, namely that of treating patients. All he can do is reinforce protective measures to prevent infection.

e. *Buddhist*

It is acceptable to make an HIV test before any surgery provided that the patient is informed. If the test is positive the surgeon still has to operate however, otherwise he is breaking the law by failing to assist a person in danger.

4. From the standpoint of agnostic morality

Routine screening for HIV is permissible, but not without the patient's knowledge.

If a patient refuses this test, the surgeon has the right not to operate. On the other hand, if the patient accepts the test and is found positive, the surgeon cannot morally refuse to operate nor can he invoke the conscience clause.

Acquired immune deficiency syndrome (Aids)

A patient who is HIV-positive requests a prosthetic operation on the penis. The urologist refuses on the grounds that the patient is HIV-positive.

1. From the standpoint of international law

The only text which deals with problems arising from Aids is Recommendation R (87) 25 adopted by the Committee of Ministers of the Council of Europe on 26.11.1987 (following Recommendations R (83) 8 and R (85) 12 concerning the screening of blood donors for Aids markers).

According to the first sub-paragraph of paragraph 2.2.3, "individuals, whether donors or not, should be informed of a confirmed positive result of a blood test".

Paragraph 2.2.3 of Recommendation R (87) 25 states that "if they take appropriate measures, health staff can usually avoid contamination; patients should, therefore, themselves be left to advise health staff of their seropositivity unless the patient has specifically authorised a doctor to pass on this information"; however, it gives no explicit reply to the question raised. See in the same connection sub-paragraph 3 of paragraph 2.4 *idem*; "staff who may have occupational exposure to infected fluids and secretions should be kept informed of sensible hygienic precautions to be taken both for themselves and for their clients". For the rest, see the reply to case 47.

2. From the ethical standpoint

According to the WMA Declaration on the treatment of Aids patients (Vienna, 1988), Aids patients and seropositive persons should receive appropriate medical care; they must not be treated with iniquity or suffer arbitrary or irrational discrimination in their everyday lives. Doctors respect the age-old tradition of treating patients afflicted with infectious diseases with compassion and courage. This tradition must be continued in the face of this Aids epidemic.

Aids patients have the right to receive appropriate medical care, administered with compassion and in respect of their human dignity. A doctor does not have a moral right to refuse to treat a patient whose disease comes within his present field of competence simply because the patient is seropositive. Medical ethics do not permit discrimination against certain categories of patient solely based on the fact that they are seropositive. A person suffering from Aids needs to be treated appropriately and with compassion. A doctor who is unable to provide the care and the services required by Aids patients must refer them to doctors and services equipped to provide this kind of care. The doctor (man or woman) must care for the patient to the best of his or her ability until the patient can be received elsewhere.

In its Declaration of Marbella (1992) on the problems posed by the HIV epidemic, the WMA adds eleven new recommendations to national medical associations, in particular the study of ways to help improve measures to control HIV infection in hospitals and other medical establishments.

3. From the standpoint of religious moralities

a. *Catholic*
There is no official position of the magisterium on this point. On the basis of the therapeutic principle,[1] supposing that the operation to insert a penile prosthesis is medically advisable and efficacious – at least in psychological terms – the urologist's refusal on the sole grounds of seropositivity seems to us morally unacceptable.

b. *Protestant*
At all events, whatever the technical answer, the fundamental question in this case concerns the use made – what for? – of the patient's sexuality. It is probable that a good exchange on this subject will lead to shared convictions. In any case, it would seem difficult in the present case to refer to some kind of "conscience clause" for the doctors.

c. *Jewish*
In this case, it seems to me difficult to give a categoric reply. Each case must be treated on its own merits. The doctor must take into account a number of factors, among them:
– the causes of the disease;
– the family situation;
– the social context.
The doctor must also take into account the fact that penile surgery is very difficult for patients psychologically, particularly for a patient who is seropositive. Also this technique is less and less popular, as it may be replaced by a papaverine injection.
At all events, if the patient is married, it is indispensable that his wife should be informed.

d. *Muslim*
In this case, the seropositive patient is aware of his condition. The surgeon is obliged to carry out the surgical operation, and it is up to him to reinforce protective measures to prevent accidental contamination for himself and for members of the hospital staff.

---

1. Pius XII, AAS 45 (1953), pp. 674-675 and AAS 48 (1956), pp. 461-462.

e. *Buddhist*

It is acceptable to do an HIV test before any surgery provided that the patient is informed. If the test is positive the surgeon still has to operate however, otherwise he is breaking the law by failing to assist a person in danger if the operation is necessary.

4. From the standpoint of agnostic morality

This is a borderline case.

The urologist can invoke the conscience clause if he considers that the operation would be very likely to favour the propagation of the disease.

277

Individual responsibility

A woman of 53 is an alcoholic; she suffers from cirrhosis and repeated haemorrhaging from oesophageal varices.
Extensive transfusions are required each time.
The patient refuses to stop drinking alcohol with a view to alleviating or eliminating these haemorrhages.
The issues are the doctors' position and the price to be paid by society for each transfusion for which the patient is herself responsible.

1. From the standpoint of international law

There are as yet no binding international legal instruments laying down the duty of each individual to protect his or her own health.

Admittedly, nobody doubts that, in western legal systems, each subjective right implies a corresponding duty on the part of its holder, but the same cannot be said of international law, particularly as there is no provision in force on which such a conclusion may be based. However, see section B of Recommendation R (80) 4 of the Committee of Ministers of the Council of Europe concerning the patient as an active participant in his own treatment.

See also point 7.vi of Recommendation 1153 adopted on 26.4.1991 by the Parliamentary Assembly of the Council of Europe on concerted European policies for health, which invites the Committee of Ministers to make "continuous effects to combat effectively addiction to and dependence on drugs, alcohol and tobacco (bearing in mind an increase in tobacco smoking among women)".

If the refusal to abstain from alcohol was brought about by deterioration of the woman's mental faculties, reference should be made to Article 5.e of the ECHR and Article 7 of the BC. According to the former, "everyone has the right to liberty and security of person. No one shall be deprived of his liberty save in the following cases and in accordance with a procedure prescribed by law: (...) the lawful detention of (...) alcoholics", and according to the second, "subject to protective conditions prescribed by law, including supervisory, control and appeal procedure, a person who has a mental disorder of a serious nature may be subjected, without his or her consent, to an intervention aimed at treating his or her mental disorder only where, without such treatment, serious harm is likely to result to his or her health". According to point 54 of the explanatory report appended to the BC, "such a risk exists, for example, when a person suffers from a suicidal tendency and is therefore a danger to himself or herself". In less serious cases, Article 6 (3) of the BC stipulates that "where, according to law, an adult does not have the capacity to consent to an intervention for his or her direct benefit (Article 6 (1) idem) because of a mental disability (or) a disease (...), the intervention may only be carried out with the authorisation of his or her representative or an authority or a person or body provided for by law. The individual concerned shall as far as possible take part in the authorisation procedure".

2. From the ethical standpoint

The doctor must not base his intervention on the patient's conduct. It his duty to inform the patient and, in this case, he is obliged to inform the patient on the risks she is running as a result of alcohol (WMA, Tokyo, Declaration on abusive drugs, 1975). But the decision on treatment does lie with the doctor (CIO, Quality of care, 1983; WMA Patients' rights, Lisbon, 1981).

The twelve principles of social security (WMA, 1963, XI) state that, in the patient's best interests, there may be no restriction on the doctor's right to prescribe drugs and to perform any other form of treatment deemed appropriate on the basis of recognised medical standards.

3. From the standpoint of religious moralities

a. *Catholic*

Every individual has the duty to keep his or her body intact and to make all kinds of efforts to keep it as it is. No one is the absolute master of his own body and mind, which means that he cannot freely dispose of himself as he likes.[1] The doctor's duty is to inform the patient of the risks of alcoholism and its consequences, and he may in extreme cases prescribe hospitalisation. However, it would not appear that he can require hospitalisation and treatment on a coercive basis, unless recourse to compulsory health treatment becomes necessary as a result of a loss of consciousness by the patient or because of danger to the public.

b. *Protestant*

Why does the patient "refuse"? No doubt she is unable to free herself from her alcoholism, which does not necessarily mean that she does not wish to do so. In any case, alcoholism is a disease made up of many components and it can only be treated by taking the person and his or her environment into account.

c. *Jewish*

Society must conduct anti-alcohol and anti-smoking campaigns and invest the necessary funds in prevention rather than in treatment of these scourges. Moral

---

1. Pius XII, *Broadcast speeches and messages*, Vol. XIV, 1952.

pressure must be exerted on these people to dissuade them from persisting in their current conduct. At all events, society must assume its responsibilities *vis-à-vis* these patients and give them the care they require, whatever the costs. These patients are victims of an evil of our societies. Society must under no circumstances stick its head in the sand and seek to ignore these unfortunate human beings.

d. *Muslim*

The doctor should inform the patient who is suffering from cirrhosis with complications of the risk to which alcohol is exposing her. A disintoxication cure should be prescribed. At all events, it is for society to conduct anti-alcohol campaigns. Where these fail, as they do for some individuals, society must assume its responsibilities and provide suitable care.

e. *Buddhist*

Society must take responsibility for the problems it causes, directly or indirectly. This type of situation cannot be governed by general rules as the problem cannot be assessed without reference to the particular individual circumstances. However, the patient must be made to face up to her responsibilities.

4. From the standpoint of agnostic morality

The doctor should not take account of the circumstances which have led the patient to the present stage of the disease but should place at her disposal all the technical resources he has available to relieve her suffering.

On the other hand, he must try to persuade her to modify her attitude so as not to aggravate the disease, this being an integral part of the treatment.

In the case of objective refusal on the part of his patient, the doctor must in no way act as judge by depriving her of part or all of the care deemed essential.

The society should permit him to exercise his art under optimal conditions.

It is only in the case of restriction of a technical or financial nature that the doctor may, in all conscience, have to make a therapeutic choice as a function of the patient's case history and motivations.

Medical examinations

A man aged 45 is contractually bound to undergo a medical check-up.
Unfavourable results are passed on to the private sector employer (Aids, drug addiction) without the patient's knowledge.
The doctor's position: respect for human rights.

1. From the standpoint of international law

Both Article 7 of the Covenant on Civil and Political Rights and Article 5 of the BC, already mentioned several times, prohibit making anybody submit to any kind of intervention in the field of health (including for diagnosis and prevention) without his free and informed consent, consent which may be withdrawn at any time. As a result, the clause requiring the worker to submit to a check-up needs to be accepted by him.

As regards the results of the check-up, the patient (Articles 10 (1) of the ECHR, 19 (2) of the Covenant on Civil and Political Rights and 10 (2) of the BC) has the right to know them, unless he has expressed the wish not to be informed (Article 10 (2) of the BC). Please note in passing that in this case, the right not to know may be subject in national law to restrictions in the interest of the patient himself. Point 70 of the explanatory report appended to the BC puts it as follows: "Furthermore, it may be of vital importance for patients to know certain facts about their health, even though they have expressed the wish not to know them. For example, the knowledge that they have a predisposition to a disease might enable them to take preventive measures. In this case, a doctor's duty to provide care, as laid down in Article 4, might conflict with the patient's right not to know. (…) It will be for domestic law to indicate whether the doctor, in the light of the circumstances of the particular case, may make an exception to the right not to know" (Article 10 (3) of the BC).

As a result, there is no doubt about the illegitimacy of communication without the patient's knowledge in international human rights law. Such communication would also violate the respect of the patient's private life protected by Article 8 (1) of the ECHR, and Article 10 (1) of the BC: "everyone has the right to respect for private life in relation to information about his or her health", unless the national law obliged the doctor, as a public authority, to ignore the wording of these provisions under the terms of Articles 8 (2) of the ECHR and 26 (1) of the BC.

As regards administrative proceedings brought for refusal to submit to an alcohol test (imposition of a fine with deprivation of freedom in the case of non-payment) see Court Decisions Nos. 328 B of 23.10.1995 in the *Umlauft* case (*Commission* v. *Austria*), 329 B, (same date) in the *Palaoro* case (*Commission* v. *Austria*) and 328 C, (same date) in the *Pfarrmeier* case (*Commission* v. *Austria*).

See also, *mutatis mutandis*, the Commission Decision of 2.12.1995 in *Z* v. *Finland* and Decision No. 306 A of 9.2.1995 in *Vereniging Weekblad Bluf!* case (*Commission* v. *France*) and the Decision (no number) of 27.3.1996 in the *Goodwin* case (*Commission* v. *United Kingdom*).

2. From the ethical standpoint

The attending doctor is bound by absolute professional secrecy (WMA, London, 1949; Geneva, 1948; Lisbon, 1981; *The twelve principles of social security*, 1963). Even the company doctor appointed by the employer must respect professional secrecy (EECSCD, 1969).

3. From the standpoint of religious moralities

a. *Catholic*

It is morally acceptable for society to satisfy itself of a worker's state of health, but the results of medical examinations must be allowed to influence only as regards fitness for the work in question and as a guarantee of the safety of other people who may be associated with this work.

b. *Protestant*

Inasmuch as the patient's condition is not likely to cause damage to third parties, the doctor is bound to respect professional secrecy. True, the patient and his employer are bound by a contract, but it is for the patient to respect it and not for another to act in his place. This applies only if the doctor is not one appointed by the employer, by whom the patient must be examined under his contract. In that case, the problem does not arise.

c. *Jewish*

A medical examination with a view to protecting the other workers from risk of contamination is certainly indispensable. In this case, the doctor is bound to inform the employing authorities of the nature of the condition if it is in any way related to the work.

d. *Muslim*

In principle, there may be no discrimination in recruitment against people who are HIV-positive or drug dependent.

However, it is common practice for candidates to undergo a medical examination prior to recruitment, the purpose being to discover whether the individual is not suffering from a morbid condition which may be dangerous for those around him. Use of hard drugs may be considered a morbid condition, particularly in certain high-risk professions. Similarly, carriers of the Aids virus may propagate the virus in certain conditions. However, while the doctor is bound by medical secrecy, respect of human rights must also be taken into consideration. Life in society imposes on each citizen limits to his rights for the sake of the security and health of all.

Consequently:

1. the candidate for employment must be warned of the test to which he is to be subjected and must give his consent;

2. the two tests (Aids, drugs) should not be carried out as a routine measure, but in relation to the real risks associated with the occupation in question;

3. the company doctor must inform the recruit of the results straight away. It shall be for the doctor to judge whether or not the candidate is capable of exercising the occupation in question, and, as a last resort, medical secrecy must be raised in certain conditions.

e. *Buddhist*

Since this medical examination is part of his contract, the results should be communicated directly to him by the company doctor, who is the only person capable of judging whether the person can continue to work in the post concerned or not.

4. From the standpoint of agnostic morality

The doctor cannot violate medical secrecy in this case, that is communicate the diagnosis to the employer. On the other hand, he must communicate to the employer the employee's fitness or otherwise to fulfil his functions. At the patient's request the doctor can tell him precisely what affliction(s) he has, and the patient is free to use this information as he thinks fit.

Compulsory treatment

A child aged 3 suffers from congenital heart malformation.
Open-heart surgery is required.
The parents (Jehovah's Witnesses) refuse their consent.
The operation is not urgent (refusal to authorise the pre-operative transfusion essential in this case).

1. From the standpoint of international law

Protection of the child's right to life (Articles 2 of the ECHR; 6 (1) of the Covenant on Civil and Political Rights; 8 (1) of the Convention on the Rights of the Child) requires that, despite such justification as may be drawn from the parents' fundamental right to freedom of religion and freedom to manifest this religion (Articles 9 (1) of the ECHR and 18 (1) of the Covenant on Civil and Political Rights) and their right to provide their children with religious and moral education in conformity with their own convictions (Articles 18 (4) of the Covenant on Civil and Political Rights and 14 (2) of the Convention on the Rights of the Child), their refusal should not be taken into account by the doctor, even if the patient's immediate survival is not at stake.

The fact is that the parents' exercise of their fundamental rights must not destroy or impair the fundamental rights of the child (Articles 9 (2) of the ECHR and 18 (3) of the Covenant on Civil and Political Rights), all the less so because the standards concerning the right to life, individual freedom and the prohibition of torture constitute the "hard core" of the international system of human rights and thus admit no exception or derogations.

The Convention on the Rights of the Child also stipulates in many places that in all decisions concerning the child, the child's interests must be paramount and, more specifically, compels the parents (or where necessary the child's legal representatives) to guide the child in the exercise of the right of freedom of conscience and religion "in a manner consistent with the evolving capacities of the child" (Article 14 (2)). As regards the BC, Article 6 contains a general provision concerning persons without the capacity to consent to a medical intervention in accordance with Article 5 (Article 6 (1)) and one specifically concerned with minors (Article 6 (2)).

The general principle laid down is that "an intervention may only be carried out on a person who does not have the capacity to consent, for his or her direct benefit" (as regards research and the removal of organs and tissues from living donors incapable of consent, reference should be made to Articles 17 and 20 *idem*, as well as to Article 26 (1) and (2) *idem*).

As regards minors in particular, Article 6 (2) stipulates that: "Where, according to law, a minor does not have the capacity to consent to an intervention, the intervention may only be carried out with the authorisation of his or her representative, an authority, or a person or body provided for by law". The problem of the refusal of authorisation is thus not dealt with *ex professo*. In fact, Article 6 (4) limits itself to adding that "The representative, the authority, the person or the body mentioned in paragraphs 2 and 3 above shall be given, under the same conditions, the information referred to in Article 5", and Article 6 (5) that "The authorisation referred to in paragraphs 2 and 3 above may be withdrawn at any time in the best interests of the person concerned", subject, however, to Article 26 (1) of the BC.

The parents' refusal alone should not suffice to prevent the essential pre-operation transfusion, even if it is not a case of emergency, the intervention and the authorisation of an authority or person or body provided for by law being essential. In the case of conflict between the parents and the authority, person or body provided for by national law, it will be for the latter to decide and to settle the problem, bearing in mind the fundamental rights of the child.

As regards alternatives to transfusion, in particular with respect to Jehovah's Witnesses, reference should be made to the reply to case 82.

As regards minors capable of understanding, Article 12 (1) of the Convention on the Rights of the Child guarantees the child the right to freely express his opinion on any matter concerning him, the child's opinion being duly taken into account according to his age and degree of maturity, and Article 6 (2) of the BC stipulates that "the opinion of the minor shall be taken into consideration as an increasingly determining factor in proportion to his or her age and degree of maturity".

In their turn, point 45 of the explanatory report notes that "the second paragraph prescribes that where a minor is not capable of consenting to an intervention, the intervention may be carried out only with the consent of parents who have custody of the minor, his or her legal representative or any person or body provided for by law. However, as far as possible, with a view to the preservation of the autonomy of persons with regard to interventions affecting their health, the second part of paragraph 2 states that the opinion of minors should be regarded as an increasingly determining factor in proportion to their age and capacity for discernment. This means that in certain situations which take account of the nature and seriousness of the intervention as well as the minor's age and ability to understand, the minor's opinion should increasingly carry more weight in the final decision. This could even lead to the conclusion that the consent of a minor should be necessary, or at least sufficient for some interventions. Note that the provision of the second sub-paragraph of paragraph 2 is consistent with Article 12 of the United Nations Convention on the Rights of the Child, which stipulates that States Parties shall assure the child who is capable of forming his or her own views the right to express those views freely in all matters affecting the child, the views of the child being given due weight in accordance with the age and maturity of the child".

Along these lines see also the Decisions of the Court Nos. 255 of 23.6.1993 in the *Hoffmann* case (*Commission* v. *Austria*) and 260 of 24.6.1993 in the *Kokkinakis* case (*Commission* v. *Greece*), as well as, *mutatis mutandis,* and Commission Decision of 22.5.1995 on the admissibility of Application No. 20948/92 (*Isiltan* v. *Turkey*).

2. From the ethical standpoint

The WMA has set out patients' rights in the Declaration of Lisbon, in which it is stated that "a doctor must always act according to his conscience and in the patient's best interests".

3. From the standpoint of religious moralities

a. *Catholic*

According to Catholic morality, it is licit for society to exercise authority to save the child's life, even against the will of the family based on religious reasons: religious freedom is subordinate to the right to physical integrity and must respect the nature and dignity of the human person.[1]

b. *Protestant*

The solution indicated above as necessary under international law seems a perfectly sound one.

c. *Jewish*

The law sees no objection to a blood transfusion where it is intended to save a patient's life or relieve his condition. "To treat a patient in danger of death, everything is allowed – except that which involves the three irremissible crimes: idolatry, debauchery and murder."[2]

d. *Muslim*

Where a surgeon finds that a child whose parents are Jehovah's Witnesses needs a surgical operation, protection of the child's rights must take precedence over any other considerations. If necessary, a blood transfusion must be carried out even if the parents object to it. In Islam, the physical and mental integrity of the individual is paramount.

---

1. Second Vatican Council, *Dignitatis Humanae,* 2, AAS 58 (1966), pp. 929-941.
2. *Pessahim,* 25 a.

e. *Buddhist*

The doctors must try to explain to the parents what is at stake and what can be done. The child must be treated even without their consent, according to the principle of providing the necessary assistance to all living creatures.

4. From the standpoint of agnostic morality

Parental authority cannot permit the child's health to be endangered by refusing to let it have a blood transfusion.

The existing decisions in fact concern only urgent or emergency situations (where the life of a minor incapable of discernment is in immediate danger).

Right to a healthy environment

A child of 10 is found to have lead in the blood.
Emissions (fumes) from a nearby chemical works.
Attitude of society.

1. From the standpoint of international law

Article 12 of the Covenant on Economic Social and Cultural Rights states that the States Parties to it "recognise the right of everyone to the enjoyment of the highest obtainable standard of physical and mental health"; paragraph 2 and its sub-paragraphs *a* and *b* of the same article specify that "the steps to be taken by the States Parties (...) to achieve the full realisation of this right shall include those necessary for: the provision for the healthy development of the child and the improvement of all aspects of environmental and industrial hygiene".

In the case put forward here, the child's health has already been damaged by emissions from the factory which is near his house; the doctors responsible for health inspections in factories and the factories inspectorate therefore have a duty to intervene so that the harmful fume emissions cease or are cleansed by appropriate technology. Moreover, since ILO Convention 139/1974 concerning Prevention and Control of Occupational Hazards caused by Carcinogenic Substances and Agents is addressed to company doctors and factory inspectors, they have a duty to implement the measures stipulated in the convention in order that any damage to workers' health should immediately cease.

Article 2 (1) of the BC stipulates that "the interests and welfare of the human being shall prevail over the sole interest of society" and Article 4 *idem* provides that "any intervention in the health field (...) must be carried out in accordance with relevant professional obligations and standards", the term "intervention" here being understood in a general sense (point 29 of the explanatory report).

Points 31 and 32 of the explanatory report appended to the BC point out, however, that "the content of professional standards (...) is not identical in all countries. The same medical duties may vary slightly from one society to another. However, the fundamental principles of the practice of medicine apply in all countries. Doctors, and, in general, all professionals who participate in a medical act are subject to legal and ethical imperatives. They must act with care and competence (...)".

See also Decision No. 303 C of 9.12.1994 in the in the *López Ostra* case (*Commission* v. *Spain*), concerning the harm caused to the applicant's health by emanations of gases, smells and pollutants from a treatment plant for waste waters contaminated with chlorine and wastes from a number of tanneries, a plant built twelve metres from the applicant's home. She alleged infringement of Article 8 of the ECHR in the first place.

"On the basis of medical reports and expert opinions produced by the government or the applicant, (...) the Commission noted, *inter alia*, that hydrogen sulphide emissions from the plant exceeded the permitted limit and could endanger the health of those living nearby and that there could be a causal link between those emissions and the applicant's daughter's ailments (...). Naturally, severe environmental pollution may affect individuals' well-being and prevent them from enjoying their homes in such a way as to affect their private and family life adversely, without, however, seriously endangering their health. Whether the question is analysed in terms of a positive duty on the state – to take reasonable and appropriate measures to secure the applicant's rights under paragraph 1 of Article 8 – as the applicant wishes in her case, or in terms of an 'interference by a public authority' to be justified in accordance with paragraph 2, the applicable principles are broadly similar. In both contexts a fair balance has to be struck between the competing interests of the individual and of the community as a whole, and in any case the state enjoys a certain margin of appreciation (...). At all events, the Court considers that in the present case, even supposing that the municipality did fulfil the functions assigned to it by domestic law (...) it need only establish whether the national authorities took the measures necessary for protecting the applicant's right to respect for her home and for her private and family life under Article 8 (...). The Court notes, however, that the family had to bear the nuisance caused by the plant for over three years before moving house with all the attendant inconveniences. They moved only when it became apparent that the situation could continue indefinitely and when Mrs López Ostra's daughter's paediatrician recommended that they do so (...). Having regard to the foregoing, and despite the margin of appreciation left to the respondent state, the Court considers that the state did not succeed in striking a fair balance between the interest of the town's economic well-being – that of having a waste treatment plant – and the applicant's effective enjoyment of her right to respect for her home and her private and family life. There has accordingly been violation of Article 8" (paragraphs 49, 51, 55 and 59 of the judgment).

See also the Commission Decision of 17.5.1990 on Application No. 13728/88 (*X* v. *France*), as well as, from the standpoint of Article 10 of the ECHR, the Commission Decision of 6.7.1995 on the admissibility of Application No. 14967/89 (*Anna Maria Guerra and thirty-nine other women* v. *Italy*).

2. From the ethical standpoint

The Declaration of São Paulo (WMA, 1976) on pollution invites doctors to devote themselves to educating the public and applying community and environment protection programmes.

3. From the standpoint of religious moralities

a. *Catholic*

Protecting children from pollution-related diseases is part of the duties of the public health authorities. It is right for society to organise an appropriate service in recognition of the human right to life and health care.[1]

b. *Protestant*

In this case, it would be wise to check whether other people in the district are not suffering from the same ills, and to take the necessary sociopolitical and economic measures.

c. *Jewish*

The Talmud denounces any source of contamination, particularly the nausea-inducing emissions which harm the good air of urban areas. The *Mishna*[2] requires that all kinds of pollution be kept away from towns, for instance dead bodies, tanneries, etc. Even barns where grain is winnowed should not be within the town boundaries because of the dust and straw.

Today, in the face of the ill effects of pollution in all its forms, the health authorities are bound to take all measures to ensure that everyone enjoys a healthy environment. They have a duty not only to protect the citizen against the dangers of all forms of pollution, but also to protect flora and fauna. Strict measures must be taken whenever they are required to guarantee society a healthy environment and in order to try to avoid disasters which can have very serious consequences for the individual in society.

d. *Muslim*

Society must take all the measures necessary to protect the health of all human beings. In the case of pollution from chemical works, for instance, which can damage the physical integrity of human beings, protection of which is a particularly sacred principle in Islam, company doctors and factory inspectors are responsible for the consequences.

e. *Buddhist*

Society must take all necessary steps to protect all people in equitable fashion and ensure that the polluter remedies the situation and assumes full responsibility for the consequences.

---

1. John Paul II, *Speech of 21 October 1980 to participants in two medical congresses of the St Luke Medico-biological Union.*
2. *Mishna Baba Batra,* 2, 9-10.

4. From the standpoint of agnostic morality

The contaminated child has the right:

– first, to be protected by action on the part of the factory to stop the emission of the chemicals concerned;

– second, to just compensation, paid by the agent responsible for the damage, or if this agent cannot pay, by the social insurance system.

Natural disasters

International aid in cases of earthquakes, tidal waves, destruction of energy sources, drug stocks or means of communication.

1. From the standpoint of international law

There are a number of European agreements providing for mutual assistance, exchanges and donations in cases of natural disaster: see European Agreement on the Exchange of Therapeutic Substances of Human Origin (Council of Europe, 15.12.1958-1.1.1959) and the Additional Protocol thereto (1.1.1983); the Agreement on the Temporary Importation, Free of Duty, of Medical, Surgical and Laboratory Equipment for Use on Free Loan in Hospitals and other Medical Institutions for Purposes of Diagnosis or Treatment (Council of Europe, 28.4.1959-29.7.1960) and the Additional Protocol thereto (1.1.1983) and the European Agreement on the Exchange of Tissue-Typing Reagents (Council of Europe, 17.9.1974-23.4.1977) and the Additional Protocol thereto (1976). See also Recommendation R (79) 5 adopted by the Committee of Ministers of the Council of Europe on 14.3.1979 concerning international exchange and transportation of human substances. Finally, see Article 2 (1) of the Covenant on Economic and Social Rights, the European Agreement on the Exchange of Blood-Grouping Reagents (Council of Europe, 14.5.1962-14.10.1962) and the Additional Protocol thereto (1.1.1983); the European Agreement on Mutual Assistance in the Matter of Special Medical Treatments and Climatic Facilities (Council of Europe, 14.5.192-15.6.1962) and Resolution (68) 32 adopted by the Ministers' Deputies of the Council of Europe on 31.10.1968 concerning the establishment in Amsterdam of a European blood bank of rare groups.

See also the documentation concerning the activities of the UN before and after the designation of the 1990s as the "International decade for natural disaster reduction" (Docs. A/44/332/Add. 1 and 2 – E/1989/114/Add. 1 and 2; A/45/271 – E/1990/78).

As regards the General Assembly, reference should also be made to resolutions:
– 2816 (XXVI) of 14.12.1971: Assistance in cases of natural disasters and other disaster situations;
– 3440 (XXX) of 9.12.1975: Assistance in cases of natural disasters and other disaster situations;
– 34/55 of 29.11.1979: Office of the UN Natural Disaster Relief Co-ordinator;
– 36/225 of 17.12.1981: Strengthening the capacity of the United Nations system to respond to natural disasters and other disaster situations;
– 39/207 of 17.12.1984: Special Economic and Disaster Assistance Office of the Natural Disaster Relief Co-ordinator;

– 41/201 of 8.12.1986: Office of the UN Natural Disaster Relief Co-ordinator;

– 42/169 of 11.12.1987: International decade for natural disaster reduction;

– 43/131 of 8.12.1988: Humanitarian assistance to victims of natural disasters and similar emergency situations;

– 43/202 of 20.12.1988: International decade for natural disaster reduction;

– 44/224 of 22.12.1989: International co-operation in the monitoring, assessment and anticipation of environmental threats and in assistance in cases of environmental emergency;

– 44/236 of 22.12.1989: International decade for natural disaster reduction and International Framework of Action for the International decade for natural disaster reduction;

– 45/100 of 14.12.1990: Humanitarian assistance to victims of natural disasters and similar emergency situations;

– 43/204 of 15.12.1990: Humanitarian assistance to victims of natural disasters and similar emergency situations;

– 46/182 of 19.12.1991: Strengthening of the co-ordination of humanitarian emergency assistance of the United Nations;

– 48/57 of 14.12.1993: Strengthening of the co-ordination of humanitarian emergency assistance of the United Nations.

As regards ECOSOC, reference should be made to documents:

– E/1992/94 of 8.7.1992: Office of the UN Natural Disaster Relief Co-ordinator: Report of the Secretary General;

– E/1993/90 of 21.6.1993: Co-ordination of humanitarian assistance: emergency relief and the continuum to rehabilitation and development.

As regards the Human Rights Committee, reference should be made to Resolutions:

– 1989.42 of 6.3.1989: Movement and dumping of toxic and dangerous products and wastes;

– 1993.90 of 10.3.1993: Movement and dumping of toxic and dangerous products and wastes;

– 1993.70 of 8.8.1993: Human rights and mass exoduses;

– 1994.65 of 9.3.1994: Human rights and the environment.

As regards the WHO, reference should be made for example to Resolutions:

– WHA 34.18 of May 1981;

– WHA 34.26 of May 1981;

– WHA 36.29 of May 1983;

– WHA 39.12 of May 1986;

– WHA 42.24 of May 1989;

– WHA 46.6 of May 1993.

As regards the ICRC, see in particular the "Basic rules of international humanitarian law" to be used by Red Cross and Red Crescent first aiders.

2. From the ethical standpoint

In disasters, calamities and nuclear wars, doctors should fulfil their obligations associated with emergencies in time of war: the doctor shall give the care immediately required without consideration of sex, race, nationality, religion or opinion.

They shall continue to give their care as long as their presence is needed (WMA, Havana, 1956).

Further, given the medical resources available, a doctor is required, for instance in case of nuclear war, to refrain from undue prolongation of life, that is extraordinary treatment which cannot be expected to provide the patient with any benefits. This does not release the doctor from the obligation to assist the dying by means of sedatives and drugs to suitably alleviate his end (WMA, Venice, 1983).

The WMA Declaration of Stockholm (1994) on medical ethics in disaster situations gives doctors precise instructions regarding priorities in the triage of victims, extreme emergencies, relations with victims, dignified management of bereavement, relations of reserve and secrecy with third parties, the duties of paramedical assistants, the need for training and reduced liability for the doctors who should receive for this mission the assistance and protection of governments, without discrimination according to race or religion.

3. From the standpoint of religious moralities

a. *Catholic*

International aid is morally compulsory and is sanctioned by the principle of subsidiarity.[1] In this way, international institutions may render enormous services to the human race and "the Church is glad to view the spirit of true brotherhood existing in all spheres between Christians and non-Christians as it seeks to intensify its untiring efforts to alleviate the enormity of human misery".[2]

b. *Protestant*

The vastness of the questions raised makes it difficult to reply in only a few lines. However, several simple principles should be recalled to mind:

1. all human beings live in the same world and all its parts are interdependent; what happens in one place necessarily has – or will have – an impact (positive or negative) elsewhere on the planet;

2. at all times, popular wisdom – echoed by the gospels – has reiterated that it is advisable to do as you would be done by: "all things whatsoever ye would that men should do to you, do ye even so to them" (Matthew, 7, v. 12; Luke, 6, v. 31);

---

1. *Gaudium et Spes*, No. 86 c.
2. *Idem*, No. 84.

3. in this system of faith, this rule of reciprocity is transcended and gives way to attitudes of giving without reward and of love;

4. too much utopia and too many appeals to man's better nature are counterproductive. A requirement or a law which cannot be met or respected throws a mortal suspicion on the very principle behind the requirement or law. We should therefore be wary of programmes which are too much of a good thing and claim to guarantee everyone unclouded happiness, as they rapidly prove illusory and devalue the very idea of possible plans and improvements, thereby proving completely counterproductive; however, conversely, it is true that nothing that is profoundly human is achieved without dreams, without hope and (...) without faith – which is always a gamble on a future which is a priori unrealistic.

5. laboriously, amidst the vicissitudes of life and history, through the complexity of the situations it faces, mankind is called to trace an – ethical – path towards an ever more human world, guided by the thoughts set out above.

c. *Jewish*

"That thy brother may live with thee"[1] is the biblical commandment which obliges us to come to the aid of our human brother in distress and to help him. The right of the poor to help and the sick to care and succour is incontestable in the biblical text.

The Hebrew word which is used to refer to the charitable duty to help those in distress is significant: *tzedaka*, from the same root as *tzedek*, which means justice, suggests a concept broader than justice.

The concept of charity-justice considered fundamental by the Bible obliges us to combat all poverty and remedy social inequalities. Assistance to a person whose life is in danger is strictly imperative. "He who sees another drowning in a river or being dragged off by a wild beast (...) has the imperative duty to save him".[2]

In all cases and whatever the system of the affected country, international health assistance must be able to do its duty to help, succour and heal. There must be no limits to this assistance. It must be given spontaneously, whatever the reason for the disaster.

d. *Muslim*

The Islamic view of international society or the human community is a pluralistic one based on coexistence in peace, co-operation and solidarity. Recognition of and respect for the other (non-Muslim) are fundamental tenets of Islam. As stated in verse 44 of Sura V, "We have sent down the law (Towrat) wherein are guidance and

---

1. Lev., 25, v. 36.
2. Sanhedrin, 73 *a*.

light (...)" the same goes for Christians; verse 47 of the same Sura is plain: "And whoso will not judge by what God hath sent down – such are the Infidels". In a general way, the Koran recommends the greatest tolerance in matters of religion, freedom and respect of all opinions. Verses to this effect abound. "Let there be no compulsion in Religion" says verse 256 of Sura II.

Moreover, the idea of the unity of the human family and an appeal to better knowledge of one another, co-operation and justice in relations between peoples are set out in two Sura of the Koran: Sura LX; verse 8, and Sura V, verse 8. Similarly, in one Hadith: it is written that "men are equal like the teeth of a comb". Finally, we may cite in the same context of human brotherhood verse 13 of Sura XLIX: "O men! Verily, we have created you of a male, and a female; and we have divided you into peoples and tribes, that ye might have knowledge one of another. Truly the most worthy of honour in the sight of God is he who feareth Him most".

e. *Buddhist*

All people are interdependent and should act in solidarity, giving aid and assistance in all circumstances, all the more so in the case of disasters.

4. From the standpoint of agnostic morality

In such a case international aid is essential. It is a manifestation of human solidarity. A very substantial and permanent global budget should be made available at international level, perhaps administered by the UN. Structural aid should be provided for all victims.

296

Free circulation of information

Databanks protected by professional secrecy.
Anonymous epidemiological statistics.

1. From the standpoint of international law

Medical databanks could, if they were not protected by professional secrecy, constitute or give rise to "arbitrary or unlawful interference with (...) privacy, family", etc., as prohibited by Article 17 (1) and (2) of the Covenant on Civil and Political Rights and Article 8 of the ECHR.

Furthermore, it is easy to imagine that unrestricted access to the data contained in computers could give rise to forms of discrimination (for instance in access to employment) prohibited by all international human rights instruments. See in particular the Convention for the Protection of Individuals with Regard to Automatic Processing of Personal Data (Council of Europe, 1981). See also the appendix to Recommendation R (81) 1 of the Committee of Ministers of the Council of Europe (23.1.1981) setting out regulations for automated medical databanks, particularly Principles 1.2, 4.1, 4.2, 4.3, 5 and 6, and the appendix to Recommendation R (83) 10 of the Committee of Ministers of the Council of Europe of 23.9.1983 on protection of personal data used for scientific research and statistics, particularly Principles 2, 3.1, 3.2 and 3.4, 4.1 and 4.3.

As regards the BC, see Article 10 (1), according to which "everyone has the right to respect for private life in relation to information about his or her health, and point 63 of the explanatory report, which reads: "the first paragraph [of Article 12] establishes the right to privacy of information in the health field, thereby reaffirming the principle introduced in Article 8 of the ECHR and reiterated in the Convention for the Protection of Individuals with Regard to Automatic Processing of Personal Data. It should be pointed out that, under Article 6 of the latter convention, personal data concerning health constitute a special category of data and are as such subject to special rules".

2. From the ethical standpoint

The various ethical positions (WMA, 1982; UEMO, Amsterdam, 1979; EEC Standing Committee of Doctors, Dublin, 1982) only express reservations *vis-à-vis* personalised computer data and have no objection to statistical scientific use subject to certain precautions: purely statistical data from which the identity of patients might be discovered must be completely separate from medical data containing information on, for example, diagnosis and treatment which must remain anonymous.

3. From the standpoint of religious moralities

a. *Catholic*

There would not seem to be a moral obligation to secrecy when the data does not concern the patients by name, but only scientific information which, if it is made public, can help scientists to make an effective contribution to the common good.[1]

b. *Protestant*

Freedom of information depends on the transparency and equal communication opportunities which determine the very health of a culture or a civilisation. It goes without saying that this freedom, like all others, ends where the freedom of others and respect for their rights begin.

c. *Jewish*

Everything that can contribute to better knowledge with a view to helping and developing medical treatment must be done. No limitation may be imposed and governments and health and social bodies must help towards this free movement. There must be exchange of information in this area, not only to help, but also and primarily to ensure that other countries do not fall victim to the same ills. However, despite this need to encourage free circulation of information, professional secrecy must be preserved. Databanks must provide general information, but never personal data. Free circulation of information is indispensable to medical progress and must therefore be fostered and encouraged as far as possible.

d. *Muslim*

Medical databanks are a source of scientific information for cognitive and epidemiological purposes. They thus serve science and the progress of knowledge in our ability to heal. Inasmuch as these data are not personalised, they may be used without reticence in the interests of society which benefits from the medical progress to which they give rise.

e. *Buddhist*

Information which can contribute to improved health and welfare for all must be shared, while taking care to protect individual privacy.

4. From the standpoint of agnostic morality

The law on computerised data and individual freedoms protects the confidentiality of files and hence, *a fortiori*, that of data which are covered by professional

---

1. Second Vatican Council, *Inter Mirifica*, 4, AAS 56 (1964), pp. 145-157.

secrecy. Access to files should be regulated by law. Epidemiological statistics must be anonymous. No direct or indirect key must permit the data source to be identified.

Need for consent

Mr X is 42-years-old, married and father of two children (12 and 7 years).
Following a viral infection, he is suffering from terminal cardiorespiratory failure.
With his consent, he has been entered on the list of patients to be given a heart-
lung transplant as a matter of acute urgency.
On the day of the transplant, while still conscious, he refuses the operation which
alone can save him.
His family, wife and children, ask the surgical team to override his refusal.

1. From the standpoint of international law

There is only one provision of international general law on human rights at present which stipulates as a general rule the obligation to obtain the patient's consent. This is Article 7 (2) of the Covenant on Civil and Political Rights, which states that "In particular, no one shall be subjected without his free consent to medical or scientific experimentation".

This provision is applicable in the present case inasmuch as the double heart-lung transplant may still be considered as "medical experimentation".

However, the principle of freely given consent is fundamental also in cases which do not constitute medical or scientific "experimentation", as the patient's right to physical integrity presupposes that any medical operation which is not purely routine (application of a stethoscope, measuring of blood pressure, administration of injections, etc.) should only take place subject to the freely given and informed consent of the person in question.

In emergencies, that is if the patient's life is in immediate danger, if the patient is not conscious or is not able to grasp the seriousness of his situation or the nature of the medical operation required, the doctor's duty to preserve the patient's life and health takes precedence. If, however, despite his very serious state, the patient is conscious and hence able to refuse the proposed medical operation or withdraw his previously given consent, freely and in full knowledge of the situation, his will should take precedence over the doctor's duty to save him. There is, however, no definite reply in international law, as the problem of renunciation of the fundamental right *par excellence*, the right to life, has not yet been resolved by texts, binding or otherwise.

As regards specific international law, Article 5 of the BC, , clearly establishes the consent rule: "An intervention in the health field may only be carried out after the person concerned has given free and informed consent to it. This person shall beforehand be given appropriate information as to the purpose and nature of the intervention as well as on its consequences and risks. The person concerned may freely withdraw consent at any time". In, and because of, an emergency situation, when the appropriate consent cannot be obtained, any medically necessary intervention may be carried out immediately for the benefit of the health of the individual concerned (Article 8 of the BC and points 56 to 59 of the explanatory report). See however Article 9 of the BC and points 60 to 62 of the explanatory report.

If patients are not capable of deciding what is in their best interest because of mental disorders of a serious nature they "may be subjected, without their consent and subject to protective conditions prescribed by law, to an intervention aimed at treating their mental disorders only where, without such treatment, serious harm is likely to result to their health" (Article 7 of the BC).

Point 52 of the explanatory report adds in this regard that "the intervention must be necessary to treat specifically these mental disorders. For every other type of intervention, the practitioner must therefore seek the consent of the patient, insofar as this is possible, and the assent or refusal of the patient must be followed (...). In other words, if persons capable of consent refuse an intervention not aimed at treating their mental disorder, their opposition must be respected in the same way as for other patients capable of understanding".

Should the patient, according to domestic law, be incapable to consent because of a mental disability, a disease or for similar reason, "the intervention may only be carried out with the authorisation of his or her representative or an authority or a person or body provided for by law" (Article 6 (3) of the BC) only if the intervention is for his or her direct benefit (Article 6 (1) of the BC). See points 41 to 45 of the explanatory report appended to the BC.

Lastly, see the summary of the facts in the Commission Decision of 17.5.1995 on Application No. 25949/94 (*Sampedro Camean v. Spain*).

2. From the standpoint of medical ethics

The physician's primary concern must be the patient's health, but the doctor must also protect and respect the patient's rights (WMA, Madrid, 1987). The patient, after being adequately informed on the treatment proposed, has the right to accept or refuse it (WMA, Lisbon, October 1981). The doctor may not allow the family's will to prevail over that of the patient.

3. From the standpoint of religious moralities

a. *Catholic*

A heart-lung transplant must be considered one of the means provided by the most advanced medical techniques. Recourse may be had to these with the patient's consent, even if they are still at the experimental stage and are not without a certain risk.

301

From the point of view of Catholic morality, it is therefore ethically permissible both for the patient's family and for the doctor not to "impose on anyone the obligation to have recourse to a technique which is already in use but which carries a risk or is burdensome".[1] It is permissible to make do with the "normal means that medicine can offer": this is not equivalent to suicide but may signify acceptance of the human condition in a wish to spare the patient the application of a medical procedure disproportionate to the results that can be expected.

b. *Protestant*

Organ transplants have not as yet given rise to the adoption of any particular stance in Protestantism. In principle nothing should oppose the practice, but closer study may reveal that the problems are more serious than often imagined. In this particular case, it is of course necessary to know what caused the patient's last-minute refusal. Was it a fundamental and duly motivated refusal (Why? How?) or simply a fleeting but very understandable fear in the face of an operation which is serious in all respects? Be this as it may, our ignorance on this point shows the extent to which taking account of the patient's words has not been sufficient. The fact is that acting ethically does not mean the blind application of ready-made standards, but lies in the way in which account is taken of all the fragility and complexity of a human situation and then deciding the appropriate action.

c. *Jewish*

The Torah imposes upon us a strict duty to take care of our health and to take all the necessary measures to combat disease. It is written in Deuteronomy (4, v. 15): "You must take great care of yourselves". For this reason, all rules can be broken to save a man's life as life is a supreme value. Consequently, a man does not have the right to renounce life or to put an end to his days. He must follow the advice of the doctors whose role is to preserve life. He may by no means rely on a miracle or let himself go without trying all the opportunities offered him by medicine. In this case, the patient was included on the list of potential transplantees. The family and children are asking for the operation. The doctors must therefore try to persuade the patient to accept the operation by trying to explain to him that it is the only way he can be saved. The doctor must do this with tact and skill and try to restore the man's courage, optimism and hope.

d. *Muslim*

One of the conditions required, as pointed out at the Second International Congress of the Society for Organ Transplants in the Middle East, held in Kuwait in

---

1. Declaration of the Congregation for the doctrine of the faith on euthanasia, No. IV.

March 1990 (see introduction) is the donor's written consent given while he was still alive, and, failing that, that of his family. No reference has ever been made to consent on the part of the recipient. In the present case, it appears that, given the physical and mental state of the recipient, who is terminally ill, his rejection of a heart and lung transplant cannot be taken into account. Inasmuch as the team of doctors and surgeons considers that the operation may save the patient's life, it should carry out the transplant, the more so since the close relatives have given their consent and the patient was formerly placed on the list of potential transplant recipients with his consent.

e. *Buddhist*

The family has a duty to obtain the patient's consent by calming him and explaining to him with compassion the justification for the operation. Given the still somewhat experimental nature of this operation, after a complete explanation of the risks and prognosis has been given to the patient and the family, the patient's decision must be respected. This is a limit situation between respect for life and relentless prolongation of life.

4. From the standpoint of agnostic morality

Nobody can override the patient's wishes. The patient's decision is a matter for his conscience alone, and his own freedom, provided of course that his choice is free and informed.

Computerised databanks

The list of patients to undergo organ transplants is available by remote access, but this requires a confidential code. Despite the guarantees of ad hoc committees, is there not a possibility of abuse of such operational files at both national and European level?
This question particularly concerns jurists.

1. From the standpoint of international law

The provisions referred to in connection with case 54, particularly Recommendation R (81) 1 adopted by the Committee of Ministers of the Council of Europe on 23.1.1981 (see in particular Principles 5.1, 5.2, 5.3, 5.4 and 8 and paragraphs 39, 41, 42, 43, 44, 45, 46, 47, 53 and 54 of the explanatory report to the above recommendation) are specifically aimed at ensuring that there are no abuses constituting "arbitrary or unlawful interference with (...) privacy", as prohibited by Article 17 (1) and (2) of the Covenant on Civil and Political Rights and Article 8 of the ECHR, as well as by Article 10 (1) of the BC, the latter being specifically concerned with information about health.

It should be noted that Recommendation R (81) 1 does not prevent states from introducing more extensive protection for persons to whom medical data refer.

2. From the standpoint of medical ethics

This is a question of law and of fact. In law as in ethics, access to such files, be it by remote data processing or any other means, is covered by professional secrecy and their use is limited by their purpose. In fact, it appears that there is no such thing as absolute security for computer files and the use of remote data processing in itself raises possibilities of easier violation of secrecy or abuse. It is for users to ensure by reinforced precautions that these means are not abused, as the need for rapid action may not allow the use of computers to be avoided. Medical databanks can under no circumstances have links with other databanks (WMA Declarations of Munich, 1973, and Venice, 1983).

3. From the standpoint of religious moralities

a. *Catholic*
There is no official position of the Catholic Church on this issue. We may draw inferences indirectly from the Church's position as regards secrecy in general and

medical secrecy in particular. In this connection, we may affirm that respect for secrecy is an ethical obligation directly linked to the eighth commandment.[1]

b. *Protestant*

The question concerns the possibilities and limits of computer techniques and the effectiveness of the legal protection of privacy, rather than ethics proper. It goes without saying that private life has to be absolutely protected.

c. *Jewish*

Computer techniques have now become an absolute necessity. They make it possible to save human lives by providing rapid and complete information. It is therefore impossible to deny ourselves such a powerful tool which, I am sure, will become increasingly indispensable.

It is our duty to ensure that every precaution is taken to ensure that professional secrecy and private data are fully protected at both national and European level.

d. *Muslim*

Although this is primarily a question for lawyers, Islam is in favour of medical staff keeping files containing health data identified by name. The purpose of such data must be the knowledge, protection and improvement of health. All staff called upon to consult the databanks are bound by medical secrecy.

e. *Buddhist*

Everything must be done to protect confidentiality.

4. From the standpoint of agnostic morality

As far as computerised files are concerned, despite the precautions taken by national legislation, unauthorised access unfortunately remains possible.

---

1. Pius XII, *Broadcast speeches and messages*, Vol. II, 1944-45, p. 194; Vol. XV, 1953-54, p. 73.

Organ transplants

Problem posed by patients in a state of brain death.
Young X, aged 19, injured in a traffic accident, shows all the clinical and
paraclinical signs of brain death.
Two members of a transplant team refuse to take part in treatment and the removal
of several organs for transplant purposes.
They invoke the conscience clause.
An exemplary disciplinary measure is requested by the doctor in charge of the
team.

1. From the standpoint of international law

Resolution (78) 29 adopted by the Committee of Ministers of the Council of Europe on 18.5.1978 on "harmonisation of legislations of member states relating to removal, grafting and transplantation of human substances" does not provide for a conscience clause. However, it does not rule it out, as it confines itself to stating that "Death must be established by a doctor who does not belong to the team which will effect the removal, grafting or transplantation" (Article 12) and that "death having occurred a removal may be effected even if the function of some organ other than the brain may be artificially preserved" (Article 11).

Points D and E of the aforementioned resolution state that member states must "intensify, by appropriate means, their efforts to inform the public and arouse the interest of doctors in the need and importance of donations of substances, while keeping the confidential character of individual operations" and "provide or encourage the preparation of practical guidelines for those entitled to decide according to paragraph 1 of Article 11 that a substance may be removed from a deceased person".

This explains the absence of any provision for a conscience clause.

As regards the BC, Article 4 refers to the relevant professional obligations and standards in force in the different Council of Europe countries, which may take the form of professional codes of ethics, other codes of medical conduct, health law or medical ethics or any other means of ensuring respect for the rights and interests of patients (points 28 to 33 of the explanatory report), as well as "the right of conscientious objection by health care professionals" (point 30 of the explanatory report).

It should be noted in passing that the BC takes into consideration organ and tissue removal for transplantation purposes from living donors only (Chapter VI, Articles 19 and 20). The content of Article 19 (2) and, above all, Article 20 (v) leads us to conclude that the notion "live donors" does not include patients in a state of brain death. Reference should also be made to Article 9 of the BC so far as the previously expressed wishes are concerned.

With regard to the conformity of disciplinary procedures before the medical councils with Article 6 of the ECHR, namely with the principle of the fair hearing, see Court Decision Nos. 33 of 23.6.1981 in the *Le Compte, van Leuven and De Meyere* case (*Commission* v. *Belgium*); 45 of the 10.2.1983 in the *Albert and Le Compte* case (*Commission* v. *Belgium*) and 325 A of 26.9.1995 in the *Diennet* case (*Commission* v. *France*).

2. From the standpoint of medical ethics

This case is rather unexpected, since the doctors referring to the conscience clause are part of a team routinely practising transplants. The objection can therefore not be related to the principle of transplantation, as these doctors would otherwise have chosen some other service. They must therefore be contesting the death of the donor. According to the ethical rules of the WMA, determination of death may not be carried out by the transplant team; death must be determined by two other doctors applying recognised scientific methods. This being so, the transplanter must consider both the donor and the recipient as his patients and defend their interests (WMA Declaration, October 1987). No doctor may perform a transplant if the patient's rights are not respected (WMA Declaration of Madrid, 1987). Consequently, the transplanter can only rely on the conscience clause if there are doubts as to the judgment of the doctors who have recognised the death or if death has only been determined by a single doctor.

3. From the standpoint of religious moralities

a. *Catholic*

There is no official position of the Church as regards evaluation of brain death as a criterion for defining a person's death. We may recall that Catholic doctrine accepts the result of experimental science as regards determination of the death of a man: "once this determination has taken place, the apparent conflict between the duty to respect a person's life and to treat or save that of another person no longer exists".[1]

However, it does not seem ethical to provide for a disciplinary penalty for those (doctors or health personnel) who rely on the conscience clause – for moral or religious reasons – and refuse to take part in treatment and removals for multi-organ transplants.

---

1. John Paul II, "Address to the participants in the Congress of the Pontifical Academy of Sciences on determination of the moment of death", *L'Osservatore Romano* of 17 December 1989.

b. *Protestant*

Here again, the precise reasons for the refusal of the two doctors are not known. The "conscience clause" in fact appears to be too vague a term which does not suffice to explain and justify an act with such serious consequences. It is therefore not sure that it can be said that disciplinary penalties can be imposed in such a complex situation. What is essential is not to be afraid to open a debate and to take part in it.

c. *Jewish*

It is quite legitimate for members of a transplant team to refuse to take part in treatment and removals for a multi-organ transplant for reasons of conscience.

The idea of imposing a disciplinary penalty seems to be aberrant and to constitute a lack of respect for the most elementary human rights. The case under consideration poses two delicate problems:

1. removal of organs;
2. definition of the time of death.

For Judaism, the sacred respect due to human life does not mean contempt for the dead body. Even after death, we owe to the human body the respect due to the soul.

Respect for human mortal remains is strikingly emphasised in the Talmud.[1] The cadaver and all the organs indelibly bear the mark of the sacred and we must behave towards them with infinite respect. Only in clearly defined circumstances are autopsies[2] and organ transplants permissible.[3]

Furthermore, certain decision-makers do not accept the criterion of brain death. For them, death is recognised by absence of movement, heartbeat and respiration. These three conditions must be met before death can be determined.

d. *Muslim*

Transplantation of organs removed from the body of a dead person is authorised in Islam subject to the following conditions:

1. establishment of brain death (see introduction) by three doctors, including a neurologist (the surgeons who are to carry out the transplant may not belong to this committee);
2. there may be no remuneration;
3. the transplant must be carried out in a centre approved by the Ministry of Health of the country concerned;

---

1. *Talmud Treaty I*, "Baba Batra", p. 154, b; "Berachot", p. 18 a.
2. Eliezer Landau, *Noda' Biyehuda Yoré Déah*, p. 210; Hatam Sofer, *Yoré Déah* p. 336.
3. Hatam Sofer, *Yoré Déah*, p. 338; *Talmud Treaty*, "Yoma", p. 85 a; "Orah Hayim", p. 330, 5.

4. the dead person made no objection to removal of organs while he lived.

In this case, two members of the transplant team object. The reason given, namely removal of multiple organs, cannot be accepted as justification, given that such transplant operations have already proved their worth.

e. *Buddhist*

Everything must be done to save the patient but relentless prolongation of life should be avoided. Once brain death has been confirmed by two independent medical teams, the conscience clause cannot be accepted. The donation of organs is accepted provided that the donor has previously given permission for altruistic reasons (see case 10).

4. From the standpoint of agnostic morality

These doctors are members of a transplant team. They must do their job. They cannot invoke the conscience clause here, because by so doing they would endanger the lives of patients waiting for transplants.

Transsexualism

The legal, ethical and moral problems posed by surgical operations related to transsexualism.

1. From the standpoint of international law

As regards rectification of official documents, opinions against are to be found in the Commission Report in the *van Oosterwijck* v. *Belgium* case (1.3.1979) from the point of view Article 8 (1) and (2) of the ECHR and the Court's Judgments in the *Rees* case (*Commission* v. *United Kingdom*) No. 106 of 17.10.1986, and in the *Cossey* case (*Commission* v. *United Kingdom*) Decision No. 184 of 27.9.1990, viewed from the same angle. It should be noted, however, that the Court decisions are strictly linked to the characteristics of the British legal system, which, while it does not allow for rectification of all civil status documents, nevertheless permits the issue of identity and other documents in conformity with the acquired sex (change of given names, photograph, etc.). In the light of this circumstance, the Court ruled as follows "The introduction of a civil status system indicating and proving present civil status has not hitherto been considered necessary in the United Kingdom. It would have important administrative consequences and would impose new duties on the rest of the population. The governing authorities in the United Kingdom are fully entitled, in the exercise of their margin of appreciation, to take account of the requirements of the situation pertaining there in determining what measures to adopt. While the requirement of striking a fair balance may possibly, in the interests of persons in the applicant's situation, call for incidental adjustments to the existing system, it cannot give rise to any direct obligation on the United Kingdom to alter the very basis thereof".

Where on the contrary national law not only does not permit the rectification of civil status documents, but does not guarantee the issue of identity and other documents in conformity with the acquired sex (as, for example, in the French system, Judgment No. 232 C of 25.3.1992 in the *B.* case – *Commission* v. *France*), the Court ruled for the violation of Article 8 (1) of the ECHR. "The disadvantages and even perturbation to which transsexuals are exposed in their everyday life when their identity and other documents do not correspond to the new conditions they have acquired in fact reach such a degree of seriousness as to be taken into account for the purposes of Article 8 (1)".

The positive obligation incumbent upon states to adopt reasonable and adequate measures to protect the rights that applicants derive from paragraph 1 of Article 8, namely the right to the effective respect of the rights that are recognised, obliges states to put an end to the situation in which transsexuals find themselves placed every day, which is incompatible with due respect for their private life.

As regards the right to marry (Article 12 of the ECHR), the Court has ruled that "the right to marry guaranteed by Article 12 refers to the traditional marriage between persons of opposite biological sex. This appears also from the wording of the article which makes it clear that Article 12 is mainly concerned to protect marriage as the basis of the family. Furthermore, Article 12 lays down that the exercise of this right shall be subject to the national laws of Contracting States as regards its exercise. The limitations thereby introduced must not restrict or reduce the right in such a way or to such an extent that the very essence of the right is impaired. However, the legal impediment in the United Kingdom on the marriage of persons who are not of the opposite biological sex cannot be said to have an effect of this kind" (*in contrario*, Commission Report 1.3.1979 quoted above).

There is no reply as regards the legal status of children born of a marriage in which one partner is a transsexual.

As regards the rights of the child born from a pregnancy resulting from fertilisation by donor in a stable couple formed by a transsexual and a woman to have the name of the (transsexual) father recorded in the register of births, even though this father remains registered as being a woman, see the Commission Decision of 27.6.1995 on Application No. 21830/93 (*X, Y and Z* v. *United Kingdom*) and the dissenting opinions appended to it. The Commission established in particular violation of Article 8 of the ECHR in the case of the third applicant, namely the child. See also Article 4 of BC and points 28 to 33 of the explanatory report appended thereto.

2. From the standpoint of medical ethics

The legal and ethical problems raised by transsexuality are associated with the scientific problem. The infringement of a person's physical integrity is justified only for therapeutic purposes. Hence, an operation must be justified by such a purpose. In the field under consideration, the operation is acceptable if, scientifically speaking, it is the only effective treatment for a severe mental disorder.

3. From the standpoint of religious moralities

a. *Catholic*

There is no official position of the Catholic Church as regards surgical operations associated with transsexuality.

Most Catholics theologians consider that a surgical operation on a subject whose organic sexuality is complete and healthy in order to treat the psychological pathology underlying transsexualism is not ethical. Indeed, the patient "is not the absolute master of himself, of his body, of his spirit (...) the patient is bound by the immanent teleology fixed by nature".[1]

b. *Protestant*

Whole works have been devoted to transsexuality, but it would not appear that official Protestant authorities have had to give an opinion. This certainly does not mean to say, of course, that Protestant theology, as a critical reflection on the human condition, has nothing to say on the subject. It will, nevertheless, refrain from hasty generalisations and will consider the problems more from the "pastoral" standpoint than the "dogmatic". It will also consider that the cases mentioned put their finger on the limits of a mentality which believes it possible to resolve all problems from an exclusively technical standpoint. If ever there were complex problems requiring the taking of multiple factors into account they are those concerning identity and sexuality.

c. *Jewish*

Surgical operations associated with transsexuality should be forbidden for the following reasons:

– to damage the body or a human organ is absolutely forbidden: it is written in Deuteronomy (4, v. 15): "You shall take care of yourselves";

– to destroy the reproductive organ is to hold the work of creation in contempt;

– to perform a surgical sex change operation is to infringe the biblical prohibition on effeminacy (Deut., 22, v. 5);

– the doctor's duty is to heal and not to use his art for this type of operation;

– it is not permitted to endanger one's life to no purpose, for any surgical operation contains an element of risk.

d. *Muslim*

Transsexuality may be defined as a deep-seated feeling on the part of an individual of belonging to the sex opposite to that which is genetically, physiologically and legally his or hers, together with the need to change his or her sexual condition and, in particular, his or her sexual anatomy. It is not always easy to distinguish this condition from intersexuality, which is accompanied by physiological anomalies which make the individual part man and part woman.

A surgical operation gives rise to legal, ethic and moral problems which are closely interlinked, and which should be addressed with caution in view of the following principles and concepts:

– in Islamic morality, there is an inviolable principle that no one can deliberately change his condition because he is the result of an act of divine creation;

---

1. Pius XII, *Broadcast speeches and messages*, Vol. XIV, 1952-53, p. 322.

hence, the individual's physical and mental integrity must remain intact. Moreover, as indicated above, the diagnosis of transsexuality is based entirely on the individual's conviction which may be highly subjective.

– the syndrome of transsexuality is a complex one made up of several sometimes discordant components; no scientific basis has been found to explain it (difficulties of defining chromosomal, morphological and psychosocial sex). For this reason, diagnosis of the transsexuality syndrome must be made by a committee of doctors made up of an endocrinologist, a surgeon and a psychiatrist, all experts in the field. The risk of a misdiagnosis is all the more serious since the surgical treatment is irreversible and the individual, who may have desired the operation very strongly, may subsequently regret it.

– one by no means negligible difficulty is the need for recognition of the sex change by the authorities. Where the change is not recognised, enormous administrative complications may attend the integration of the individual who has undergone the operation, particularly where he or she has children.

To sum up, we may conclude that:
– in the absence of cast iron scientific bases, transsexuality is difficult to diagnose;
– as regards the administrative aspect of a change in civil status, legislation on transsexuality exists in a few countries only, and is always subject to various conditions;
– there are irreversible complications from the psychological and the social point of view;
– the physical integrity of the individual, a divine creation, is violated.

For this reason, a surgical operation associated with transsexuality is proscribed in Islam until such time as scientific progress brings greater understanding and more detail on this pathological state, which gives rise to a host of complications of all kinds.

e. *Buddhist*
Every individual should be able to find his balance and it could be that such operations may help.

4. From the standpoint of agnostic morality

Under the law any mutilation is a criminal offence, and the consent of the victim has never freed the offender from liability.

From the moral standpoint it appears difficult to condemn a person's free and informed request to adapt his body to what he considers to be his or her personality.

Despite the prohibition in principle, where this intervention is considered necessary for the fulfilment of the individual authorisation is given, but this is only in exceptional circumstances.

However, considerable reflection is required for defining the new civil status.

313

Medically assisted procreation

Childless woman, now post-menopause, 60, in good health, hearing about successful cases of late in vitro *fertilisation and zygote intra-fallopian transfer (ZIFT) in Italy, wishes to attempt it despite the opposition of her spouse.*

1. From the standpoint of international law

Since the woman is married, the prior informed consent of the husband, to whom the birth of a child would in fact be attributed by the legislation of the majority of Council of Europe member states unless he brought an action to disown it, must be sought and obtained under the terms of Articles 5, Protocol 7 to the ECHR and 23 (4) of the Covenant on Civil and Political Rights, which stipulate equality of civil rights and responsibilities of the spouses between themselves and *vis-à-vis* the children.

In the case of an unmarried woman linked to a partner by a stable relationship, while the consent of the partner is often not required by national law, the birth of a child not giving rise *per se* to any legal relationship between the new-born child and the biological father/partner of the mother, Article 8 (1) ECHR and the respect of the family's right to family life, nevertheless, do require it.

Concerning this particular case, and in the same sense, see points D and E of the preamble and point 10, paragraphs 3 and 4, Resolution 372/88 of the European Parliament on artificial insemination *in vivo* and *in vitro*.

See also, *mutatis mutandis*, points 10, 11, and 13 Recommendation 1100 (1989) of the Parliamentary Assembly of the Council of Europe on the use of human embryos and foetuses in scientific research.

With respect to Resolution 372/88, "*in vivo* and *in vitro* artificial insemination should be used for therapeutic purposes (to remedy infertility)" (point 9), "whereas the causes of infertility are often inexplicable" (paragraph A of the preamble). Point 1 "confirms the need for extensive and appropriate research into the causes of infertility and methods of prevention and cure: this should include research into the replacement of substances causing low fertility or infertility with harmless substances". Point 3 "considers that adoption procedures should be harmonised and simplified as much as possible". Infertility caused by age is thus not considered.

Reference should also be made to the decisions of the Commission cited in the reply to case 1 *in fine*, as well as to Article 4 of the BC, and to points 28 to 33 of the explanatory report.

Lastly, it should be noted that by a resolution of May 1995, the Council of the Italian Federation of Doctors decided to prohibit making menopausal women pregnant.

2. From the ethical standpoint

Without the husband's agreement the request cannot be acceded to. What is more, since the woman is post menopausal the idea cannot be considered acceptable.

The WMA adopted a declaration on the subject in Madrid in 1987 and more recently in Bali in 1995.

The WMA Declaration of Madrid takes account of the philosophical sensibilities and the legal requirements, notably as regards filiation, and indicates to the doctor the prudence he must exercise in taking his decision.

3. From the standpoint of religious moralities

a. *Catholic*

The late ZIFT that the ageing, menopausal, sterile woman with no children wants to try is a particular case of heterological ZIFT. According to Catholic morality it is "contrary to the unity of the marriage, the dignity of the spouses, the true vocation of parents and the rights of the child conceived and born in the marriage".[1] It is also stressed that "these techniques have high failure rates", exposing the human embryo "to the risk of death in a generally very short time".[2] In addition, in this particular case, the "break between genetic relationship, gestational parenthood and educational responsibility"[3] is even more flagrant.

b. *Protestant*

Virtually all Protestant thinking on the subject opposes giving in to such a desire: out of concern for the equilibrium of the child which may be born, concern for the proper use of the society's health care resources, and because it is never good to "try to play God". And the woman is no longer young and there must already be a number of problems involved in accepting this fact in a positive way.

c. *Jewish*

Medically assisted procreation techniques can concern only a married couple, whether it is a matter of fertilisation *in vitro* or *in vivo*. Only the fertilisation of the female ovule by the husband's sperm is permitted, and this only under well-defined conditions. Any other method is formally forbidden from the religious standpoint, because it would cause too many problems for the unity of the couple and with respect to the legal position regarding the identity of the child.

---

1. Congregation for the doctrine of the faith, *Teachings on the respect of newly-born human life and the dignity of procreation*, II, 2; Pius XII, AAS 41 (1949), p. 559 and AAS 45 (1953), pp. 674-675.
2. John Paul II, *Evangelium Vitae*, 25 March 1995, No. 14.
3. Congregation for the doctrine of the faith, op. cit.

Knowledge of the child's identity with no risk of error is in fact a vital factor for Judaism. The durability of the Jewish people depends on this knowledge of identity. The imprecision as to the child's identity constitutes a source of serious problems for Jewish law.

In the present case there is also the problem of the opposition of the husband and the fact that the wife is 60 and post-menopausal.

There is an age for everything. A successful family life cannot be built with a father and mother who are over 60 and who would in most cases soon leave the child an orphan.

d. *Muslim*

According to Muslim morality, IVF can be used only if two conditions are fulfilled:

– the egg which will produce the embryo formed by the fertilisation *in vitro* of the ovule by the spermatozoid is acceptable only if the two gametes (ovule and spermatozoid) come from a couple legally united in marriage;

– the mutual free and informed consent of the married couple is necessary.

For this reason IVF here (and in particular so late in life) cannot be in conformity with Muslim morality, given the opposition of one of the spouses.

e. *Buddhist*

The lack of a common desire to generate a child may lead to imbalances in its development. Furthermore, the advanced age of the mother may make it difficult to bring the child up normally.

4. From the standpoint of agnostic morality

Quite apart from the risks to the woman's health, we are not in favour of the use of such a technique because it is contrary to natural morality.

Furthermore, given the mother's age, what would become of the child?

Medically assisted procreation

Post-menopausal widow, 55, childless, presents herself for IVF and ZIFT (in vitro fertilisation and zygote intra-fallopian transfer).

1. From the standpoint of international law

No specific reply. See, however, point D of the preamble of Resolution 372/88 of the European Parliament, in the terms of which: "the main criteria governing this area [*in vivo* or *in vitro* artificial insemination] are the (...) respect of the rights and interests of the child, namely the right (...) to a family, the right to be looked after by the parents" and point E *idem*, in the terms of which: "it is to the child's advantage to have a common 'biological', 'legal' and 'emotional' bond with both father and mother".

See also Articles 3 (1), 9 (1) and 18 (1) of the Convention on the Rights of the Child, Article 3 of Resolution 41/85 of 3.12.1986 of the UN General Assembly concerning the Declaration on the social and legal principles applicable to the protection and well-being of children, envisaged above all from the standpoint of adoption and family placement practices at national and international level, and Articles 4 and 5 (2) of the BC, namely appropriate prior information as to the purpose and nature of the intervention as well as on its consequences and risks, as well as point 30 of the referring to national law, codes of medical ethics, health legislation (...) which may (also) take account of any right of conscientious objection by health care professionals.

2. From the ethical standpoint

The request should not be acceded to because of the relatively advanced age of the woman and the absence of any father. What is more, since the woman is post menopausal the idea cannot be considered acceptable.

The WMA adopted a declaration on the subject in Madrid in 1987 and more recently in Bali in 1995.

The Declaration of Madrid takes account of the philosophical sensibilities and the legal requirements, notably as regards filiation, and indicates to the doctor the prudence he must exercise in taking his decision.

3. From the standpoint of religious moralities

a. *Catholic*

This is a case of heterological ZIFT where there is donation of either the ovocyte or the spermatozoid: in fact the woman, a menopausal widow, could never be

317

the genetic mother, but only, possibly, the gestational mother. The same moral considerations apply here as in the previous case. In addition, the father figure is lacking from the outset and this is just as irreplaceable for the development and growth of the child as the mother figure: at least this is what the psychological sciences say, quite apart from the moral aspect. The child has a right "to be conceived, carried, brought into the world and brought up by its own parents".[1]

b. *Protestant*
Same case as the above.

c. *Jewish*
Same reply as for case 59.

d. *Muslim*
IVF in the case of a post-menopausal widow can be performed only if the embryo has been preserved by freezing in accordance with Muslim morality and is the product of two gametes from the couple. The consent of the spouses is required.

e. *Buddhist*
Technical progress is opening up new possibilities which bring new desires on the part of menopausal women, young lesbians, male homosexual couples, etc., who want to have children using these new techniques. The advice given, without containing any moral judgment, should take account of the motivation of the people concerned. In any event, the absence of the father or mother will make the child's development unbalanced.

4. From the standpoint of agnostic morality

This request should be refused for moral reasons concerned with the child to be born and to protect the woman's health.

---

1. Congregation for the doctrine of the faith, *Teachings on respect for newly-born human life and the dignity of procreation*, II, 3.

Medically assisted procreation

Young lesbian, 30, presents herself to benefit from the donation of an embryo.

1. From the standpoint of international law

See points D and 10 (1) of Resolution 372/88 of the European Parliament, and point IV, 7 of Recommendation 1046 (1986) of the Parliamentary Assembly of the Council of Europe (24.9.1986) on the use of human embryos and foetuses for diagnostic, therapeutic, scientific, industrial and commercial purposes: prohibition of the creation of children from people of the same sex.

See also the reply to case 4.

2. From the ethical standpoint

The request should be refused because of the absence of any father and the fact that the maternal ovules are not used.

The doctor should be able to refuse to associate himself with an operation he considers in all conscience to be unacceptable. The best interests of the child yet to be born require that they benefit from a normal family, which is based on a couple.

The Declaration of Madrid takes account of the philosophical sensibilities and the legal requirements, notably as regards filiation, and indicates to the doctor the prudence he must exercise in taking his decision.

3. From the standpoint of religious moralities

a. *Catholic*

The natural place for procreation is the family based on marriage between a man and a woman: "The family has always been considered as the first and fundamental expression of the social nature of man (...). The family is born of conjugal communion, which the Vatican II Council qualified as 'alliance', in which the man and the woman 'mutually give and receive themselves'."[1] Furthermore, the procreative act must be the expression of the conjugal communion of the spouses.[2]

In the present case, for the child to be born there is no possibility of a family or a stable heterosexual couple, because the gestational mother is a lesbian. The words of John Paul II apply in cases of this type: "Sexuality, too, is depersonalised

---

1. John Paul II, *Letters to families* (2 February 1994), No. 7.
{30} Congregation for the doctrine of the faith, *Teachings on the respect for newly-born human life and the dignity of procreation*, II, 1.

and exploited: instead of being sign, place and language of love, that is the giving of oneself and the welcome of the other in all the richness of the person, it is becoming increasingly the occasion and instrument of the affirmation of the self and the egotistical satisfaction of desires and instincts."[1]

b. *Protestant*
Since a child has the right to have a father and mother and to be brought up in an environment which offers the best chances for balanced development, there is no reason why society – through care services – should "aid and abet" a project which does not offer proper guarantees of balance and health.

c. *Jewish*
The child should be the object of love. This is why this woman should be refused the donation of an embryo which she would like for this would deprive the transmission of life of its character of sanctity, making it a scientific exploit pure and simple.

This young lesbian can make one or more unfortunate children happy by adopting them. In this way she can save a child doomed to death and hunger and at the same time satisfy her maternal instinct in a legitimate fashion.

As from the technical standpoint this operation can be entirely successful, competition between medical teams must be avoided at all cost. In our countries at the leading edge of progress and where the results in this field are among the best in the world, we must be particularly vigilant and not fall into the temptation of permitting everything.

Ethics committees must do everything to avoid a "science with no conscience" which carries the risk of becoming "the ruin of the soul".

d. *Muslim*
According to Muslim morality the donation of an embryo cannot be accepted in this case (young lesbian) because the conditions set out in case 59 are not fulfilled. The case is aggravated here by the fact that the couple is a homosexual one whose existence is considered immoral by Islam.

e. *Buddhist*
See case 60.

4. From the standpoint of agnostic morality

We must first assume that this young woman of 30 is informed, free and conscious of the implications of the request.

---

1. John Paul II, *Evangelium Vitae*, 25 March 1995, No. 23.

If this is the case, then taking account of the maternal love which inspires her choice and despite the fact that the child will be fatherless, this request can be accepted, but only after thorough discussion with the doctor implanting the embryo and a psychiatrist.

Medically assisted procreation

A candidate surrogate mother, sponsored by a male homosexual couple, presents herself at a clinic specialising in medically assisted procreation, offering her ovocytes.

1. From the standpoint of international law

See the replies to cases 3 and 61.

Reference should again be made to point 11 of Resolution 372/88 EEC, in the terms of which "in general, any form of surrogate motherhood should be rejected. The procuring of surrogate mothers for gain should be punishable by law. Undertakings carrying on such activities should be banned and trade in embryos and gametes should be prohibited". Reference should also be made to Article 4 of the BC and points 30 to 32 of the explanatory report, including "right of conscientious objection by health care professionals".

See also Article 21 of the BC, worded: "The human body and its parts shall not, as such, give rise to financial gain", as well as points 131 to 134 of the explanatory report.

2. From the ethical standpoint

The request should be refused because of the absence of a mother.

The doctor should be able to refuse to associate himself with an operation he considers in all conscience to be unacceptable. The best interests of the child yet to be born require that he benefit from a normal family, namely based on a couple.

The Declaration of Madrid takes account of the philosophical sensibilities and the legal requirements, notably as regards filiation, and indicates to the doctor the prudence he must exercise in taking his decision.

3. From the standpoint of religious moralities

a. *Catholic*

The would-be surrogate mother not only offers herself for gestation, but also offers her ovocytes. In fact, the woman would be surrendering – presumably under a contract and for reward – her own child, which is such from both the genetic and gestational standpoints, even though conceived outside any family perspective or conjugal act. The object of the contract and/or purchase and sale is not only the woman's uterus but also and above all the child.

This type of maternity is ethically unacceptable "for the same reasons which lead to the refusal or heterological artificial insemination: it is in fact contrary to the unity of the marriage and the dignity of procreation of the human being".[1]

Another truth is relevant here: the child will never be the child of both members of the homosexual couple, but only one, for even if the sperm of both is mixed, the spermatozoid that fertilisers the ovocyte is always single and unique.

The Catholic Church, while respecting the individual rights of the homosexual person, does not recognise the right to or licitness of forming a natural couple or adopting a child.[2]

b. *Protestant*

Protestant morality cannot accept the commercialisation of the human body – or parts of it – or that the child's identity is heavily burdened from the outset, or that the human body should be seen as a kind of "kit" in which parts are interchangeable.

c. *Jewish*

Any system which consists of "lending the uterus" as a surrogate mother for an infertile wife is totally forbidden. All the more so when as in the present case a homosexual couple is involved. Besides the series of prohibitions which appear in the replies to earlier cases, we must always bear in mind the mother-foetus relationship, which cannot be dissociated, because pregnancy is not a simple "mechanical carrying", and in the course of it powerful links are established between the foetus and the mother bearing it.

In the case of the surrogate mother, the child is treated by their mother as a means and not as an end. The child thus becomes a good, subject to the laws of supply and demand, and in the present economic situation the child risks becoming a potential object of violence.

d. *Muslim*

IVF in this case implies that the embryo produced by fertilisation *in vitro* is foreign to the couple, which is contrary to Muslim morality. As in the reply to case 61, the problem is aggravated by homosexuality, considered immoral by Islam.

---

1. Congregation for the doctrine of the faith, *Teachings on the respect for newly-born human life and the dignity of procreation*, II, 3.
2. Congregation for the doctrine of the faith, *Persona Humana*, 29 December 1975, No. 8; "Letter to Catholic Bishops on the pastoral of homosexuals", 1 October 1986; *The Cathechism of the Catholic Church*, III, section 2, Nos. 2357-2359.

e. *Buddhist*
See case 60.

4. From the standpoint of agnostic morality

Agnostic morality is opposed to procreation using substitute mothers.

Medically assisted procreation

A young couple, in which the husband is sterile, presents itself at an authorised medically assisted procreation centre in order to benefit from the Belgian (Van Steirteghein) method of intracytoplasmic injection of spermatozoids.

1. From the standpoint of international law

This case seems to involve a problem of experimentation in the field of assisted procreation, rather than assisted procreation itself.

In this connection, points B.i and B.ii of Recommendation 1100 (1989) of the Parliamentary Assembly of the Council of Europe on the use of human embryos and foetuses in scientific research (2.2.1989) invite the governments of member states "to set up as a matter of urgency the national or regional multidisciplinary bodies mentioned in Recommendations 934 (1982) and 1046 (1986), also entrusting them with the task of informing society and the public authorities of scientific and technological advances in embryology and biological investigation and experimentation, of guiding and monitoring the potential applications thereof, evaluating results, benefits and drawbacks, notably in general terms, that is including also the dimension of human rights, human dignity and other ethical values, and authorising, provided there are appropriate regulations or delegations of authority, specific projects of scientific investigation or experimentation in these fields", and "to take steps to guarantee that society is informed simply, accurately and sufficiently of activities involving techniques of assisted fertilisation and related techniques".

In its turn, point B.iv invites the governments of member states "to promote investigations aimed at (...) improving technical procedures of assisted fertilisation, strictly as and where permitted".

It should also be recalled that in the terms of Recommendation R (90) 3 of 6.2.1990 adopted by the Committee of Ministers of the Council of Europe concerning medical research on human beings "medical research may not be carried out unless satisfactory evidence as to its safety for the person undergoing research is furnished" (Principle 10).

As for the BC, Article 4 stipulates that: "Any intervention in the health field, including research, must be carried out in accordance with relevant professional obligations and standards". Points 30 and 31 of the explanatory report read as follows: "All interventions (the term "intervention" being understood in a broad sense, i.e. covering all medical acts, in particular interventions performed for the purpose of preventive care, diagnosis, treatment or rehabilitation or in a research context) must be performed in accordance with the law in general, as supplemented and developed by professional rules (i.e. codes of medical conduct, health legislation, medical ethics or any other means of guaranteeing the rights and interests of the patient). Doctors and, in general, all professionals who participate in a medical act are subject to legal and ethical imperatives. They must act with care and competence, and pay careful attention to the needs of each patient and which may take account of any right of conscientious objection by health care professionals". Point 32 adds to this that "competence must be determined primarily in relation to the scientific knowledge and clinical experience appropriate to a profession or speciality at a given time. The current state of the art determines the professional standard and skill to be expected of health care professionals in the performance of their work. In following the progress of medicine, it changes with new developments and eliminates methods which do not reflect the state of the art. Nevertheless, it is accepted that professional standards do not necessarily prescribe one line of action as being the only one possible: recognised medical practice may, indeed, allow several possible forms of intervention, thus leaving some freedom of choice as to methods or techniques. Further, a particular course of action must be judged in the light of the specific health problem raised by a given patient. In particular, an intervention must meet criteria of relevance and proportionality between the aim pursued and the means used".

In application of the rule of consent of the couple (Articles 5 of Protocol 7 to the ECHR and 23 (4) of the Covenant on Civil and Political Rights), they must first be informed of the "relevant facts", that is all the factors that might influence the choice, including, possibly, any alternatives to the intervention proposed and/or the danger of the intervention failing. This information must be sufficiently clear and suitably worded. The wife, in particular, being the person most concerned with the pregnancy according to the European Commission of Human Rights, must be put in a position, through the use of terms she can understand, to weigh up the necessity or usefulness of the aim and methods of the intervention against the risks and the discomfort or pain it will cause (Article 5 (2) of the BC and points 35 to 37 of the explanatory report appended to the BC).

Lastly, reference should be made to point 32 of Resolution 327/88 EEC of 16.3.1989 concerning the ethical and legal problems of genetic manipulation, and also the reply to case 1.

2. From the ethical standpoint

The WMA has not yet considered the ethics of this technique.

It should be mentioned, however, that contrary to the ethical principles of experimentation applicable to human beings, no experimentation on animals and no test evaluation preceded the rapid and widespread implementation of the method, under the pressure of couples wanting a child at any price.

It has not yet been proved that the introduction of spermatids into the ovocyte through the pellucid wall is harmless in the long term.

Authorisation will be given if both parents agree after their attention has been drawn to the possible risks of this new technique for the health of their future child, risks which are often a secondary consideration compared with the couple's desire to have a child.

3. From the standpoint of religious moralities

a. *Catholic*

Since it is supposed that such a method permits the use of the husband's spermatozoids, the fertilisation thus effected would be homologous; however, it takes place outside an authentic conjugal act and thus remains negative in the judgment of the Church: "(...) even in the case where every precaution is taken to avoid the death of human embryos, homologous ZIFT dissociates the acts which are destined for human fertilisation through the conjugal act (...). Homologous ZIFT is performed outside the bodies of the spouses, by the acts of third persons whose competence and technical activity determine the success of the operation; it places the life and the identity of the embryo in the power of doctors and biologists, and institutes the domination of technology over the origin and destiny of the human being. Such a relationship of domination is in itself contrary to the dignity and equality which should be common to the parents and the children (...). Thus in homologous ZIFT (...) the generation of the human being is objectively deprived of proper perfection: that of being the term and fruit of a conjugal act".[1]

b. *Protestant*

There are three questions here: is the husband totally sterile, hence the necessity to resort to the sperm of a third party, or is he a hypofecund man from whose sperm a spermatozoid can be extracted? In the second case, there is generally no fundamental problem for Protestantism, which considers it to be simply a technical aid. The first case, AID, is less straightforward in that it complicates the question of the child's filiation. It can therefore be undertaken only with prudence, after discussion and mature reflection. But intracytoplasmic injection techniques raise the question of sorting the spermatozoids and the choice of gametes, leading to latent forms of eugenics, which is unacceptable. What is more, from the purely technical standpoint, these methods seem to give relatively uncertain results.

---

1. Congregation for the doctrine of the faith, *Teachings on respect for newly-born human life and the dignity of procreation*, II, 5.

c. *Jewish*

The Belgian Van Steirteghein method of intracytoplasmic injection of spermatozoid consists of the intra-ovular injection of a spermatozoid.

This method seems entirely lawful provided that the sperm is that of the husband. It is a method which gives a higher rate of success.

In this case it must, nevertheless, be stressed that every precaution must be taken to prevent any confusion of sperm from different donors (substitution due to manipulation errors or the mixing of sperm in the technique of activating a defective sperm by associating it with that of a healthy donor).

d. *Muslim*

Medically assisted procreation is impossible here because the spermatozoid would necessarily have to come from a person outside the couple, the husband being sterile.

e. *Buddhist*

Since this technique has not yet been sufficiently tried and tested, no opinion can be expressed at present.

4. From the standpoint of agnostic morality

This request is acceptable.

Medically assisted procreation

A team of non-medical researchers, wishing to study possible deviant behaviour in children issuing from artificial insemination by donor (AID), obtains a file of names from a private sperm bank.

1. From the standpoint of international law

Reference should be made to the Convention on the Protection of Individuals with Regard to Automatic Processing of Personal Data (Council of Europe, 28.11.1981-1.9.1982), as well as to Recommendation R (81) 1 of the Committee of Ministers of the Council of Europe to member states on regulations for automated medical databanks (23.1.1981), in particular points 1.1 ; 1.5 ; 3 ; 4.2 ; 5.1 ; 5.2 ; 5.3 and 5.4, both texts stemming from the principle set out in Article 8 (1) of the ECHR.

See also Article 10 (1) of BC and point 63 of the explanatory report appended thereto.

2. From the ethical standpoint

Contrary to medical ethics. The sperm bank file is covered by public law medical secrecy.

The WMA adopted a very clear position on this subject – involving a databank – in the Declaration of Munich of 1973 which was amended in Venice in 1983.

The Declaration of Madrid takes account of the philosophical sensibilities and the legal requirements, notably as regards filiation, and indicates to the doctor the prudence he must exercise in taking his decision.

3. From the standpoint of religious moralities

a. *Catholic*

First of all a negative moral judgment must be expressed at the existence of a sperm bank, public or private, in so far as it aims to achieve heterological fertilisation. In any event, the violation of the personal secrecy of those who are born by assisted procreation procedures does not appear justified in the light of the general duties stemming from the eighth commandment.[1] However, individual medical reasons may authorise the lifting of this secrecy, if the persons concerned agree.

---

1. Pius XII, *Speech of 12 November 1944 to the St Luke Medico-biological Union.*

b. *Protestant*

One of the constitutive principles of AID lies in the confidentiality – or strict anonymity – of data concerning the donor. There can be no derogation from this rule, the case of the child himself wishing to know his biological origins being reserved.

c. *Jewish*

It is legitimate to study any possible deviant behaviour in children issuing from AID in order to be better able to treat it or even prevent it.

However, this must be done by a team of doctors specialised in the field and under the conditions laid down by the medical ethics committee.

However, in this particular case, it is a non-medical research team, hence subject to neither professional secrecy nor to the various additional controls.

What is more, it obtains a file with names from a private sperm bank. It is possible today for any medical practice to set up as a fertility centre, with no health guarantees. Legislation is required to make the approval of such centres subject to the required quality standards and to regulate sperm banks which, in the present legal vacuum, do not make the population safe from the risk of accidental consanguinity.

d. *Muslim*

There are two factors opposing the proposed study:

– the researchers are outside the medical profession;

– there is no sperm bank in a country governed by Muslim morality, according to which the spermatozoid must come from the partner legally united by marriage, thus making artificial insemination by donor (AID) impossible.

e. *Buddhist*

Negative opinion.

4. From the standpoint of agnostic morality

Such access to a file would be an intolerable infringement of the right to private life.

This file cannot be transferred or communicated, and only persons authorised by the law are allowed access to it.

A research team should be allowed access only with the agreement of an ethics committee.

Medically assisted procreation

In order to increase the chances of implantation, an authorised medically assisted procreation centre transfers four or five embryos and commonly practices embryonic reduction.

1. From the standpoint of international law

See point 4 of Resolution 372/88 EEC, in the terms of which the European Parliament "recognises the value of life and more especially the human being's right to protection and therefore expresses its concern at the 'waste' of embryos which *in vitro* fertilisation can entail; and hopes that techniques and practices will be employed to eliminate this risk".

Points 5 and 6 of the same text should also be recalled, in the terms of which the European Parliament "calls therefore for the number of egg cells fertilised *in vitro* to be limited to the number that can actually be implanted" and "considers that embryos should only be frozen to keep them alive where immediate transfer *in utero* is impossible for any reason occurring during fertilisation".

On this last subject see also point 8 of the same resoluiton as well as point 39 of Resolution 327/88 EEC (17.4.1989) on the ethical and legal problems of genetic manipulation. As far as the BC is concerned, reference should be made to Articles 1, 4 and 5 (as well as Articles 11, 12, 13, 14 and 26(1) and (2)).

2. From the ethical standpoint

The generally accepted figure is three, without reduction. Account should be taken of the circumstances however.

Details were given by the WMA in its Declaration of Madrid (1987) and more recently in Bali in 1995.

The Declaration of Madrid takes account of the philosophical sensibilities and the legal requirements, notably as regards filiation, and indicates to the doctor the prudence he must exercise in taking his decision.

3. From the standpoint of religious moralities

a. *Catholic*

Embryonic reduction is nothing other than deliberate abortion. The aim of increasing the changes of success of ZIFT in no way justifies the method used, that is direct and selective abortion. "Human life is sacred and inviolable in all the moments of its existence even in the initial period which precedes

birth."[1] "Direct abortion, namely desired as an end or a means, always constitutes a serious moral offence as the deliberate murder of an innocent human
being. This doctrine is based on natural law and on the written Word of God; it
is transmitted by Church tradition and taught by the ordinary and universal magisterium".[2] In addition, "under the pretext of scientific or medical progress, in
reality [this technique reduces] human life to a mere 'biological material' which
can be freely disposed of".[3]

b. *Protestant*

For a great many Protestants the embryo can be considered a "potential human
being". For this reason it should be considered neither as sacred or taboo, nor as
simple biological matter, and must be treated with caution and respect. For this reason it is necessary to seek a proper compromise between a technique which places
the least strain on the woman and an approach which consists of producing
embryos with no thought to what will happen to them.

c. *Jewish*

The fact of embryonic reduction is intended to protect the future of the baby and
its mother (neurological sequels, premature birth, etc.). But implanting four or five
embryos creates a situation in which there must necessarily be reduction, which is
nothing other than selective abortion, something to be condemned out of hand.

d. *Muslim*

The transfer of four or five embryos and embryonic reduction can be practised
according to Muslim morality provided that the conditions for IVF are fulfilled, as
set out in case 59.

e. *Buddhist*

The fact of relying on embryonic reduction as a way of controlling the number
of children to be born is counter to the Buddhist ethic, which is to preserve all living creatures from suffering.

4. From the standpoint of agnostic morality

The therapeutic procedure is acceptable if the woman agrees.

---

1. John Paul II, *Evangelium Vitae*, 25 March 1995, No. 61.
2. *Idem*, No. 62.
3. *Idem*, No. 14.

Medically assisted procreation

A non-sterile woman from a family at risk requests in vitro *fertilisation and transfer of the embryo with pre-implantation diagnosis.*

1. From the standpoint of international law

Reference should be made to Resolution 327/88 EEC (17.4.1989) on the ethical and legal problems of genetic manipulation, in particular paragraph D; points 2 and 4 *idem*; and also points 12.*a*; *b*; *c* and *f*; 22; 24; 25; 26; 29; 31 and 32. See also point 7 of Resolution 372/88 EEC.

As regards the BC, Article 18 stipulates that "1. Where the law allows research on embryos *in vitro*, it shall ensure adequate protection of the embryo; 2. The creation of human embryos for research purposes is prohibited". Article 12 adds that "Tests which are predictive of genetic diseases or which serve either to identify the subject as a carrier of a gene responsible for a disease or to detect a genetic predisposition or susceptibility to a disease may be performed only for health purposes or for scientific research linked to health purposes". Reference should also be made to the appended explanatory report, namely to point 83, according to which "Article 12 as such does not imply any limitation of the right to carry out diagnostic interventions at the embryonic stage to find out whether an embryo carries hereditary traits that will lead to serious diseases in the future child".

Attention should also be drawn to Articles 13, 14 and 4 of the BC (and to Article 26 (1) and (2) of the same), as well as to Article 1 of the BC, and to point 19 of the explanatory report appended thereto, and to Article 11 of the BC and to points 74 and 75 of the explanatory report.

2. From the ethical standpoint

Yes, if the father is the donor and he agrees. The premeditated choice of sex is contrary to medical ethics.

The WMA has expressed its views in detailed fashion on the human genome in a declaration adopted in Marbella (Spain) in 1992.

The Declaration of Madrid takes account of the philosophical sensibilities and the legal requirements, notably as regards filiation, and indicates to the doctor the prudence he must exercise in taking his decision.

3. From the standpoint of religious moralities

a. *Catholic*

First of all the judgment is negative as regards the methodology itself. In addition, pre-implantation diagnosis is based – even if carried out for health reasons

– on a principle of embryo selection, becoming "too often an occasion for proposing and provoking abortion".[1] Pre-implantation diagnosis thus violates the respect which is owed to all humans from the moment of their conception.[2]

b. *Protestant*

What kind of risk is involved? A major risk or a "minor" one? Generally speaking, the answer should be a firm "no". In order to avoid any drift towards eugenics, because wanting to give life means also being able to take certain risks. But the specific case may deserve to be submitted to an ethics committee to determine whether it is purely a matter of convenience or a case of real distress.

c. *Jewish*

Pre-implantation diagnosis should be a technique strictly limited to families at risk.

On no account must pre-implantation diagnosis on demand be authorised. This would become selection, with all the dangers this term implies.

d. *Muslim*

ZIFT can be practised on a non-sterile woman from a family at risk if the conditions required by Muslim morality are fulfilled (see case 59). If the pre-implantation diagnosis reveals no risk the ZIFT can go ahead.

e. *Buddhist*

The opinion will be a function of the type of risk and the possibilities for diagnosing the disease by other means. If these techniques permit the woman to give life, they may be envisaged.

4. From the standpoint of agnostic morality

This practice is considered suitable. We are in favour of its use.

---

1. John Paul II, *Evangelium Vitae*, 25 March 1995, No. 61.
2. See the Charter of the Rights of the Family published by the Holy See, Article 4; Congregation for the doctrine of the faith, *Teachings on the respect for newly-born human life and the dignity of procreation;* 22 February 1987, I, 8 and II, 8; *Catechism of the Catholic Church,* Nos. 2270 and 2378.

Medically assisted procreation

A medically assisted procreation centre offers a woman of 30, sterile because of ovulation difficulties, ovules collected from foetuses obtained by abortion.

1. From the standpoint of international law

See points B.vi.*a* and B.vi.*d* of Recommendation 1046 (24.9.1986) of the Parliamentary Assembly of the Council of Europe on the use of human embryos and foetuses for diagnostic therapeutic, scientific, industrial and commercial purposes and points D.9; 10 and 12; E.12 and 13; F.16; H.20; 22 and 23 Recommendation 1100 (1989) on the use of human embryos and foetuses in scientific research.

See also point 10 of Resolution 372/88 EEC.

Lastly, see Article 22 of the BC: "When in the course of an intervention any part of a human body is removed, it may be stored and used for a purpose other than that for which it was removed, only if this is done in conformity with appropriate information and consent procedures", as well as Articles 4 and 5 (2) of the BC. Reference should also be made to Article 21 of the BC and to points 35 and 36 of the explanatory report.

2. From the ethical standpoint

The collection and use of not yet mature ovules has not so far been experimented on animals and has not been proved harmless for the future child, like indeed those taken from corpses or from tissues which produce ovules. This collection is therefore not ethical.

Any use of organs or of human embryonic procreation should be exceptional, because of possible pressure for planned abortions. It should be duly supervised by an ethics committee.

3. From the standpoint of religious moralities

a. *Catholic*

This case concerns first of all heterological fertilisation, which is "contrary to the unity of marriage, the dignity of the spouses, the true vocation of the parents and the right of the child to be conceived and brought into the world in marriage".[1] But it is even more immoral because it connects the artificial fertilisation with induced

---

1. Congregation for the doctrine of the faith, *Teachings on respect for newly-born human life and the dignity of procreation*, II, 2; Pius XII, AAS 41 (1949), p. 559 and AAS 45 (1953), pp. 674-675.

abortion, namely with "an act which is intrinsically illicit in the heart of all men [and which] no circumstance, no purpose, no law in the world will ever be able to make licit".[1] Furthermore, the cadavers of human embryos and foetuses, deliberately aborted or not, should be respected like the remains of other human beings. In particular, "the foetus cannot become the object of experimentation or organ transplantation if the abortion has been deliberate".[2]

b. Protestant

This proposal is morally somewhat irresponsible for we do not know all the imaginings and harm that its implementation may lead to both for the woman concerned and for the future child if he should learn the truth.

c. Jewish

In any event, this donation is to be refused because it is a case of a foetus (beyond fifteen weeks).

It all boils down to the same thing. Either the abortion is performed because of genetic malformation, in which case the ovule collected cannot be used because nobody is going to implant an ovule with a genetic malformation, the risk being unacceptable. On the other hand, if there is no genetic malformation there is no justification for the abortion.

d. Muslim

Since the conditions for the realisation of MAP in accordance with Muslim morality are not fulfilled (case 59), the sterile woman cannot accept the proposal made by the MAP centre.

e. Buddhist

There are simpler ways of solving ovulation difficulties, without using methods which have not yet proved themselves.

4. From the standpoint of agnostic morality

There is no moral reason to oppose such a treatment.

---

1. John Paul II, *Evangelium Vitae*, 25 March 1995, No. 62.
2. Pontifical Council for the Pastoral of Health Services, Charter of health personnel, No. 146, Vatican City 1995.

Medically assisted procreation

A doctor in an authorised medically assisted procreation centre systematically carries out pre-implantation diagnosis on his patients.

1. From the standpoint of international law

See points G and H of the preamble, as well as points 31 ; 32 ; 36 (and 37) of Resolution 327/88 EU, and points B.i ; B.ii and B.v of Recommendation 1046 (24.9.1986) of the Parliamentary Assembly of the Council of Europe.

See also Articles 5, 11, 12, 13 and 14 of the BC, as well as points 34 to 40 and points 74 to 94 of the explanatory report appended thereto.

2. From the ethical standpoint

If the aim is the premeditated choice of sex, it is contrary to medical ethics. If, on the other hand, the aim is to detect a hereditary pathological condition, the informed consent of the parents is required.

The Declaration of Madrid takes account of the philosophical sensibilities and the legal requirements, notably as regards filiation, and indicates to the doctor the prudence he must exercise in taking his decision.

3. From the standpoint of religious moralities

a. *Catholic*

For Catholic morality pre-implantation diagnosis is immoral because it leads to selective abortion. In fact the sole aim of pre-implantation diagnosis is to prevent the transfer to the maternal uterus of an embryo which presents genetic anomalies or faults, because at present there is no possibility of genetic therapy for the benefit of the embryo. In addition, "any directive or programme (...) which would favour in any way the connection between prenatal diagnosis and abortion"[1] should be condemned as a violation of the embryo's right to life.

Lastly, the general moral responsibilities of the MAP centre must not be forgotten, and in particular those of the doctor who systematically carries out pre-implantation diagnosis. We deduce from the brief text that pre-implantation diagnosis is not even proposed each time to the patient and carried out with her consent, but

---

1. Congregation for the doctrine of the faith, *Teachings on the respect for newly-born human life and the dignity of creation* (22 February 1987), I, 2.

forms part of the protocol adopted by the doctor concerned, disregarding the moral obligation of informed consent.

b. *Protestant*

It would be a good thing to have legislation on this subject – if such is not already the case – and for the doctor to comply with it. The systematic practice of pre-implantation diagnosis is undesirable, because it leads to the expectation of "normal" children and tends towards eugenics.

c. *Jewish*

The doctor in this approved MAP centre who systematically carries out pre-implantation diagnosis on his patients is acting improperly. He favours the abusive selection of ovocytes which will become an à la carte choice.

What is more, this test is not justified. The fact is that the risk of chromosomic malformation is now 1-in-1 000 for women under 30. To avoid this 1 in 1 000 risk this centre is destroying 5 per cent of the ovocytes.

d. *Muslim*

Pre-implantation diagnosis is acceptable according to Muslim morality only if performed for a medical reason.

e. *Buddhist*

Since this technique causes problems – it sacrifices a potential life – it can be justified only through the desire to protect a life.

4. From the standpoint of agnostic morality

This pre-implantation diagnosis is acceptable since it contributes to the development of a predictive medicine.

Medically assisted procreation

A medical research team, in order to improve the survival rate of embryos, has just cloned a human embryo, despite numerous warnings on ethical grounds by European bodies.

1. From the standpoint of international law

See Recommendation 1046 (24.9.1986) of the Parliamentary Assembly of the Council of Europe on the use of human embryos and foetuses for diagnostic, therapeutic, scientific, industrial and commercial purposes, in particular points 10; 11; 12 and 14. A.iv.1.

See also the prohibition set out in Article 18 (2) of the BC.

2. From the ethical standpoint

The danger of mutation and the temptation to multiply copies are too great for it not to be considered that to take this risk would be contrary to medical ethics.

This is the case with the ethical rules in the Declaration of Marbella of 1992 on the human genome.

The Declaration of Madrid takes account of the philosophical sensibilities and the legal requirements, notably as regards filiation, and indicates to the doctor the prudence he must exercise in taking his decision.

3. From the standpoint of religious moralities

a. *Catholic*

"Attempts or hypotheses made to obtain a human being without any connection with sexuality , by 'gemellary fission', cloning, parthenogenesis, are to be considered contrary to morality, for they are in opposition with the dignity of both human procreation and conjugal union."[1]

b. *Protestant*

Cloning is strictly prohibited. This practice should be denounced and punished.

---

1. Congregation for the doctrine of the faith, *Teachings on the respect for newly-born human life and the dignity of procreation*, 22 February 1987, I, 6.

c. *Jewish*

Cloning a human embryo opens the door to all sorts of abuses. Such procedures should be legally banned. Everybody knows where nazi theory led humanity. What defence would we have if such research fell into the hands of bloody dictators who decided to build a race of men and women with blond hair and green eyes?

Medical science can exist only if it is based on professional ethics. We must banish and combat any science applied without conscience.

We all know the errors of the men who built the Tower of Babel. What mattered for them was performance – they wanted to reach God. The Midrash tells us that when a man fell from the top of the tower everyone remained indifferent, another man would immediately come to replace him, but when a stone fell they wept, crying "who will bring a new stone so that construction will not be halted?". The consequence of their action was the confusion of values which brought the destruction of humanity. Man must not play the apprentice sorcerer.

Judaism accepts science, of course, but a channelled science which respects ethical and moral standards.

d. *Muslim*

The restrictions on cloning a human embryo are those set out in case 59.

e. *Buddhist*

Any manipulation of the living being is a certain form of violence and hence contrary to Buddhist ethics.

4. From the standpoint of agnostic morality

Assuming that such cloning is possible – diploid or polyploid embryo – the embryo which provided the sample must not pass the vital stage of the fifteenth day, and this with the conscious, free and informed consent of the mother.

Acquired immune deficiency syndrome (Aids)

A young accident victim, admitted to a hospital emergency service with serious injuries, refuses a human immune deficiency virus (HIV) test, which makes some of the medical team reluctant to treat him.

1. From the standpoint of international law

Article 4 of the BC stipulates that "any intervention in the health field, including research, must be carried out in accordance with relevant professional obligations and standards".

In addition, point 2.4, paragraph 3, of Recommendation R (87) 25 on a common European health policy to fight the acquired immune deficiency syndrome (Aids), adopted on 26.11.1987 by the Committee of Ministers of the Council of Europe, states that "staff who may have occupational exposure to infected fluids and secretions should be kept informed of sensible hygienic precautions to take for themselves". Point 2.2.3 stipulates that "if they take appropriate measures, health staff can usually avoid contamination; patients should, therefore, themselves be left to advise health staff of their seropositivity unless the patient has specifically authorised a doctor to pass on this information".

If the patient admitted for emergency treatment for serious injuries is conscious, he is free to accept or refuse the HIV test (Article 7 of the Covenant on Civil and Political Rights and Articles 5 (1) and 10 of the BC).

However, should the HIV test be "medically necessary", as a preliminary act, for the benefit of the health of the person concerned, Article 8 of the BC permits it in emergency situation, even if the appropriate consent cannot be obtained (see points 56 to 59 of the explanatory report appended to the BC).

Refusal of the test cannot lead to the refusal of emergency treatment (Article 8 of the BC and point 58 of the explanatory report), i.e. of medically necessary interventions which cannot be delayed.

If the test should finally be accepted, point 2.2.1 of Recommendation R (87) 25 cited above stipulates that the rules of confidentiality must be scrupulously observed. See also Article 10 (1) and (2) of the BC and points 63 to 70 of the explanatory report, in the case where the patient should turn out to be infected with the disease.

2. From the ethical standpoint

The refusal of care is contrary to medical ethics. On the other hand, if it is not an emergency, the doctor may refuse to the extent that by refusing this test or another the patient does not permit him to freely use the methods he deems necessary for making his diagnosis.

3. From the standpoint of religious moralities

a. *Catholic*

The doctor cannot refuse to accept and treat for illnesses other than Aids the seropositive person or the person carrying risk,[1] because:
– there is a moral duty to treat patients without discrimination;
– there are valid precautions which are sufficient to prevent contagion.

Obviously the patient who knows he is seropositive should warn the doctor and the carers so that they can take the appropriate precautions for themselves and for the other patients.

In fact, "receiving and treating patients, whatever the origin of their disease, is a duty. Protecting oneself against Aids is a good thing. It is a social, family and personal necessity".[2] "It is right that specific precautions should be taken to avoid any unnecessary risk of contracting the disease. Furthermore, from the moral standpoint, one of the most serious duties is that of taking the appropriate measures to prevent the propagation of the virus. But in taking these precautions it is necessary to take account of the human dignity and the needs of the patients; while trying to isolate the disease, care must be taken not to create humiliating situations or make ill-considered refusals. From the Christian standpoint, all patients, and these no less than the others, deserve attention and a treatment full of love and mercy".[3]

b. *Protestant*

It is necessary to talk to the patient, ask the reasons for his refusal and explain the carers' reservations. It is then for the patient to choose which of the two evils he prefers: receive care marked by suspicion and reservation, or submit to the test.

c. *Jewish*

The attitude of members of a medical team who are reluctant to treat a young accident victim who refuses the HIV test is incomprehensible.

Do they have the same reluctance in the face of other contagious diseases? Must a young accident victim be left to die because the doctor whose vocation is to prolong life refuses to take the necessary precautions and prefers to let him die in

---

1. See Administrative Commission of Catholic Bishops of the United States, "The different faces of Aids: an evangelical response", 24 December 1987, in *Il Regno – Documenti*, 1988, 45, pp. 170-177.
2. Communication concerning Aids information campaigns issued by the Conseil permanent de la Conférence Episcopale française, in *La documentation catholique*, 1 March 1987, p. 328.
3. Pastoral note on Aids by the Spanish bishops, Madrid, 12 June 1987, in *Dolentium Hominum*, 1987, No. 6, p. 26.

indifference? If so, then this doctor cannot do his job properly and should resign and retrain for something different.

We now have a whole series of measures to protect people against infectious diseases. It is for the medical team to take the necessary precautions.

d. *Muslim*

The doctor has the duty to convince the young accident victim admitted to the emergency service with serious injuries to agree to an HIV test. This test should be carried out, with the consent of the patient, who will have been informed of the consequence and the desire to avoid contaminating members of the medical team if he should be seropositive.

Exposing a person to a serious risk is a possible violation of his physical integrity, an essential principle of Muslim morality.

e. *Buddhist*

All medical personnel have the obligation to treat everybody regardless of the their situation, and normal aseptic measures are sufficient to protect these personnel.

4. From the standpoint of agnostic morality

The young victim's refusal must be overridden and the HIV test carried out in order to ensure the particularly necessary and sufficient protection of the medical team.

Acquired immune deficiency syndrome (Aids)

A young HIV-positive pregnant woman wishes to keep her child.

1. From the standpoint of international law

According to the decisions of the Commission (see for example Application No. 8416/79 – *X* v. *United Kingdom*), the woman being the person most concerned by the continuation or termination of the pregnancy, the wish expressed by her should prevail, with or without the consent of the husband/partner, notwithstanding the wording of Article 5 of Protocol 7 to the ECHR and Article 8 (1) of the ECHR.

Moreover, no medical intervention (here abortion) can be carried out without the free and informed consent of the person concerned (Articles 7 of the Covenant on Civil and Political Rights; and 4, 5 and 10 (1) of the BC), after he or she has been given appropriate information as to the purpose and nature of the intervention (or the reasons for non-intervention) as well as on its consequences and risks (Article 5 (2) of the BC).

2. From the ethical standpoint

The doctor must comply with the patient's decision.

In all circumstances, a mentally capable patient has the right to refuse the treatment proposed by the doctor.

The WMA adopted a clear position on this matter in its Declaration of Lisbon on patients' rights in 1981, completed and revised in Bali in 1995.

3. From the standpoint of religious moralities

a. *Catholic*

The HIV-positive pregnant woman should not have pressure put on her because of her desire to keep her child and hence refuse abortion. "It is true also that, in certain cases, prejudice is caused to important goods that it is normal to wish to safeguard",[1] but "life is far too fundamental a good to be put in balance in this way, even with very serious disadvantages".[2] Abortion would be all the more unjustified in that, on the basis of scientific knowledge relating to the mother-foetus transmission of the Aids virus, we know that only some 15-20% of the children born to seropositive mothers contract the disease.

---

1. Pontifical Council for the Pastoral of Health Services, Charter of health personnel, No. 146, Vatican City, 1995.
2. Congregation for the doctrine of the faith, Declaration on induced abortion, 28 June 1974, No. 14.

b. *Protestant*

She is surely not going to have the child aborted by force. On the other hand, she should be informed in the most appropriate way of the risks entailed, and of the chances the child may have of not carrying the virus, and on the probable future that her condition may bring for herself, those around her, and the child. She will then be able to take a duly informed decision, which will be her own and which must be scrupulously respected.

c. *Jewish*

The patient is aware of her condition. She knows that she can transmit Aids to her baby and that he risks losing his mother, but she nevertheless wishes to keep the child. This is her right, all the more so because science progresses every day and we are certain that what is impossible today will be done tomorrow. Hope must never be dashed. This is indeed the purpose of medicine and the role of the doctor.

d. *Muslim*

In the case where a pregnant woman is found to be HIV positive before the hundredth day, the doctor must convince the young woman of the consequences of the risk of probable contamination of the unborn child. Termination before the hundredth day of pregnancy for medical reasons is tolerated in Muslim morality. The result of the test should, nonetheless, be covered by medical secrecy if the patient turns out to be HIV-positive.

e. *Buddhist*

The opinion is positive, all the more so because there is only a one-in-five chance of the baby being seropositive.

4. From the standpoint of agnostic morality

The seriousness of the risk of contamination of the child by Aids is so great that a therapeutic abortion should be advised and recommended to the mother, but she still retains her freedom of decision.

345

Acquired immune deficiency syndrome (Aids)

An odontologist requires a patient to have an HIV test before making two major extractions.

1. From the standpoint of international law

See Article 7 of the Covenant on Civil and Political Rights and Articles 4, 5 (1) and 10 (1) of the BC, as well as Recommendation R (87) 25 of the Committee of Ministers of the Council of Europe (26.11.1987).

Possible reference to Article 26 (1) of the BC as regards, in particular, the physician's right to health.

2. From the ethical standpoint

If the patient refuses the test the doctor can exercise his right to refuse care. Free choice exists for the doctor as well as the patient, unless the latter's life is in immediate danger.

For this case see the reply to case 70 completed by that to case 71, which is also based on the Declaration on patients' rights.

3. From the standpoint of religious moralities

a. *Catholic*

The orthodontist's demand does not seem morally acceptable, because the doctor and the other carers can take every precaution to prevent infection, whether they know the patient is HIV-positive or not. Thus the odontologist's refusal to extract teeth if the patient refuses an HIV test is not acceptable. John Paul II says: "Let your solicitude know no discrimination. Know how to receive, interpret and develop the confidence placed in you by your suffering brother."[1]

b. *Protestant*

This odontologist should know that a negative test result is no guarantee that the patient has not very recently become infected. His desire to protect himself is perfectly understandable, but the way he goes about it is surprising and technically ineffective.

---

1. John Paul II, "Speech to participants in the 4th International Congress organised by the Pastoral for Health Services", in *L'Osservatore Romano*, 16 November 1989.

c. *Jewish*

This odontologist has no right to insist on an HIV test. He should take all the necessary precautions before making the extractions but can certainly not insist on a test that the patient refuses.

d. *Muslim*

The odontologist should convince the patient to have an HIV test before making the extractions. As in the previous case, medical secrecy must be respected.

e. *Buddhist*

If the practitioner respects the normal asepsis procedures there is no risk of infection. In our opinion therefore there is nothing to justify his insisting on an HIV test.

4. From the standpoint of agnostic morality

It is acceptable for the odontologist to require the test, but he cannot refuse treatment if the result is positive.

Acquired immune deficiency syndrome (Aids)

A life assurance company recommends policyholders to submit to HIV tests in order to qualify for more favourable conditions.

1. From the standpoint of international law

See Articles 7 of the Covenant on Civil and Political Rights; 8 (1) and 10 (2) of the ECHR; 5 (1) and 10 (1) of the BC, concerned in particular with information about the health of the person concerned.

2. From the ethical standpoint

Only the future insured patient has the right to decide.

An insurance contract is an accord between two parties who agree together to accept it. It therefore cannot exist if one of the parties does not agree. It is a legal problem, not an ethical one.

3. From the standpoint of religious moralities

a. *Catholic*

There are no specific references to this theme on the part of the Catholic magisterium. In general, the fact that the company "advises" HIV tests for the persons interested goes against the respect of the individual and the protection of his private life. In addition, it goes against the principle of subsidiarity.

b. *Protestant*

To be prohibited, for it would then open a Pandora's box of dubious competing offers endangering the principle of equality. The very meaning of life assurance would be seriously affected.

c. *Jewish*

Under all circumstances the practice of sending HIV test results to obtain better life assurance conditions is to be condemned. Starting with such practices would lead in the longer term to making them compulsory for everybody. Seropositive people would then find themselves not only afflicted by an incurable disease, but also automatically excluded from insurance cover.

What is more, if we accept the principle of HIV tests today, tests for other diseases will be required tomorrow. Then where would it stop?

Lastly, what is to become of the data held by these insurance companies? They could be sold or exchanged for other data. What will become of medical secrecy?

It is necessary not only to condemn such practices, but also to inform people about the risks involved in them and tell them never to be tempted into accepting such insidious offers. It is necessary above all to introduce appropriate legislation in our countries to prohibit such offers.

d. *Muslim*

Two factors are involved in making an adequate reply from the standpoint of Muslim morality:

– the problem of insurance, and more particularly life assurance, which was long considered to be risky business not tolerated by Muslim morality. For some years now however, insurance of all kinds has been authorised by a derogation (*fatwa*), in the same way as bank interest;

– the HIV test may be carried out in order to obtain better conditions from the life assurance company, with the consent of the person assured and provided that medical secrecy is respected.

e. *Buddhist*

The very principle of life assurance is called into question here; it seems to us that everybody should be able to be insured under the same conditions.

4. From the standpoint of agnostic morality

This request is acceptable provided that it does not lead to refusal to insure or to an unreasonable surcharge.

Acquired immune deficiency syndrome (Aids)

An employer in a high-risk branch requires employees to take an HIV test.

1. From the standpoint of international law

See Articles 7 of the Covenant on Civil and Political Rights; 8 (1) and 10 (2) of the ECHR; 5 (1), 10 (1) and 26 (1) of the BC, should this Article be relevant in the case. See also the reply to case 45.

2. From the ethical standpoint

It is necessary to know and assess the risks involved in the occupation.

In principle, the employer cannot have access to this type of information. The WMA has defined its ethical rules on this subject in three declarations: in 1987 in Madrid, where it affirmed the necessity for the patient's consent for the diagnostic test; in Vienna in 1988; and in Marbella in 1992.

3. From the standpoint of religious moralities

a. *Catholic*

There are no specific references to this theme on the part of the Catholic magisterium. It does not seem justified to submit employees to compulsory screening because it is possible to take every precaution to prevent infection, regardless of whether a person is known to be HIV-positive or not.

b. *Protestant*

Same reaction as with case 72: a negative test result is no guarantee for a third party of the present and future "innocuousness" of a given person. It is therefore much better to appeal to the employee's sense of responsibility and discuss with him how to best meet the challenges which could arise. What is more, while the need to protect the health – and the life – of third parties is well understood, it is necessary to assess the extent to which the "risks" in question are not more imaginary than real. In this case the employee's right to respect of his private life should be evoked and respected.

c. *Jewish*

Same reply as in case 74.

The HIV test result forms part of the individual's medical history. It is to be known only to the doctor, who is bound by professional secrecy.

In no case can the employer impose such a test before hiring an employee.

If the fact of being seropositive risks endangering the life of fellow workers or other persons, the case becomes more complex.

It would then be necessary for the requirement to comply with criteria laid down by medical ethics.

d. *Muslim*

The HIV test may be carried out at the request of an employer in a high-risk field with the consent of the employee. The doctor has the duty of convincing the employee to submit to the test and warning him of the risks involved in the case of accidental contamination. Lastly, the doctor is bound by medical secrecy.

e. *Buddhist*

It is not possible to give an answer without knowing the nature of the activity and what risks are involved and for whom.

4. From the standpoint of agnostic morality

Imposing the test is acceptable, but it is necessary to ensure that the results are confidential so as not to infringe the rights and freedoms of an HIV carrier.

351

Experimentation on vulnerable persons

A team of European paediatricians seek authorisation from the guardians of orphans between 7 and 15 to test the effects of a new molecule for treating infantile epilepsy.

1. From the standpoint of international law

The general principle of the free and informed consent of the patient being established by Article 7 of the Covenant on Civil and Political Rights, specific rules will help reply to this case.

Reference should thus be made first to Recommendation R (90) 3 adopted on 6.2.1990 by the Committee of Ministers of the Council of Europe concerning medical research on human beings. This recommendation, after stating that "for the purpose of application of these principles, medical research means any trial and experimentation carried out on human beings, the purpose of which or one of the purposes of which is to increase medical knowledge", sets out some fundamental principles: "in medical research the interests and well-being of the person undergoing medical research must always prevail over the interests of science and society. The risks incurred by a person undergoing medical research must be kept to a minimum. The risks should not be disproportionate to the benefits to that person or the importance of the aims pursued by the research"; "No medical research may be carried out without the informed, free, express and specific consent of the person undergoing it. Such consent may be freely withdrawn at any phase of the research and the person undergoing the research should be informed, before being included in it, of his right to withdraw his consent" (Principles 2 and 3 (1)). Principle 3 (2) goes on to stipulate that "the person who is to undergo medical research should be given information on the purpose of the research and the methodology of the experimentation. He should also be informed of the foreseeable risks and inconveniences to him of the proposed research. This information should be sufficiently clear and suitably adapted to enable consent to be given or refused in full knowledge of the relevant facts". Lastly, Principle 3 (3) stipulates that "The provisions of this principle should apply also to a legal representative and to a legally incapacitated person having the capacity of understanding, in the situations described in Principles 4 and 5".

Thus "a legally incapacitated person may not undergo medical research unless it is expected to produce a direct and significant benefit to his health" (Principle 5 (1)). This condition is not sufficient however: the medical research must be authorised by "his legal representative or an authority or an individual authorised or designated under his national law, must consent. "If the legally incapacitated person is capable of understanding, his consent is also required, and no research may be undertaken if he does not give his consent" (Principle 4).

"By way of exception, national law may authorise research involving a legally incapacitated person which is not of direct benefit to his health when that person offers no objection, provided that the research is to the benefit of persons in the same category and that the same scientific results cannot be obtained by research on persons who do not belong to this category" (Principle 5 (2)).

In any event, "if the person undergoing research is legally incapacitated, his legal representatives should not receive any form of remuneration whatever, except for the refund of their expenses" (Principle 13 (2)) and "persons undergoing medical research and/or their dependants should be compensated for injury and loss caused by the medical research" (Principle 14 (1)). "Terms and conditions which exclude or limit, in advance, compensation to the victim should be considered null and void" (Principle 14 (3)).

Lastly, "potential subjects of medical research should not be offered any inducement which compromises free consent" (Principle 13 (1)).

The same broad lines emerge as regards removal of substances which cannot regenerate from legally incapacitated persons, for which Article 6 (2) of Resolution (78) 29 adopted by the Committee of Ministers of the Council of Europe on 11.5.1978 on harmonisation of legislation of member states relating to removal, grafting and transplantation of human substances requires that: 1. the donor must be capable of understanding; 2. he must give his consent; 3. his legal representative must also give his consent and authorisation must also be obtained from an appropriate authority.

The consent of the guardians is therefore not sufficient *per se* to permit the experimentation.

Article 3 (1) of the Convention on the Rights of the Child stipulates that "in all the decisions concerning children, whether made by public institutions or private social protection bodies, courts, administrative authorities or legislative organs, the child's best interests must be the prime consideration" and Article 3 (3) adds: "States Parties shall see that the working of institutions, services and establishments which have the charge of children and assure their protection are in conformity with the standards fixed by the competent authorities, particularly in the field of safety and health and as regards (...) the existence of appropriate control".

Lastly, Article 12 states that: "States Parties shall assure to the child who is capable of forming his or her own views the right to express those views freely in all matters affecting the child, the views of the child being given due weight in accordance with the age and maturity of the child. For this purpose, the child shall in particular be provided the opportunity to be heard in any judicial and administrative proceedings affecting the child, either directly, or through a representative or an appropriate body, in a manner consistent with the procedural rules of national law", and Article 36 adds that "States Parties shall protect the child against all other forms of exploitation prejudicial to his or her well being".

For European case-law, see the decision of the Commission in Application No. 15853/89.

As regards the BC, the general rule (Article 15) being that scientific research in the field of biology and medicine shall be carried out freely subject to the provisions of this convention and (the) other legal provisions ensuring the protection of the human being, Article 17 of the DBC (F) is specifically concerned with the protection of persons not able to consent to research.

In detail: Article 17 (1) states that research on persons without the capacity to consent as stipulated by Article 5 may be undertaken only if all the following conditions are met: i. the conditions laid down in Article 16, sub-paragraphs i to iv, are fulfilled; ii. the results of the research have the potential to produce direct benefit to his or her health; iii. research of comparable effectiveness cannot be carried out on individuals capable of giving consent; iv. the necessary authorisation provided for under Article 6 has been given specifically and in writing; and v. the person concerned does not object".

Article 17 (2) adds that "exceptionally and under the protective conditions prescribed by law, where the research has not the potential to produce results of direct benefit to the health of the person concerned, such research may be authorised subject to the conditions laid down in paragraph 1, sub-paragraphs i, iii, iv and v above, and to the following additional conditions: i. the research has the aim of contributing, through significant improvement in the scientific understanding of the individual's condition, disease or disorder, to the ultimate attainment of results capable of conferring benefit to the person concerned or to other persons in the same age category or afflicted with the same disease or disorder or having the same condition; ii. the research entails only minimal risk and minimal burden for the individual concerned". Attention should also be drawn to Article 26 (2) and 24 of the BC, as well to the comments to case 76.

2. From the ethical standpoint

It is necessary to comply with the amended WMA Declaration of Helsinki, which in its eleventh basic principle states unequivocally that: "When the minor is capable of giving his consent, this must be obtained in addition to the consent of his legal guardians."

354

3. From the standpoint of religious moralities

a. *Catholic*

During the experimentation phase, namely when research findings are being tested on man, the good of the person, protected by ethical standards, "requires the respect of prior conditions essential for informed consent".[1] This consent may be given by the legal representative of the patient who is incapable of taking this decision, provided that it is for the benefit of the patient himself and provided that it is therapeutic experimentation.

b. *Protestant*

The question as stated is too succinct. In most countries now any research on human beings is possible only after submission of a dossier in good and due form to an *ad hoc* committee (ethics committee or committee on the protection of individual rights). These committees give an opinion only as a function of certain precise criteria, including respect of the Helsinki Charter and Recommendation R (90) 3 of the Committee of Ministers of the Council of Europe, stipulating that: "No medical research may be carried out without the informed, free, express and specific consent of the person undergoing it." This recommendation also stipulates that a legally incapacitated person (in our case a minor) may not undergo medical research unless it is expected to produce a direct and significant benefit to his health. However, "by way of exception, national law may authorise research involving a legally incapacitated person which is not of direct benefit to his health when that person offers no objection, provided that the research is to the benefit of persons in the same category and that the same scientific results cannot be obtained by research on persons who do not belong to this category". In this case the legal representative of the person concerned has to give his consent and: "If the legally incapacitated person is capable of understanding, his consent is also required".

Protestant morality here approves the autonomy and consistency of public sector action and has nothing to add to these rules.

c. *Jewish*

It is legitimate for a team of medical researchers to seek to experiment the effects of a new molecule to treat infantile epilepsy. It is also necessary to seek authorisation before carrying out such experiments.

But why do they have to choose orphans?

It all boils down to the same thing. Either the research is in no way prejudicial to the physical and mental health of the children, in which case why not make it

---

1. Pontifical Council for the Pastoral of Health Services, Charter of health personnel, No. 76, Vatican City, 1995.

available to all children of 7 to 15; or, if it represents the slightest danger, it is certainly forbidden to carry out experimentation on anybody at all, and particularly not on orphans who have already been disadvantaged.

What is shocking in this case is the discrimination made between normal children and orphans.

d. *Muslim*

Experimenting with a new molecule to study the effects on orphans of 7 to 15 suffering from epilepsy poses a serious ethical problem *vis-à-vis* their guardians from whom authorisation is sought. In the first place, this type of experimentation cannot be carried out if the molecule is very different from those already known in the treatment of epilepsy, since secondary effects may have irreversible effects, which is contrary to Muslim morality, one of the essential principles of which is the maintenance of the physical integrity of the individual.

e. *Buddhist*

Any attempt to experiment on vulnerable persons is to be prohibited.

4. From the standpoint of agnostic morality

Assuming that the experimentation involves no danger, it is necessary to have the agreement of the guardian, the supervisory authority and a hospital ethics committee for such a practice to be acceptable.

Experimentation on vulnerable persons

A medical research team seeks authorisation from the head of a psychiatric establishment to experiment with a new molecule in phase I, with no direct therapeutic value.

1. From the standpoint of international law

In the terms of Principle 10 of Recommendation R (90) 3 of the Committee of Ministers to Council of Europe member states concerning medical research on human beings (6.2.1990), "medical research may not be carried out unless satisfactory evidence as to its safety for the person undergoing research is furnished". Principle 11 adds that "medical research that is not in accordance with scientific criteria in its design and cannot answer the questions posed is unacceptable even if the way it is to be carried out poses no risk to the person undergoing research" (on this point, see also Principle 1).

Lastly, Principle 2 (1) stipulates that "in medical research the interests and well-being of the person undergoing medical research must always prevail over the interests of science and society" and Principle 16 states that "any medical research which is unplanned, or contrary to any of the preceding principles or in any other way contrary to ethics or law, or not in accordance with scientific methods in its design and cannot answer the questions posed should be prohibited or, if it has already begun, stopped or revised, even if it poses no risk to the person(s) undergoing the research".

As regards the question of consent in particular, Principle 3 (1) of Recommendation R (90) 3 speaks of "informed, free, express and specific consent of the person undergoing" medical research, who should be given information "sufficiently clear and suitably adapted to enable consent to be given or refused in full knowledge of the relevant facts" (Principle 3 (2)). The same is true of Article 5 (1) of the BC and points 34 to 40 of the explanatory report, being the word 'intervention' understood in its widest sense, as in Article 4, that is to say, it covers all medical acts, in particular interventions performed for the purpose of preventive care, diagnosis, treatment, rehabilitation or research. The patient's consent is considered to be free and informed if it is given on the basis of objective information from the responsible health care professional as to the nature and the potential consequences of the planned intervention (...), in the absence of any pressure from anyone (...). The information must include the purpose, nature and consequences of the intervention and the risks involved. Information on the risks involved in the intervention (...) must cover not only the risks inherent in the type of intervention contemplated, but also any risks related to the individual characteristics of each patient, such as age or the existence of other pathologies (...). Moreover, this information must be sufficiently clear and suitably worded for the person who is to undergo the intervention. The patient must be put in a position, through the use of terms he or she can understand, to weigh up the necessity or usefulness of the aim and methods of the intervention against the risks and the discomfort or pain it will cause. Consent may take various forms. It may be express or implied. Express consent may be either verbal or written. Article 5, which is general and covers very different situations, does not require any particular form of consent. The latter will largely depend on the nature of the intervention. It is agreed that express consent would be inappropriate as regards many routine medical acts. The consent may therefore often be implicit, as long as the patient is sufficiently informed. In some cases, however, for example, invasive diagnostic acts or treatments, express consent may be required. Moreover, the patient's express, written consent should normally be sought for participation in research. Freedom of consent implies that consent may be withdrawn at any time and that the patient's decision shall be respected once he or she has been fully informed of the consequences."

In the case of persons not able to consent (whether legally incapacitated or not) Article 6 is the other general rule provided for by the BC (together with points 41 to 49 of the explanatory report appended thereto).

The BC has three other provisions concerning specifically scientific research and the protection of persons undergoing research, i.e. Articles 15, 16 and 17 and points 89 to 114 of the explanatory report.

The principle of freedom of research in the field of medicine and biology being set in Article 15 "subject to the provisions of this convention and the other legal provisions ensuring the protection of the human being", Article 16 stipulates the conditions which have to be met in order to carry out research on a person. Said conditions are the following: "i. there is no alternative of comparable effectiveness to research on humans; ii. the risks which may be incurred by the person are not disproportionate to the potential benefits of the research; iii. the research project has been approved by the competent body after independent examination of its scientific merit, including assessment of the importance of the aim of the research, and multidisciplinary review of its ethical acceptability; iv. the persons undergoing research have been informed of their rights and the safeguards prescribed by law for their protection; v. the necessary consent as provided for under Article 5 has been given expressly, specifically and is documented. Such consent may be freely withdrawn at any time".

According to Article 17(1), a few other conditions have to be met if the person undergoing research is without the capacity to consent as stipulated in Article 5. Said additional conditions are the following: "(...); ii. the results of the research have the potential to produce real and direct benefit to the person's health; iii. research of comparable effectiveness cannot be carried out on individuals capable of giving consent; iv. the necessary authorisation provided for under Article 6 has been given specifically and in writing and v. the person concerned does not object." The general rule with regard to research on a person who is not able to consent being namely that the research must be potentially beneficial to the health of the person concerned, that the benefit must be real and follow from the potential results of the research, while the risk must not be disproportionate to the potential benefit, Article 17(2) provides exceptionally for the possibility of waiving its direct benefit rule on certain very strict conditions. "Were such research to be banned altogether, progress in the battles to maintain and improve health and to combat diseases only afflicting children, mentally disabled persons or persons suffering from senile dementia would become impossible. The group of people concerned may in the end benefit from this kind of research" (point 107 of the explanatory report).

Thus, under the protective conditions prescribed by law, Article 17(2) stipulates that "where the research has not the potential to produce results of direct benefit to the health of the persons concerned, such research may be authorised subject to the conditions laid down in paragraph 1, subparagraphs i, iii, iv and v above, and to the following additional conditions: i) the research has the aim of contributing, through significant improvement in the scientific understanding of the individual's condition, disease or disorder, to the ultimate attainment of results capable of conferring benefit to the person concerned or the other persons in the same age category or afflicted with the same disease or disorder or having the same conditions; ii) the research entails only minimal risk and minimal burden for the individual concerned."

Reference should also be made to case 75.

For the rest, reference should be made to the provisions mentioned in the reply to case 10, in particular Article 5 (2) of Recommendation R (83) 2 adopted by the Council of Europe (22.2.1983), concerning the legal protection of persons suffering from mental disorder placed as involuntary patients.

2. From the ethical standpoint

It is necessary to comply with amended WMA Declaration of Helsinki, which in its eleventh basic principle states that: "In the case where a physical or mental incapacity makes it impossible to obtain informed consent, the authorisation of the close relatives replaces that of the subject, with the same reserve.

3. From the standpoint of religious moralities

a. *Catholic*

The patient "must be informed as to the experimentation, its aims and its possible risks, so that he can give or refuse his consent in full knowledge and freedom".[1] As a result, those who are incapable of giving consent cannot be subjected to experimentation which requires informed consent: only therapeutic experimentation can be practised on them, after all other available therapeutic resources have been exhausted.

b. *Protestant*
Same reply as in the preceding case.

c. *Jewish*
The experimentation concerned in this case is of no direct therapeutic value. I therefore do not understand why this team of medical researchers wishes to carry it out.

If the experimentation is of direct therapeutic interest, it is necessary to be certain that it presents no danger to the patients.

But here again, I wonder why there should be discrimination between people? Why choose mentally ill patients in psychiatric hospitals who cannot defend themselves?

d. *Muslim*
Experimenting with new molecules with no direct therapeutic value directly on psychiatric patients is contrary to Muslim morality because there is a risk of impairing their physical or mental integrity, two of the essential principles of Muslim morality.

e. *Buddhist*
Since the patients are unable to make an informed decision due to their mental condition, it would appear dangerous to agree to such a request.

4. From the standpoint of agnostic morality

A favourable opinion must be sought and obtained from a hospital ethics committee.

---

1. John Paul II, "Address to the participants in two medical and surgical conferences, 27 October 1980", in *Insegnamenti*, III/2, 1009, No. 5, 16 November 1989.

Transplants

A surgical team seeks authorisation to make intracerebral grafts of viable mesencephalic tissues from embryos and foetuses of six to nine weeks for experimentation on a number of people suffering from Parkinson's disease.

1. From the standpoint of international law

This case raises two problems: the consent for the graft of viable embryo and foetus tissues, and consent for experimentation on Parkinson's disease patients.

Regarding the first question, Recommendation 1046 (1986) adopted on 24.9.1986 by the Parliamentary Assembly of the Council of Europe on the use of human embryos and foetuses for diagnostic therapeutic, scientific, industrial and commercial purposes distinguishes between embryos and foetuses living *in utero* or outside the uterus and dead embryos and foetuses.

As regards the latter, point B of the appendix to this recommendation, which sets out the "rules governing the use of human embryos or foetuses and the removal of their tissues for diagnostic and therapeutic purposes", stipulates in paragraph vi that "the use of dead embryos or foetuses must be an exceptional measure, justified in the present state of knowledge by the rare nature of the illness treated, the absence of any equally effective therapy and a manifest advantage (such as survival) for the person receiving treatment; it must comply with the following rules: a. the decision to terminate pregnancy and the conditions (date, technique, etc.) must under no circumstances be influenced by the possible or desired subsequent use of the embryo or foetus; b. any use of the embryo or foetus must be undertaken by highly qualified teams in approved hospitals or scientific centres supervised by the public authorities; to the extent that national legislation foresees, these centres must possess multidisciplinary ethical committees; c. total independence between the medical team terminating pregnancy and the team which might use the embryos or foetuses for therapeutic purposes must be guaranteed; d. embryos and foetuses may not be used without the consent of the parents or gamete donors where the latters' identity is known; e. the use of embryos, foetuses or their tissues for profit or remuneration shall not be allowed".

(It should be noted in passing that point B.v of Recommendation 1100 (1989) of the Parliamentary Assembly of the Council of Europe on the use of human embryos and foetuses in scientific research invites the governments of member states "to draw up national or regional registers of accredited and authorised centres where research or experiments are undertaken on reproductive material – be it human gametes, embryos or foetuses or cells, tissues or organs – and to monitor and evaluate such activities, and to require that the biomedical and scientific teams are properly qualified and authorised to perform such activities and have the necessary resources".)

In application of the principles laid down in Recommendation 1046 (1986), Recommendation 1100 (1989) cited above stipulates in point F.15 of the appendix that: "before proceeding to any intervention on dead embryos or foetuses, centres or clinics shall ascertain whether death is partial (when the embryo is clinically dead (its cells, tissues or organs may still remain alive for several hours) or total (when clinical death is matched by death of the cells)". Possible application, by analogy, of Articles 11 (1) and 12 (3) of Resolution (78) 29 on harmonisation of legislation of member states relating to removal, grafting and transplantation of human substances, adopted by the Committee of Ministers of the Council of Europe on 11.5.1978.

In its turn, point 16 of Recommendation 1100 adds that "the use of biological matter from dead embryos or foetuses for scientific, preventive, diagnostic, therapeutic, pharmaceutical, clinical or surgical purposes shall be permitted within the framework of the rules governing investigation, experimentation, diagnosis and therapy, in accordance with the terms of this recommendation".

Lastly, paragraph H of the same appendix (points 20 to 24) stipulates that "the donation of human embryological material shall be authorised solely for scientific research or diagnostic, preventive or therapeutic purposes. Its sale shall be prohibited. The intentional creation and/or keeping alive of embryos or foetuses, *in vitro* or *in utero*, for any scientific research purpose, for instance to obtain genetic material, cells, tissues or of the organs therefrom, shall be prohibited. The donation and use of human embryological material shall be conditional on the freely given written consent of the donor parents. The donation of organs shall be devoid of any commercial aspect. The purchase or sale of embryos or foetuses or parts thereof by their donor parents or other parties, and their importation or exportation, shall also be prohibited".

With respect to the BC, Chapter VI (Articles 19 and 20) is specifically concerned with organ and tissue removal from living donors for transplantation purposes.

In the case of living embryos or foetuses *in utero*, the expression "living donor" does not, *per se*, permit us to know whether the donor is the pregnant woman or the embryo or foetus itself. As a result, the problem of the express and specific consent, given in writing or before an official body (Article 19 (2)) remains unsolved. Attention should be drawn, however, to the terms of Article 19 (1): "the therapeutic benefit of the recipient and where there is no suitable organ or tissue available from a deceased person and other alternative therapeutic method of comparable effectiveness" and the same expression "alternative of comparable effectiveness" appears in Articles 16 and 17 concerning respectively the protection of persons undergoing research and the protection of persons not able to consent to research.

In the contrary case of living embryos *in vitro*, reference should be made, as regards research, to Article 18 (1) of the BC: "where the law allows research on embryos *in vitro,* it shall ensure adequate protection of the embryo", in accordance with Article 1 of the BC and points 18 and 19 of the explanatory report appended thereto. Consequently, Article 18 (2) of the BC adds that "the creation of human embryos for research purposes is prohibited". According to point 20 of the explanatory report, "each Party shall take in its internal law the necessary measures to give effect to the provisions of the Convention (…). The internal law of the Parties shall conform to the Convention. Conformity between the Convention and domestic law may be achieved either by applying directly the Convention's provisions in domestic law or by enacting the necessary legislation to give effect to them. With regard to each provision, the means will have to be determined by each Party in accordance with its constitutional law and taking into account the nature of the provision in question. In this respect, it should be noted that the Convention contains a number of provisions which may, under the domestic law of many states, qualify as directly applicable ("self-executing provisions")." See also points 115 and 116 of the appended explanatory report.

Possible application, by analogy, of Article 6 (2) and (3) of Resolution (78) 29 on harmonisation of legislation of member states relating to removal, grafting and transplantation of human substances, adopted by the Committee of Ministers of the Council of Europe on 11.5.1978.

As for the consent of the Parkinson's disease patients themselves to the proposed experimentation on them, this consent is required according to the terms and principles set out in the reply to case 76.

2. From the ethical standpoint

Grafts of tissue from the ventral part of the mesencephalon of an embryo or foetus, not yet differentiated by potential producers of dopamine, on the deficient striata of Parkinson's disease patients have been successfully experimented on rats for some time. Experiments have been carried out in several countries, in particular in Europe, under the control of ethics committees, but so far no convincing results have been achieved. Uncertainty as to the optimum age of the embryos and foetuses is probably the reason, but it is obviously unethical to experiment with this.

The use of tissues from embryos and foetuses must remain exceptional, only in cases where there is no other palliative, and under the strict control of ethics committees, because of possible pressure for planned abortions, which could increase due to clinical demand.

One solution might be to try to obtain a culture of dopamine-producing embryonic cells, which could even indicate the way to go for the serotonin essential for Alzheimer's disease.

Same reply as for cases 75 and 76.

The Declaration of Helsinki of 1964 was amended and completed in Tokyo in 1975, Venice in 1983 and Hong Kong in 1989.

3. From the standpoint of religious moralities

a. *Catholic*
Catholic morality condemns "the procedure which exploits still living human embryos and foetuses – sometimes 'produced' precisely for this purpose of fertilisation *in vitro* – or as a 'biological material' to be used or as donors of tissue to be transplanted for the treatment of certain diseases. In reality, killing innocent human creatures, even if it is for the advantage of others, constitutes an absolutely unacceptable act".[1]

b. *Protestant*
From whom is the authorisation sought? According to what protocol and what criteria? The question cannot be answered as it stands and the promoters of the research would really have to have extremely good reasons, together with a maximum of guarantees for the patients, for the taking account of their project even to be envisaged.

c. *Jewish*
Intracerebral grafts of viable mesencephalic tissues from embryos and foetuses of six to nine weeks for experimentation on a number of patients suffering from Parkinson's disease gives rise to the following problem: can tissue from aborted embryos and foetuses be used?

If there is some link between termination of pregnancy and the problem of removing viable mesencephalic tissues from embryos, this removal must be prohibited because it risks becoming the cause for the termination of pregnancy.

If, on the other hand, we consider the two problems to be independent of one another, and that the woman has decided to terminate her pregnancy anyway, then the foetus may have the status of a cadaver, which in certain circumstances[2] may then be used to treat the disease of certain patients and permit them to return to a normal life.

It is clear that this removal can be carried out only on the express condition that the doctors who operate proceed in a dignified and honourable way worthy of the dead and give the body and the parts of the body to the undertakers for burial.

---

1. John Paul II, *Evangelium Vitae*, 25 March 1995, No. 63.
2. See the cases relating to autopsies and the removal of organs.

It is also necessary to take the appropriate ethical precautions. Among these I would cite in particular some of the ethical rules which NECTAR (Network of European Central Nervous System Transplantation and Restoration) intends to publish in the *Journal of Neurology*:

– tissues for experimental or clinical transplantations may be obtained only from dead embryos or foetuses;

– it is not permitted to keep embryos artificially alive in order to be able to remove tissue later;

– abortion cannot be induced for the purpose of making transplants even if the patients who would benefit are extremely ill. The decision to abort must precede any discussion as to the potential use of the foetus. There must be no link between the donor and the receiver and no designation of the receiver by the donor;

– the planning or procedure of the abortion may not be influenced by the necessities of a transplantation activity;

– the acquisition of foetus embryos or their tissues must not give rise to any profit or remuneration;

– foetal tissue must be treated with the same respect as that surrounding other tissue coming from human cadavers.

d. *Muslim*

To the extent that intracerebral grafts of viable mesencephalic tissues from embryos and foetuses of six to nine weeks are likely to be of therapeutic value in treating Parkinson's disease and are practised on people suffering from Parkinson's disease, Muslim morality could accept them provided that the experimentation does not carry any serious risk of irreversible effects and have every chance of not impairing the physical and mental integrity of the patients, whose free and informed consent must also be obtained.

e. *Buddhist*

Any manipulation on foetuses gives rise to serious problems.

4. From the standpoint of agnostic morality

If the patient gives his conscious, free and informed consent, the experimentation is acceptable.

Transplants

A hospital service refuses haemodialysis or inclusion on the waiting list for renal transplants for a man of 71 suffering from an evolutive bilateral renal sclerosis, budgetary considerations imposing other priorities.

1. From the standpoint of international law

While all the international legal texts, binding and non-binding, concerning the fundamental rights and freedoms stipulate that member states "shall secure to everyone within their jurisdiction the rights and freedoms defined" therein, and in particular the right to life, (for all these see Article 1 of the ECHR) with no discrimination for reasons of sex, race, colour, language, religion, political or other opinion, national or social origin, association with a national minority, property, birth or other status (see for example Article 14 of the ECHR), the international instruments concerned with economic and social rights (for all see Article 2 (1) of the Covenant on Economic, Social and Cultural Rights) state that "each state undertakes to act, through its own efforts and through international assistance and co-operation, notably economic and technical, to the maximum of its available resources, with a view to ensure progressively the full exercise of the rights recognised in the text by all appropriate means, including in particular the adoption of legislative measures". The principle of non-discrimination is also recognised (see for example Article 2 (2) of the Covenant on Economic, Social and Cultural Rights).

The right to health being one of the economic and social rights, its implementation often comes up against national budgetary difficulties concerning either the administration of health care as such, or because of the existence of other government expenditure priorities.

This situation being fairly widespread in our European societies, the BC deals, *ex professo*, with the problem of equitable access to health care in Article 3, which is worded as follows: "Parties taking into account health needs and available resources shall take appropriate measures with a view to providing, within their jurisdiction, equitable access to health care of appropriate quality". In their turn, points 23 to 27 of the explanatory report state that: "this article defines an aim and imposes an obligation on states to use their best endeavours to reach it. The aim is to ensure equitable access to health care in accordance with the person's medical needs. 'Health care' means the medical services offering diagnostic, preventive, therapeutic and rehabilitative interventions, designed to maintain or improve a person's state of health or alleviate a person's suffering. This care must be of a fitting standard in the light of scientific progress and be subject to continuous quality assessment. Access to health care must be equitable. In this context, 'equitable' means first and foremost the absence of unjustified discrimination. Although not synonymous with absolute equality, equitable access implies effectively obtaining a satisfactory degree of care. The Parties to the Convention are required to take appropriate steps to achieve this aim as far as the available resources permit. The purpose of this provision is not to create an individual right on which each person may rely in legal proceedings against the state, but rather to prompt the latter to adopt the requisite measures as part of its social policy in order to ensure equitable access to health care. Although states are now making substantial efforts to ensure a satisfactory level of health care, the scale of this effort largely depends on the volume of available resources. Moreover, state measures to ensure equitable access may take many different forms and a wide variety of methods may be employed to this end."

Having presented the above by way of preamble, it should be added that in the terms of Article 2 of the BC, "the interests and welfare of the human being shall prevail over the sole interest of society or science" and that point 156 of the explanatory report states that: "defending the economic well-being of the country (...) and national security are not included amongst the general exceptions referred to in the second paragraph of Article 26, unlike Article 8 of the ECHR. It did not appear desirable, in the context of this convention, to make the exercise of fundamental rights chiefly concerned with the protection of a person's rights in the health sphere subject to the economic well-being of the country (...) or to national security. The economic aspect is, however, referred to in Article 3, by the words 'available resources'; however, within the meaning of this article this notion does not represent a reason for allowing for an exception to the rights secured in other provisions of the Convention".

Possible reference to Article 23 of the BC: "the Parties shall provide appropriate judicial protection to prevent or to put a stop to an unlawful infringement of the rights and principles set forth in this Convention at short notice". See also point 76 of the explanatory report appended to the BC, in terms of which "the prohibition of discrimination set out thus applies to all areas included in the field of application of this Convention, as well as point 77 of the same, in terms of which whereas the term "discrimination" has usually a negative connotation in French, this is not necessarily the case in English (where one must use the expression "unfair discrimination"), it has, however, been decided to keep the same term in both languages, as it is in the ECHR and in the case-law of the Court. Discrimination here must, therefore, in French as in English, be understood as unfair discrimination."

2. From the ethical standpoint

This refusal has to be assimilated to euthanasia for economic reasons, the only victims of which are the poor. It is thus totally contrary to medical ethics.

367

Reference should be made to the Declaration on euthanasia adopted by the WMA in Madrid in 1987. It is very short and leaves no room for any doubt on this subject.

3. From the standpoint of religious moralities

a. *Catholic*
In our welfare states there is a "utilitarist mentality which makes the increasing numbers of aged and infirm people appear very burdensome and intolerable. They are very often [considered] almost exclusively as a function of productive efficiency criteria, according to which an irreversible incapacity deprives a life of any value".[1] Therefore, though this economic criterion cannot be ignored, exclusive reference to it cannot be accepted as a moral principle, because the final reference value can but be the life of each individual.

b. *Protestant*
It seems strange that haemodialysis and inclusion on the waiting list for a kidney transplant should be refused. While the latter is not so much a budgetary problem but more one of a tragic shortage of kidneys, access to haemodialysis comes under the right to treatment. It is true that recent studies have shown that the management of treatment resources does not always meet the required standards of rigour and transparency. There therefore still remains much to be done.

c. *Jewish*
It is inadmissible to discriminate between citizens and have a two-tier medical system.

Every person has a right to the health care he needs.

It is inadmissible that budgetary reasons should lead to the refusal to treat a patient.

Budgetary reasons may never be invoked when a human life is at stake. To allow this is once again to open the door to all the abuses. Tomorrow, there will be no more care for old people, and after that it may be the turn of immigrants and foreigners, etc.

This patient of 71 should be admitted to the hospital service and given the dialysis he needs. He should also be added to the waiting list for renal transplants if the conditions required for this transplant are fulfilled.

d. *Muslim*
To refuse haemodialysis for a 71-year-old patient is shocking, to put it mildly. Furthermore, the budgetary problem cannot be a reason for not including him on

---

1. John Paul II, *Evangelium Vitae*, 25 March 1995, No. 64.

the waiting list for a renal transplant. The Koran (Sura II, v. 211) recommends succouring one's neighbour, and Sura V, v. 32, states that "He who saveth a life, shall be as though he had saved all mankind alive".

e. *Buddhist*
The patient's age does not justify his being denied the benefit of modern techniques which could help him.

4. From the standpoint of agnostic morality

Given the patient's tragic situation a hospital service cannot refuse either haemodialysis or inclusion on the list of patients awaiting a kidney transplant.

369

Human genetics

*A suspicious father approaches a genetic identification laboratory
for a filiation test.*

1. From the standpoint of international law

Point 12.*f* of Resolution 327/88 EEC on the ethical and legal problems of
genetic manipulation adopted on 16.3.1989 by the European Parliament
requires that "knowledge resulting from genetic analyses carried out must
be absolutely reliable and provide precise information on clearly defined medical facts the knowledge of which is of direct interest for the health of the people
concerned".

In its turn, point 21 stipulates that "genetic analyses may be imposed in legal
proceedings only in exceptional cases and may be ordered by the judge in very
restricted fields; in this connection, only the parts of the genetic analysis relevant to
the case may be used, and no conclusions are to be drawn from the total genetic
information".

Lastly, point 33 states that "screening can be carried out on new-born babies
only to detect curable diseases and on a voluntary basis and non-participation must
not entail any disadvantage". The communication of these data shall be prohibited
under criminal law (point 34).

Reference should be made also to Article 10 (1) and 26 (1) of the BC, in the
terms of which everyone has the right to respect for private life in relation to information about his or her health and "No restrictions shall be placed on the exercise
of the rights and protective provisions contained in this Convention other than such
as are prescribed by law and are necessary in a democratic society in the interest of
public safety, for the prevention of crime, for the protection of public health or for
the protection of the rights and freedoms of others". Reference should also be made
to points 152 and 87 of the explanatory report appended to the BC, as well as to
point 159 of the same.

2. From the ethical standpoint

This question concerns the father's rights as defined by the law, not medical
ethics.

The doctor may comply with the request if he first obtains the child's informed
consent.

The WMA Declaration on genetics stresses, as with other delicate ethical questions, the obligation to respect the doctor's conscience clause.

3. From the standpoint of religious moralities

a. *Catholic*

In this case we see two ethical problems: first, the respect of the rights of the child; second, the respect for private life and family intimacy. The results of these examinations may constitute a threat to the family; as a result, genetic examinations to determine paternity should be reserved to public institutions with experience and authority, and practised only at the request of the court or a consultative institution for legitimate purposes laid down by the law or to favour family union.

b. *Protestant*

It is well known that there are considerable differences in the legislation in European countries on whether it is permitted to proceed to biological identification. But in any event, while it is understandable that a child may seek to determine his exact filiation, the reverse appears immoral and it is inadmissible that a "father" should proceed to a test without the specific consent of the child, and even the idea of wishing to obtain this consent appears reprehensible.

c. *Jewish*

Nothing can prevent a suspicious father from approaching a genetic identification laboratory for a filiation test.

If there is reason to doubt this filiation I would even say that it is essential to make this test, for a whole series of consequences may result from the religious standpoint.

d. *Muslim*

The filiation test requested by the suspicious father cannot be carried out without the consent of the mother.

e. *Buddhist*

What is important in filiation is the link established between the child and the person who cares for it with love and helps it to successfully enter adulthood.

4. From the standpoint of agnostic morality

Respect of the suspicious father's freedoms means that he should not be refused such an analysis, but the law should prohibit him from deriving any kind of advantage from it.

Human genetics

A research team working on population genetics seeks the parents' authorisation to take a sample from a minor and transmit the result to a deoxyribonucleic acid (DNA) bank.

1. From the standpoint of international law

Resolution 327/88 EEC cited above establishes the fundamental principle of the self-determination of the patient (point 12.*c*: "genetic analyses and genetic consultations must be solely for the good of the subjects, be based exclusively on voluntary action; if those concerned desire it, the results of the examination must be communicated to them. This principle stems from the formulation of point 33, in the terms of which "screening can be practised on new-born babies only to detect curable diseases and on a voluntary basis and non-participation must not entail any disadvantage".

In addition, point 12.*f* stipulates that "knowledge resulting from genetic analyses carried out must be absolutely reliable and provide precise information on clearly defined medical facts the knowledge of which is of direct interest for the health of the people concerned".

Lastly, point 12.*d* places among the essential preconditions for recourse to genetic analyses the prohibition of communication, collection, storage or evaluation of genetic data by public authorities or private organisations.

As a result, there is no need to discuss here the problem of the consent of the parents or of minors capable of understanding.

As regards the BC, Article 12 stipulates that "tests which are predictive of genetic diseases or which serve either to identify the subject as a carrier of a gene responsible for a disease or to detect a genetic predisposition or susceptibility to a disease may be only performed for health purposes or for scientific research linked to health purposes, and subject to appropriate genetic counselling". As for the explanatory report, points 80 and 88 state that: "the right to know as well as the right not to know and proper informed consent are (…) of particular importance in this field since problems may clearly arise for the individual from tests predictive of genetic disease for which there is currently no effective treatment. A further complicating factor is that tests predictive of genetically determined disease may also have implications for members of the family and the offspring of the person who has undergone testing. It is essential that appropriate professional standards are developed in this field" and that "according to Article 5, a genetic test may only be carried out after the person concerned has given free and informed consent. Article 12 adds a supplementary condition which is that predictive tests must be accompanied by appropriate genetic counselling." To this it must be added, in terms of point 82 of the explanatory report appended to the BC, that "because of the particular problems which are related to predictive testing, it is necessary to strictly limit its applicability to health purposes for the individual. Scientific research likewise should be carried out in the context of developing medical treatment and enhancing our ability to prevent disease."

See also Articles 16 and 17 (1) and (2) of the BC, the latter referring to Article 6 of the BC, as well as points 103 to 114 of the explanatory report appended thereto. Reference should also be made to Article 8 of the ECHR, 6 of the Convention for the Protection of Individuals with regard to Automatic Processing of Personal Data, as well as to Article 10 (1) of the BC.

2. From the ethical standpoint

If the child is capable of understanding, his agreement is just as essential as that of the parents.

This reply is based on the eleventh basic principle of the WMA Declaration of Helsinki.

3. From the standpoint of religious moralities

a. *Catholic*

"In the research phase, ethical standards require orientation towards the promotion of human well-being. Any research contrary to the true good of the person would be immoral. To invest energy and resources in it would contradict the humane ends of science and its progress".[1] As regards taking samples of biological tissues or liquids from a minor for the purposes of research, once it is established that this entails no risk, the taking of the sample requires the informed consent of the parents and of the minor, if he is capable of understanding. The general considerations regarding secrecy in general and the professional secrecy of doctors and geneticists in particular also apply here. It can rightly be said that the respect of secrecy is a duty directly connected with the eighth commandment.[2]

b. *Protestant*

Here again, more details of the case are required. On the face of it, why not, provided that the minor also gives his consent and that anonymity is strictly preserved.

---

1. Pontifical Council for the Pastoral of Health Services, Charter of health personnel, No. 76, Vatican City, 1995.
2. Puis XII, *Broadcast speeches and messages*, Vol. II, 1944-45, p. 194; Vol. XV, 1953-54, p. 73.

c. *Jewish*

For this sample to be permissible, it is first of all necessary to be certain of the confidential nature of the results obtained. It is also necessary to know the precise aim of this research team. Lastly it is necessary to be certain that taking this sample exposes the child to no danger.

d. *Muslim*

In the case where the minor's parents are in favour of the taking of the sample and transmission of the result to a DNA bank, this operation is not contrary to Muslim morality, all the less so as this is considered to be a contribution to knowledge and scientific progress.

e. *Buddhist*

The opinion is positive provided that confidentiality is respected and anonymity preserved.

4. From the standpoint of agnostic morality

Assuming that it is indeed an epidemiological study, it is essential to obtain the parents' authorisation after a favourable opinion (obligatory) has been obtained from a hospital ethics committee.

Human genetics

The European Patent Office in Munich considers an as yet unknown human gene extract to be patentable, if it has an industrial application, contrary to many ethical opinions which consider it to be a discovery.

1. From the standpoint of international law

No specific reply in international human rights law at present. The guiding principle in all the international instruments, binding and non-binding, enforceable or not, in the field of human health is and remains, however, the interest and well-being of the individual and of the human being, the respect of his dignity, his identity and his integrity, which must always prevail over economic interests.

The rule of the prohibition of financial gain from the human body and its parts is reaffirmed by Article 21 of the BC and underlined by the wording of Article 26 (2).

See also Articles 23 and 25 of the BC.

2. From the ethical standpoint

It is indeed a discovery belonging to the scientific heritage of the human community, not to the commercial company.

This position is clearly expressed in the Declaration of Marbella on the human genome, which states: "no patent must be issued for the human genome, even partially".

The WMA Declaration on genetics stresses, as with other delicate ethical questions, the obligation to respect the doctor's conscience clause.

3. From the standpoint of religious moralities

a. *Catholic*

There are no specific references to this theme on the part of the Catholic magisterium. In the moral evaluation it must, nevertheless, be considered that while a knowledge of the human gene is useful for science, this gene cannot be patented, even if it has an industrial application, and it must remain under public control. Furthermore, any patent of a human gene represents an unacceptable appropriation of the human body.

b. *Protestant*

A sound creation doctrine rejects any attempt to patent the human genome as immoral. What is more, this is not of the order of invention but rather of discovery, namely something which belongs to all.

c. *Jewish*

The extraction of a hitherto unknown human gene, even if it has an industrial application, must always be considered a discovery and benefit the whole scientific world with no restriction. The strength of scientific research lies in the fact that it lies outside financial and commercial interests. This also to a large extent helps it to advance and progress.

d. *Muslim*

The human body and its products, and in the present case its genes, cannot be used for commercial purposes.

e. *Buddhist*

This operation is at present contrary to French legislation.

4. From the standpoint of agnostic morality

The human body is not tradable and it is outside all the rules of property.

Any discovery concerning human material is thus the property of the human race and cannot be appropriated for commercial purposes.

It should be remembered that any organised society should make the necessary technical and financial resources available to the medical sciences.

Selective refusal of blood transfusions (Jehovah's Witnesses)
Informed consent and selective choice of therapy

Patient of 37, Jehovah's Witness, married and father of two children, hospitalised for major digestive haemorrhage with a haemoglobin count of less than 5 g/dl. Emergency fibroscopic examination shows renewed outbreak of ulcerous disease. Transfusion recommended by the duty anaesthetist; refusal (in writing) by the conscious patient. Emergency transfer to a centre for surgery without transfusion. Administration of recombinatory human erythropoietin and intravenous iron; proton pump inhibitor for the ulcerous growth. Because of the risk of a haemorrhagic relapse a preventive thoracoscopic vagotomy is carried out.

1. From the standpoint of international law

In the terms of Article 10.iii of Recommendation 1134 (1990) adopted on 1.10.1990 by the Parliamentary Assembly of the Council of Europe on the rights of minorities (ethnic, linguistic, religious or other) "the special situation of a given minority may justify special measures in its favour". This is what has been done in the case presented here, with alternative treatment being given instead of the refused transfusion.

With respect to the thoracoscopic vagotomy, if the underlying legal problem is that of the patient's informed consent, reference should also be made to the many binding and non-binding provisions already cited several times concerning patient's consent in emergency and other situations, including Articles 5, 8 and 9 of the BC.

If the legal problem is that of the problem of the selective choice of therapy, reference should be made to Article 10.iii of Recommendation 1134 (1990) cited above, as well as to Article 4 of the BC.

As regards European case-law concerning Jehovah's Witnesses, see Decision No. 255 of 23.6.1993 in the *Hoffmann* case (*Commission v. Austria*) and Decision No. 260 of 25.5.1993 in the *Kokkinakis* case (*Commission v. Greece*).

As regards other Churches or religions, see the Commission's decisions in Application Nos. 12587/86; 13975/88; 14524/89 and 17522/90, and also the observation of 7.12.1991 of the International Human Rights Committee concerning Communication No. 446/1991.

Lastly, as regards sects and new religious movements, reference should be made to Recommendation 1178 (1992) adopted on 5.12.1992 by the Parliamentary Assembly of the Council of Europe.

2. From the ethical standpoint

Every patient has the right to refuse a treatment. He must be correctly and completely informed about the risks to his life if he refuses.

This treatment is perfectly acceptable if the patient refuses any other treatment: it is his decision. But there can be no obligation on the doctor to effect a particular treatment if he does not wish to.

This is a principle affirmed in the Lisbon Declaration on patients' rights adopted by the WMA in 1981.

3. From the standpoint of religious moralities

a. *Catholic*

"When called upon to intervene medically on a patient, the health professional must be in possession of his consent, (...) he can act only if his patient explicitly or implicitly authorises it."[1] Respect of the religious freedom of the patient who refuses certain types of care obliges the doctor to resort to alternative methods from which the patient's health may benefit.

b. *Protestant*

The case is presented more in the form of a summary than a question offering alternatives. It is clear that the patient's conscious and clearly expressed refusal cannot be ignored.

c. *Jewish*

For Jewish tradition, the consumption of blood is prohibited. This prohibition finds its origin in Leviticus, 3, v. 17: "eat neither fat nor blood".

Mosaic law is extremely strict with regard to the sin of consuming blood. Therefore the elimination of every last trace is ensured by many regulations and the laws for slaughtering according to the rite, salting the meat, etc. "Only be sure that thou eat not the blood: for the blood is the life; and thou mayest not eat the life with the meat. Thou shalt not eat it; thou shalt pour it upon the earth as water. Thou shalt not eat it; that it may go well with thee and with thy children after thee" (Deut., 12, vs. 23-25).

This prohibition concerns only consumption through the mouth, however. Blood transfusion for medical purposes is not considered by the Rabbis of the Talmud to be consumption and is therefore permitted.

---

1. Pontifical Council for the Pastoral of Health Services, Charter of health personnel, No. 146, Vatican City, 1995.

In addition, it is important to recall that for Jewish tradition the defence of life is a supreme value. The respect of human life is absolute, sacred and inviolable. Human life has an infinite value because it is a gift of God and because man is made in the image of God. The Commandments must not be applied in a way that endangers life (Yoma 85.b). In the case of danger of death it is permitted to transgress a great many commandments of the Torah.

As regards the present case, not being a Jehovah's Witness it is difficult for me to give any judgment on it.

d. *Muslim*
No reply can be given in cases concerning Jehovah's Witnesses, Islam being opposed to their existence.

e. *Buddhist*
The patient being major and conscious, his decision must be respected.

4. From the standpoint of agnostic morality

If the patient is conscious, free and informed about his condition, he has the right to refuse the proposed blood transfusion.

379

Migrants

A Turkish woman gives birth to a child with no right ventricle. It is known that the child will live for only a few days. The child is taken from the mother and placed in an incubator in the paediatric department, with a nasogastric feeding tube, and treatment is administered by electric syringe. He moans with pain.
The mother remains in the maternity department, separated from him.
Receiving treatment herself although he cannot live, the mother suffers because her attachment to the child grows from day to day.
Dilemma: separating the child from his mother is not human in view of the diagnosis and prognosis for the child, given that leaving him with his mother would not prejudice any treatment.

1. From the standpoint of international law

The United Nations Convention on the Rights of the Child stipulates in Article 6 (1) and (2) that "States Parties recognise that every child has the inherent right to life" and that they "shall ensure to the maximum extent possible the survival and development of the child".

This convention also provides that "In all actions concerning children, whether undertaken by public or private social welfare institutions, courts of law, administrative authorities or legislative bodies, the best interests of the child shall be a primary consideration" (Article 3 (1)).

It is for this reason that Article 3 (2) goes on to say that "States Parties undertake to ensure the child such protection and care as is necessary for his or her well-being, taking into account the rights and duties of his or her parents" and Article 9 (1) stipulates that "States Parties shall ensure that a child shall not be separated from his or her parents against their will, except when competent authorities subject to judicial review determine, in accordance with applicable law and procedures, that such separation is necessary for the best interests of the child".

If the nutrition and treatment (disregarding the problem of the boundary between palliative care and relentless prolongation of life and the problem of the legitimacy of the latter in international human rights law) of the child are possible if the child is with the mother, then he should be able to remain with her.

Along the same lines, see Article 1.f of Recommendation R (79) 17 of the Committee of Ministers of the Council of Europe to member states concerning the protection of children against ill-treatment: "in order to ensure effective prevention it would be appropriate (...) to devote particular attention to the perinatal period in order to promote the establishment of emotional bonds between the parents and newborn child by (...) encouraging rooming in the maternity wards".

See also Article 1.*g* of this recommendation, according to which, "when low birthweight or sick new-born babies, particularly handicapped babies, are in special care units, to encourage maximum contact between parents and infants and especially to ensure support and counselling by nurses, doctors and others".

Reference should also be made to Article 4 of the BC with regard to the careful attention to be paid to the woman's needs (point 31 of the explanatory report).

2. From the ethical standpoint

The decision, positive or negative, must be on the basis of the mother's psychological and emotional state.

3. From the standpoint of religious moralities

a. *Catholic*

The cardiac malformation will not permit the child to live very long.

If a heart transplant, the only possible therapy, is envisaged, and if the parents agree to it – this being a therapy entailing high risk and therefore not obligatory – then in this case keeping the baby in an intensive care treatment is justified, using all means required to prolong its life until it is possible to effect the transplant, and the isolation of the child is also justified.

If the transplant is not possible or if the proposal is not accepted, then only ordinary care should be administered (alimentation, hydration, etc.) and the suffering should be eased while awaiting death, avoiding any painful therapies.

"In the imminence of inevitable death despite the methods employed, it is permissible in all conscience to take the decision to renounce treatments which would bring only a precarious and painful reprieve, though without interrupting the normal care due to a patient in such a situation. The doctor could not then reproach himself of non-assistance to a person in danger."[1]

"As for the parents, they should be informed about the ordinary treatment and involved in the decisions concerning extraordinary and optional treatments."[2]

"Death belongs to life as its final phase. It should therefore receive care like any other moment of life (...). Whenever it is possible, and if the person concerned agrees, he should be given the possibility of finishing his days together with his family with appropriate medical assistance."[3]

---

1. Congregation for the doctrine of the faith, Declaration on euthanasia, 5 May 1980, Part IV.
2. Pontifical Council for the Pastoral of Health Services, Charter of health personnel, No. 74, Vatican City, 1995.
3. *Idem*, No. 116.

In this particular case, the mother should be allowed to have the baby with her, both because she has the right to assist her child and because this would in no way interfere with ordinary care.

"It is urgent (...) that we should be able to get away from any narrow, nationalistic attitude";[1] any form of discrimination towards the mother because she is a foreigner seriously breaches the principle of respect of the dignity due in equal measure to each member of the human family. "Members of humanity share the same nature and hence the same dignity, with the same fundamental rights and duties and with an identical supernatural destiny."[2]

b. *Protestant*
Since the human being should be considered as a being dependent on relationships – that with the mother being the real matrix – and not simply a piece of biological clock-work, the mother's wishes should be acceded to, while providing the necessary care. Since this mother is doomed to suffer the loss of her child, so she needs particular support, all the more so since as a foreigner she is in a specially vulnerable situation.

c. *Jewish*
This case raises two different problems.

First, it is inhuman to separate the child from its mother when it is known that there is no medical reason for not leaving it with her. It is on the contrary important that the mother should be with child, above all because of the seriousness of its condition.

Second, why treat this child and make it moan with pain when it is known that it will live for only a few days? It should be accorded the right to live and die in decent conditions.

But there still remains the question of why cardiac surgery is excluded from the outset.

d. *Muslim*
Any mother will admit that saving the child deserves the sacrifice of her attachment (reference to the Judgment of Solomon, common to the Jewish, Christian and Muslim cultures).

e. *Buddhist*
It is important to avoid relentless prolongation of life, which is a form of aggression, and permit the mother to be with the baby in its last moments, so that she can express her love to it.

---

1. Paul VI, *Octogesima Adveniens*, 1 May 1971, No. 17.
2. *Idem*, No. 16.

4. From the standpoint of agnostic morality

To the extent that leaving the baby with its mother is not incompatible with treatment this should be done.

Migrants

After his wife has given birth normally, Mr X comes to collect her from the maternity service and refuses in the name of Allah to leave without the icteric new-born baby who needs a few more days of ultraviolet treatment.
The couple leave the hospital with the baby against the advice of the doctor and the nurse, and at the risk of neurological sequels for the baby.
Dilemma: in view of the danger that the parents are making this baby run, and taking into account the United Nations Declaration on the Rights of the Child, a decision is called for.

1. From the standpoint of international law

The answer stems from Article 9 (1) of the United Nations Convention on the Rights of the Child cited in case 83, separation being essential for the protection of the best interests of the child.

It should be noted that in the terms of this same article, such separation "may be necessary in a particular case such as one involving abuse or neglect of the child by the parents", where the child's health may be neglected or endangered.

In any proceedings aimed at having the child hospitalised for appropriate treatment, "all interested parties shall be given an opportunity to participate in the proceedings and make their views known" (Article 9 (2) of the convention).

It should be pointed out that according to Article 9 (3) of this United Nations Convention on the Rights of the Child "States Parties shall respect the right of the child who is separated from one or both parents to maintain personal relations and direct contact with both parents on a regular basis".

It should also be pointed out that according to Article 9 (2) of the ECHR (but the same applies with all international human rights instruments) "freedom to manifest one's religion or beliefs shall be subject only to such limitations as are prescribed by law and are necessary in a democratic society in the interests of public safety, for the protection of public order, health or morals, or for the protection of the rights and freedoms of others" (here the child's right to health). This applies to third parties as well as the parents, the latters' right to "ensure the religious and moral education of the children in conformity with their own convictions" (Article 18 (4) of the Covenant on Civil and Political Rights) cannot interfere with the child's fundamental right to health (and to medical care).

As regards the BC, see Article 6 (1), (2) and (4), the parents' authorisation or refusal of authorisation not being sufficient, *per se* (see the reply to case 16).

The ultraviolet ray treatment being a "medically necessary" intervention, i.e. having direct and immediate benefit of the child concerned, though not strictly necessary for the person's survival, for which no delay is acceptable, see also Article 8 of the BC and points 57 and 58 of the explanatory report appended thereto, should "the doctor be unable to contact an incapacitated person's legal representative who would normally have to authorise an urgent intervention".

2. From the ethical standpoint

The doctor has the duty to defend and protect the patient, even against its parents.

3. From the standpoint of religious moralities

a. *Catholic*

The parents' refusal to allow the child to be treated, even though it is for religious reasons, seriously violates the child's right to recuperation and the improvement of its state of health.

"Both before and after their birth, children have the right to special protection and assistance."[1]

The carers, if the attempt to convince the parents remains unsuccessful, have the duty to call on the children's judge in order to overturn decisions prejudicial for the minor and authorise the action necessary to treat the child. "All possible treatments from which the patient's health may benefit are due to the patient";[2] "those responsible for treating the sick must do it with diligence and procure for them the remedies they deem necessary or useful".[3]

b. *Protestant*

Why does the father act in this way? Is he inaccessible to reasoning which will show him the benefit to his child of staying in hospital for a few more days? Dialogue and persuasion are called for. Recourse to a third party (mullah or elder for example) may be useful. Otherwise, it should always be possible to play for time, diplomacy being by no means exclusively reserved to international institutions.

c. *Jewish*

In this case we are confronted with the principle of "demanded discharge", so that the doctor cannot legally oppose Mr X in any way.

---

1. Holy See, Charter of the rights of the family, 22 October 1983, Article 4 *(d)*.
2. Charter of health personnel, No. 63.
3. Congregation for the doctrine of the faith, Declaration on euthanasia, 5 May 1980, in AAS 72/1980, p. 549.

All that remains to the doctor is the power of persuasion. He must do everything to explain to the parents the dangers they are making their son run and try by every possible means to make them change their minds.

If they refuse, the doctor should appeal to a Muslim religious counsellor to convince them of the necessity not to endanger the child's life.

d. *Muslim*

See case 83. The parents' attitude is a response to discrimination; if they had been considered "the same as everyone else" they would not have paraded their "popular belief".

e. *Buddhist*

Technical progress cannot be understood by everybody and explanations should be given to the parents to try to make them understand the need for treatment to protect the baby's future neurological state and happiness.

4. From the standpoint of agnostic morality

In the interest of the child, the doctors and nurses must keep it in hospital for the few days required for the necessary treatment, despite the parents' attitude dictated by their religion.

Migrants

A patient from a developing country, Mrs X, is brought to Europe for treatment which normally costs a great deal, the costs of which are born by a humanitarian association. She is housed by a host family and treated as an outpatient of a teaching hospital. The specialist provides her over a period of some months with medicines which have passed the use-by date, telling the host family that there is no risk involved. The patient's condition stabilises and a month later she returns to her home country with a further stock of such medicine to continue the treatment.

Dilemma: denounce the misrepresentation of the quality of service provided by the humanitarian association or take action with this association to ensure that it fully accepts its responsibilities.

1. From the standpoint of international law

No specific reply in international law as to which approach should be taken.

In any event, see Article 4 of the BC, according to which "any intervention in the health field, including research, must be carried out in accordance with relevant professional obligations and standards". Prescribing drugs which are known to have passed their use-by date certainly does not meet the requirements of "legal and ethical imperatives" mentioned in point 31 of the explanatory report appended to the BC, nor the requirements of the other relevant points of this report. This is still true even if, for the moment, no negative consequences for the patient are apparent. Furthermore, any undue damage resulting from the prescription and administration of out-of-date drugs (which could appear at a later stage, after the patient has returned to her home country) entitles the person suffering it to fair compensation (Article 24 of the BC), but the absence of such damage does not exempt the doctor from liability for violating legal and professional obligations and standards.

The duty of the High Contracting Parties to provide for appropriate sanctions to be applied in the event of infringement "of the provisions contained in this convention" is stipulated by Article 25 of the BC as well as by point 147 of the explanatory report.

See also, mutatis mutandis, Decision No. 30 of 26.4.1979 in the Sunday Times case (Commission v. United Kingdom) and Article 10 (1) of the ECHR.

2. From the ethical standpoint

It is necessary to denounce both the deception and take action with the humanitarian association.

3. From the standpoint of religious moralities

a. *Catholic*

From the standpoint of Catholic morality there is a violation of the Fifth Commandment ("Thou shalt not kill") which prohibits not only homicide, but also prejudice to health ; the medicines concerned may in fact harm the woman's health and even put her life at risk. Furthermore, there is a violation of the Eighth Commandment ("Thou shalt not bear false witness"), which prohibits deceit.

Lastly, even foreigners have the right to appropriate and necessary care, "for it is a matter, when possible, of helping men, women, and families, to live decently and in peace on their land (...). Economic or technical support is very often essential for progress, together with, I insist, unfailing respect of the dignity of persons and families, of their traditions, of their health, of their right to live and to give life".[1]

b. *Protestant*

The terms employed in the presentation do not tell us exactly who, the specialist or the humanitarian association, is responsible for the deception. This can be unambiguously denounced and legal proceedings may be envisaged. There is no dilemma between denunciation and formal notice to the association to accept its responsibilities. The action to take is a matter of expediency.

c. *Jewish*

All men have the right to the same treatment and it is unacceptable to treat them differently. Making a distinction between patients is – it seems to me – a discriminatory act. We are all children of Adam created in the image and likeness of God. Making a difference between patients is to open a breach which threatens to endanger the fundamental principle of the Declaration of Human Rights which states that all men are free and equal. It is therefore natural that if a medicament bears a use-by date this date should be respected. It is thus the doctor's duty to approach the humanitarian association to make it fully accept its responsibilities and stop engaging in this deception.

However, it must be taken into account that the use-by date is above all a problem of an economic nature. In this particular case, there has been an improvement in the patient's health. Perhaps the humanitarian association received these medicaments as a gift and those in charge preferred to use the available funds to buy other products which could save other human lives.

---

1. John-Paul II, to the International Catholic Committee for Migration, in *Insegnamenti*, Vol. XIII, No. 2, 1990, Libreria Editrice Vaticana, p. 58.

What would be unacceptable in any event would be for the doctor to charge the full price for a medicament which has passed the use-by date and take advantage of the fact that the patient comes from a developing country.

d. *Muslim*

This problem was raised in the national ethics committee in 1986 with respect to the right of asylum for health reasons. Chairman Brunswick replied that there was no right to "health asylum", but only to "political asylum".

e. *Buddhist*

There is apparently no major problem if the medicines are really effective (verification by the specialist with the laboratory concerned). If this is not the case, the doctor and the humanitarian organisation will be liable.

4. From the standpoint of agnostic morality

The question that matters is whether, assuming good faith, the drugs which have passed the official use-by date are not still effective, since they are supplied by a consultant in a teaching hospital.

The facts should, nevertheless, be put before the humanitarian association.

Migrants

Mrs X, 19, comes from Mali. She has been in France for six months and speaks no French. She is her husband's second wife and is three months pregnant.
Admitted to the digestive medicine unit for vomiting which cannot be controlled with AEG, and loss of weight, the nurse's diagnosis is family isolation.
When setting up a drip the nurse discovers traces of blows (lacerations) on the arms and then on the body.
Knowing that in the Mali culture the wife is totally subject to the authority of the husband, the medical team is confronted with a case of ill-treatment of a legally adult person, but if action is taken there is a risk of her being repudiated by her husband and sent back to Mali under conditions which will be catastrophic for her and her child.
The nurse starts by telling the doctor, but he refuses to do anything.
Dilemma: allow the continuation of a situation which is likely to harm the health of the mother and her child in the longer term, or act in the interest of their physical and mental health without taking into account the medium-term consequences for the conjugal life?

1. From the standpoint of international law

Under the criminal law of most European countries, finding evidence of assault and bodily harm on the patient's body obliges the doctor to report it to the judicial authorities, and in this case all the more so because they are evidence of inhuman and degrading treatment in the terms of Article 3 of the ECHR (see Articles 4; 10 and 26 of the BC, as well as the relevant points of the explanatory report appended thereto).

The husband's liability having been legally proven, no expulsion measure could be decided by the host state authorities simply on the grounds of the repudiation. The fact is that although the ECHR does not, *per se*, confer the right not to be expelled or extradited (concerning expulsion, see nonetheless Article 1 of Protocol 7 to the ECHR, signed in Strasbourg on 22.11.1984 and come into force on 1.11.1988), according to Judgment No. 161 of the European Court of Human Rights of 7.7.1989 in the *Soering* case (*Commission* v. *United Kingdom*), member states are not relieved of the liability for all or part of the foreseeable consequences which expulsion leads to outside their jurisdiction, namely damage to the health of the mother and of the child to be born.

We would also recall that in the terms of Recommendation R (85) 4 on violence in the family, adopted by the Committee of Ministers of the Council of Europe on 26.3.1985, governments of member states are recommended to "arrange for and encourage the setting up and support the work of agencies, associations or foundations whose aim is to help and assist the victims of violent family situations, with due respect to the privacy of others".

Lastly, we would point out that in the terms of Recommendation R (79) 10 of the Committee of Ministers of the Council of Europe to member states concerning women migrants (points i.*a* and *b*) governments are recommended "to assist women migrants to adapt to the social environment of the receiving country, notably by providing better reception facilities such as housing, hostels, crèches, schools, etc., suited to their needs and those of their families", and "to inform women migrants and particularly unmarried mothers, widows and divorcees, through all appropriate channels and during their residence in the receiving country, about their legal rights and obligations, as well as the related legal machinery (...) that may protect and assist them with the necessary administrative formalities".

For European case-law, see Decision Nos. 94 of 25.5.1985 in the *Abdulaziz, Cabales and Balkandali* case (*Commission* v. *United Kingdom*); 138 of 21.6.1988 in the *Berrehab* case (*Commission* v. *Netherlands*); 193 of 16.2.1991 in the *Moustaquin* case (*Commission* v. *Belgium*); 234 A of 26.3.1992 in the *Beldjoudi* case (*Commission* v. *France*); 258 C of 28.6.1993 in the *Lamguindaz* case (*Commission* v. *United Kingdom*); 201 of 20.3.1991 in the *Cruz Varas and others* case (*Commission* v. *Sweden*); and 216 of 30.10.1991 in the *Vilvarajah* case (*Commission* v. *United Kingdom*).

2. From the ethical standpoint

See and try to reason with the husband and envisage the second possibility only if the psychotherapy of the husband should fail.

3. From the standpoint of religious moralities

a. *Catholic*

Two moral principles are involved: on the one hand, the respect of the dignity of each human being, in this case of the woman and child and, on the other, the safeguard of the family unity.

In order to respect both principles, and also take account of the child yet to be born (since the blows given to the mother may provoke a miscarriage), if the doctor refuses to take any action, it is necessary above all that the nurse request the intervention of the family counsellor to safeguard the woman's psychophysical integrity and make her aware of her rights as wife and mother.[1]

---

1. See John Paul II, *Letter to women*, 29 June 1995.

The family counselling centre will have the duty of involving the husband to make him aware of his duties as husband and father on both the moral and legal planes and of the consequences in the case of transgression. If this proves insufficient, he will have to be denounced to the authorities. In fact "marriage and family counsellors, through their specific action of counselling and preventive action, dispensed in the light of an anthropology in harmony with the Christian conception of the person, of the couple and of sexuality, thus constitute valuable aids for rediscovering the meaning of love and of life, and for supporting and accompanying each family in its mission of 'sanctuary of life'".[1]

b. *Protestant*
As in case 86 it is advisable to call in a third party, an association for the defence of women or a "traditional" authority recognised within the group. It would not be a bad idea either to try to let the wife explain her view on these issues.

c. *Jewish*
In this case, only the best interest of the mother and child should be taken into consideration. A husband who beats his wife is not only guilty *vis-à-vis* the law but also in the eyes of religion. In Jewish tradition, respecting and honouring his wife more than himself is one of the first duties of the husband.

The role of the doctor is to summon the husband to explain the risk he is running *vis-à-vis* the law and the danger to which he is exposing his future child.

If there should be any further occurrence, the doctor should act in the interest of the physical and mental equilibrium of the mother and child without considering the medium-term consequences for conjugal life.

d. *Muslim*
Same decision as in the case of European battered wives (consult their associations). Act in the interest of these women's physical and mental well-being (Koran II. 231).

e. *Buddhist*
Faced with the doctor's refusal, the nurse should inform the legal authorities if all dialogue with the Malian woman's husband proves impossible. The husband should be addressed with patience, sympathy and compassion, to try to make him aware of the violence of his acts.

If he refuses however, the young woman must not be left to her fate, first of all out of compassion and humanity, and second because from the legal standpoint it would be a case of "failure to assist a person in danger".

---

1. John Paul II, *Evangelium Vitae*, 25 March 1995, No. 88.

4. From the standpoint of agnostic morality

This ill-treatment must be denounced. The possible repudiation of the wife has no effect in France.

Family

*A doctor aged 80 is placed in the retirement home in which he used to practise
as a result of a fall at home and temporal and spatial disorientation.
His children are not in agreement on the choice of establishment and none of
them have asked the opinion of the patient.
Dilemma : the person's right to information and self-determination must be
respected in all cases.*

1. From the standpoint of international law

In international human rights law, the patient's right to information and self-determination is provided for by Article 7 of the Covenant on Civil and Political Rights and Article 10 (1) of the ECHR, already evoked several times.

In addition, Article 8 (1) of the ECHR stipulates that everyone has the right to his private life, and the constant case-law of the European Court of Human Rights has been that the concept of "private life" includes private life proper, professional and commercial activity, human relations with other people and the physical and mental integrity of the individual. As a result, the patient has the right to decide in which establishment he should be placed, taking account, of course, of the type of care he needs. Article 5 of the BC leads to the same conclusion.

If the temporal-spatial disorientation from which the patient is suffering is to be qualified as impairment of his mental faculties, Article 6 of the BC permits interventions only for the direct benefit of the patient (6 (1)) and only with the authorisation of the patient's representative or an authority or a person or body provided for by the law (6 (2)). Article 6 (2) adds to this that the individual concerned shall as far as possible take part in the authorisation procedure. See also points 43 and 46 of the explanatory report appended to the BC.

Article 7 of the BC is not applicable, the temporal-spatial disorientation which caused the fall not coming into the category (it would appear) of "serious mental disorder".

2. From the ethical standpoint

Agreed.

3. From the standpoint of religious moralities

a. *Catholic*
The subject "should be put in a situation of being able to choose personally and

not have to accept the decisions and choices of others".[1]

It is necessary to ensure the respect of the individual's right to take part in decisions which concern his life and health. If the old man is not capable of participating in the decision, his children, as those responsible for their father's health, cannot take the decision to place him in the retirement home unless they all agree.

b. *Protestant*

If it is only a case of temporary disorientation, the patient will soon be able to express his own point of view. The staff of the home concerned will also have their view. What is required is a responsible decision, namely an informed one respecting the desires of each – and of the person most concerned of course – according to the possibilities available.

c. *Jewish*

In the first place it is necessary to seek the opinion of a psychiatrist to know whether the patient is capable of taking a decision. It would certainly also be useful to obtain the opinion of the family doctor who often knows a great deal about the psycho-social context of his patients.

If it turns out that the patient cannot take a decision, the doctor should not take a stance if he does not know the background. He should propose solutions in the patient's interest after seeking the opinion of the family doctor. He should then leave the family to take the action which suits them best, provided there is no risk to the patient.

d. *Muslim*

Islam obliges children to take their parents into their homes and give them active care and attention (Sura XL VI, 15-18). The rights to information and self-determination must be respected.

e. *Buddhist*

In any event, the patient must be kept informed. His opinion must predominate if he is capable of formulating one. Otherwise account should be taken of any wishes he may have expressed before his accident.

4. From the standpoint of agnostic morality

This doctor should be left in the retirement home with which he is most familiar.

---

1. John Paul II, "Address to the World Congress of Catholic Doctors", 3 October 1982, in *Insegnamenti*, V/3, p. 673, No. 4.

Family

A man of 75, hospitalised for his poor general state, totally incontinent, does not eat. Has removed his nasogastric feeding tube on several occasions. The doctor says he must be strapped in his bed and the tube must be replaced. The patient becomes aggressive towards the carers (kicks them). The family is satisfied and concludes that he is being well cared for.
Dilemma : care or torture at the request of the family ?

1. From the standpoint of international law

The family (a concept that has not in fact been defined in international human rights law) does not have the right to decide the suspension or repetition of attempts to feed the patient, or the treatment to be given.

As regards the behaviour of the doctor and health professionals in general, Article 4 of the BC stipulates that "Any intervention in the health field, including research, must be carried out in accordance with relevant professional obligations and standards".

"Doctors and, in general, all professionals who participate in a medical act are subject to ethical and legal imperatives. They must act with care and competence, and pay careful attention to the needs of each patient (...). Competence must be determined primarily in relation to the scientific knowledge and clinical experience appropriate to a profession or speciality at a given time. The current state of the art determines the professional standard and skill to be expected of health care professionals in the performance of their work. In following the progress of medicine, it changes with new developments and eliminates methods which do not reflect the state of the art. Nevertheless, it is accepted that professional standards do not necessarily prescribe one line of action as being the only one possible : recognised medical practice may, indeed, allow several possible forms of intervention, thus leaving some freedom of choice as to methods or techniques. Further, a particular course of action must be judged in the light of the specific health problem raised by a given patient. In particular an intervention must meet criteria of relevance and proportionality between the aim pursued and the means used" (points 31 to 33 of the explanatory report appended to the BC).

If there is some way of feeding the patient adequately without causing him the discomfort of the probe, which makes him aggressive, this method is to be preferred. If not, then in accordance with the medical practice and the state of the art, the probe must be inserted. Any mention of "torture" is quite out of place.

2. From the ethical standpoint

The tube should not be left in place, but should be inserted only when necessary to force-feed the patient.

3. From the standpoint of religious moralities

a. *Catholic*

In themselves "alimentation and hydration, even artificial, should be classified as normal care always due to a patient if they are not dangerous for him. Their unjustified suspension could amount to veritable euthanasia".[1]

However, due regard must always be paid to the patient's wishes: "When they have to take medical action on a patient, health professionals should be in possession of his express or tacit consent."[2]

Thus if the patient is capable of expressing consent, but refuses the feeding tube as in this case, all the health professional can do, with the aid of the family, is to establish a calm dialogue on the importance of the intervention, provide the patient with correct information on the instruments used and help him bear the psychological burden of a situation of infirmity; he can never constrain him by force, going against his wishes. Except in the case where the patient is not capable, "the patient cannot be made the object of a decision he does not take himself".[3] If in fact the patient is not capable of intending and wishing "the health professional may, and in extreme situations, must, presume consent for therapeutic interventions which in all knowledge and conscience he considers necessary in the case of temporary absence of consciousness and will, by virtue of the principle of therapeutic confidence, namely the original confidence which made the patient put himself in the professional's hands".[4]

b. *Protestant*

Care. The reality of torture can never be envisaged, but is this really the right term to use here?

c. *Jewish*

The fact that a lucid patient removes his feeding tube must be considered an appeal for help. The patient is certainly uncomfortable. It is therefore necessary to talk to him, try to find out what the trouble is and propose an alternative treatment.

If he is not lucid and does not know what he is doing, it is for the carers to take the most appropriate decision.

The family can sometimes clarify certain points for the doctor, but it is for the care team to take the final decision.

---

1. Charter of health personnel, No. 120.
2. *Idem*, No. 72.
3. Pontifical Council *Cor Unum*, "Some ethical questions relating to seriously ill and dying persons", 27 June 1981, in *Enchiridion Vaticanum*, No. 7, Official documents of the Holy See, 1980-1981, EDB, Bologna, 1985, p. 1137, paragraph 2.1.2.
4. Charter of health personnel, No. 73.

d. *Muslim*

See the reply to case 89 and accept the doctor's decision. In any event, the intention (*Nya* in Arabic) counts more than the deed according to the Koran and Muslim tradition.

e. *Buddhist*

Any form of aggression (and strapping a person to a bed is one) must be avoided, even if it is intended to be for the patient's good.

It is preferable to adopt a more conciliatory attitude, speaking to the patient with compassion.

4. From the standpoint of agnostic morality

The feeding tube must not be inserted against his will and he should be fed only if he wishes it.

Family

Mrs X, 70, has cancer of the pancreas, but does not know it and does not know that she is being treated with opiates.
Her son requests all the carers not to reveal this information to her. The doctor respects this request. The patient is constantly asking the nurses what is causing her pain and why she is not allowed to go home.
Dilemma: drawing the line between the purely professional constraint and silence by constraint as a support for an inhuman and violent procedure.

1. From the standpoint of international law

Regarding the patient's right to information, see Articles 10 (1) of the ECHR and 10 (2) of the BC, according to which "individuals are entitled to know any information collected about their health", unless they have expressed the wish not to be informed, in which case "the wishes of individuals not to be so informed shall be observed".

Since the reasons for the lack of information in this case are not explained, the son's request having no legal value for the doctor, see also Article 10 (3) of the BC, according to which, in exceptional cases, restrictions may be placed by law, in the interests of the patient, on the exercise of the right to know and the right not to know.

Points 69 and 70 of the explanatory report appended to the BC state in fact that "in exceptional cases domestic law may place restrictions on the right to know or not to know in the interests of the patient's health (for example, a prognosis of death which might, in certain cases if immediately passed on to the patient, seriously worsen his or her condition). In some cases, the doctor's duty to provide information which is also covered under Article 4 conflicts with the interests of the patient's health. It is for domestic law, taking account of the social and cultural background, to solve this conflict. Where appropriate under judicial control, domestic law may justify the doctor sometimes withholding part of the information or, at all events, disclosing it with circumspection (therapeutic necessity). Furthermore, it may be of vital importance for patients to know certain facts about their health, even though they have expressed the wish not to know them. For example, the knowledge that they have a predisposition to a disease might be the only way to enable them to take potentially effective (preventive) measures. In this case, a doctor's duty to provide care, as laid down in Article 4, might conflict with the patient's right not to know. (...) Here too it will be for domestic law to indicate whether the doctor, in the light of the circumstances of the particular case, may make an exception to the right not to know".

As regards the administration of opiates, the patient's consent should have been obtained, even if she had asked not to know her state of health (Article 5 of the BC). Point 67 of the explanatory report states in fact that "the patient's exercise of the right not to know this or that fact concerning his health is not regarded as an impediment to the validity of his consent to an intervention; for example, he can validly consent to the removal of a cyst despite not wishing to know its nature". This is so despite the fact that point 65 of the same report states that "the right to know is of fundamental importance in itself but also conditions the effective exercise of other rights such as the right of consent set forth in Article 5".

Lastly, as regards the nurses' obligations *vis-à-vis* both the patient and the doctor, see the references to professional obligations and standards in Article 4 of the BC and the relevant points of the explanatory report appended thereto.

2. From the ethical standpoint

Inform the patient in a way which does not deprive her of all hope.

3. From the standpoint of religious moralities

a. *Catholic*

"A person has a right to be informed about his own state of health. This right does not disappear in the presence of a diagnosis and prognosis of an illness which will cause death, but other factors are also involved. The fact is that this information implies important responsibilities which cannot be escaped. There are responsibilities connected with the treatment, which has to be given with the informed consent of the patient."[1]

The magisterium of the Catholic Church thus states that the information has to be communicated with "discretion and humane tact",[2] and should be adapted to the capacity of the person concerned to benefit from it.[3]

Even treatment by opiates thus requires the authorisation of the patient who may in any event renounce it "to retain his full lucidity and, if he is a believer, participate consciously in the Passion of the Lord".[4]

b. *Protestant*

From the human standpoint, the truth is never purely technical or mathematical. It is built on the respect of the real, of course, but also as a function of other

---

1. Charter of health personnel, No. 125.
2. *Idem*, No. 126.
3. *Idem*, No. 127.
4. John Paul II, *Evangelium Vitae*, No. 65.

parameters (value judgments, profiles and psychological antecedents, etc.). This is one of the lessons which can be drawn from the affirmation of Christ in the form of "the path, the truth and the life" (John, 14, v. 6): the truth on the existential level is a person, who reveals himself along a common path, which is life itself.

c. *Jewish*

As a general rule, if the patient wants to know what the diagnosis is, he should be told the truth, because very often patients then participate more in their cure.

In this particular case, the patient wants to know, and she is lucid.

It is necessary to ask what family reasons make the son refuse to have the patient told the truth.

If these reasons are not considered adequate, an attempt must be made to make him change his mind, all the more so because these days it is increasingly difficult to hide the truth from patients.

d. *Muslim*

See the replies to cases 87 and 88. According to the Prophet of Islam, the principle of medical secrecy and the authority of the practitioner take precedence in all decisions, for it is necessary to address people according to what they can understand in a field of science or knowledge.

e. *Buddhist*

The fact that the patient asks questions about her state of health is probably an expression of her worrying about the seriousness of her illness. Discussing the matter with the son should make it possible for him to face the situation more calmly.

4. From the standpoint of agnostic morality

The administration of opiates is necessary to ease the pain. This patient should be told that her serious, but not hopeless, condition means that she must remain in hospital, assuming that she cannot be treated at home.

Family

A woman of 56 has a cancer of the colon in terminal phase. An operation seems medically necessary to prolong her life. Her husband agrees but she refuses. The operation is carried out and she dies seven weeks later.
Dilemma: act against the confusion between the status of a sick woman and that of her being a minor in the eyes of the husband and doctor who operate against her wishes, or accept this inhuman treatment on the pretext that the patient has not the right to refuse to live.

1. From the standpoint of international law

The operation is illegal without the patient's consent or, *a fortiori*, against her will or without her knowledge (Articles 7 of the Covenant on Civil and Political Rights, and 5 of the BC). Furthermore, since it is an invasive intervention, express consent may be required (see point 37 of the explanatory report appended to the BC). Point 34 of the explanatory report stresses that "human beings must be able freely to give or refuse their consent to any intervention involving their person" and that "this rule makes clear patients' autonomy in their relationship with health care professionals and restrains the paternalist approaches which might ignore the wish of the patient". To this point 35 adds that "the patient's consent is considered to be free and informed if its is given on the basis of objective information from the responsible health care professionals as to nature and potential consequences of the planned intervention or of its alternative, in the absence of any pressure from anyone", with the sole exception of the circumstances provided for in Articles 6 (3); 7; 10 (2); 10 (3) and 26 (1) of the BC.

Nevertheless, it should be pointed out that the problem of the legitimacy of the renunciation of the right to life not yet has been resolved or even considered by international human rights law.

The wishes of the spouse cannot affect, from the legal standpoint, the patient's wishes or her right to self-determination.

2. From the ethical standpoint

Every patient has the right to refuse treatment. If the patient cannot be convinced the treatment must be renounced.

3. From the standpoint of religious moralities

a. *Catholic*
It is necessary above all to assess the nature of the operation to be carried out.

"It is certain that the moral obligation to treat oneself and to have oneself treated exists, but this obligation must be seen in relation to specific situations; that is it is necessary to determine whether the therapeutic resources available are objectively in proportion to the prospects for improvement."[1]

"In the imminence of inevitable death despite the methods employed, it is permissible to take the decision to renounce treatments which would bring only a precarious and painful reprieve, though without interrupting the normal care due to a patient in such a situation. The doctor could not then reproach himself for non-assistance to a person in danger."[2]

"The renunciation of extraordinary or disproportionate measures is not equivalent to suicide or euthanasia; it is more a case of the acceptance of the human condition when faced with death."[3]

In this specific case the woman's wishes should have been taken into consideration, all the more so because there was no obligation to submit to the operation since she was in the terminal phase, in which the operation could even make things worse. It was therefore a risky operation.

b. *Protestant*

The patient's informed consent (or refusal) is paramount. But we always find the same problem of communication: has she been asked her reasons for refusing the operation, and has everything been discussed with her?

c. *Jewish*

Ideally, everything ought to have been done to convince the patient to accept the operation, demonstrating the positive points, namely: prolonged life and better quality of life.

d. *Muslim*

The medical act which might save a life, carried out in all conscience and according to the state of the art, takes precedence over any other consideration.

e. *Buddhist*

Relentless prolongation of life, which is a form of aggression, must be avoided. If the patient had expressed a wish, in full awareness of the implications, not to be operated on, this wish should have been respected.

---

1. John Paul II, *Evangelium Vitae*, No. 65.
2. Congregation for the doctrine of the faith, Declaration on euthanasia, 5 May 1980, Part IV.
3. John Paul II, *Evangelium Vitae*, No. 65.

4. From the standpoint of agnostic morality
The patient's wishes should have been respected.

Family

A sterile female laboratory assistant of 45 has an adopted daughter of 4 and has applied to adopt another child. An incapacitating sarcoma is discovered by chance, resistant to chemotherapy, very painful and calmed by large doses of intravenous morphine. The husband requests that the patient not be informed of her condition, and continues with the adoption application, being informed of the likely onset of handicap and the general prognosis.
Dilemma: inform the adoption organisation of the change in circumstances, or take steps to have the wife informed of her condition to make her able to manage her life and her illness in informed concert with her husband.

1. From the standpoint of international law

As regards the patient's right to be informed, as well as the right not to be informed, see Articles 10 (1) of the ECHR, 12 (2) and 10 (2) and (3) of the BC, as well as the reply to cases 89 and 90. Moreover, the administration of any kind of therapy without the knowledge and consent of the patient infringes, *per se*, Article 7 of the Covenant on Civil and Political Rights, as well as Article 5 (1) and (2) of the BC, unless conditions provided for by Article 6 (3) and/or 10 (2) of the BC are met.

As regards informing the adoption organisation, there is an obligation to respect the private life of the husband (Article 8 (1) of the ECHR) and the duty not to divulge confidential information (Article 10 (2) of the ECHR).

Lastly, as regards the nurses' behaviour, see Article 4 of the BC and the professional obligations and standards in the country concerned, *vis-à-vis* both the patient and the doctor.

2. From the ethical standpoint

Make the adoption procedure drag on.

3. From the standpoint of religious moralities

a. Catholic

"A person has a right to be informed about his own state of health (...). The fact is that this information implies important responsibilities which cannot be escaped (...), the responsibility to accomplish precise tasks concerning relations with the family, the settlement of any professional matters, the resolution of differences with third parties."[1]

---

1. Charter of health personnel, No. 125.

Health personnel therefore have the duty not so much to act independently by informing the organisation of the difficulties with respect to the adoption, but to make the husband understand that the respect of the patient requires that she should be fully informed about her own state of health, so that she can manage her own life and her own illness in full awareness of the responsibilities and in harmony with her husband,

Then together they will be able to assess the advisability of informing the adoption organisation of the new situation, thus satisfying the need for transparency and acting for the good of a family capable of accepting the child from all aspects.

b. *Protestant*

It is not possible to condone action based on a deception, in this case the idea that the wife would make a good mother without any problem. But the deception seems to be twofold here because it is requested that the patient herself should not be informed of her condition. It is therefore appropriate to take steps to have the wife informed of her condition to make her able to manage her life and her illness in informed concert with her husband. It could be that the social services, informed in their turn, may have no formal objection to some form or other of adoption after all.

c. *Jewish*

It is necessary to take action to have the wife informed about her disease so that she can manage her life and her disease in concert with her husband. It is also necessary to try to convince the wife that she should put an end to the adoption procedure and accept responsibility together with her husband.

d. *Muslim*

See the reply to case 89 and act on a case-by-case basis.

e. *Buddhist*

Action must be taken to have the woman informed about her illness so that she can manage her life and the disease in informed concert with her husband.

4. From the standpoint of agnostic morality

Take steps to inform the patient about her condition so that she can manage her life and her illness in informed concert with her husband.

Family

Mr X, father of the head of a hospital nursing service, is hospitalised because of persistent hiccough and asthenia in the establishment where his daughter works. The doctor diagnoses cancer of the lung and performs an operation. Twenty-four hours later the patient exhibits septicaemia in the intensive care service, he is intubated and ventilated. A few days later he exhibits major hypertension and septic shock, with cardiac and renal complications. He is unconscious after several days of treatment. Renal dialysis is initiated. All this is done with the agreement of the daughter.
The nurses see in this situation relentless prolongation of life. Some time later, given no change in the patient's state, it is decided to stop the dialysis and undertake no further therapeutic action. Three days later a resumption of diuresis is noted, leading to a resumption of intensive care, with the daughter's agreement. The cardiac and renal conditions improve, though the patient is still in deep coma, then after a few days there are signs of a return to consciousness and significant improvement. After two-and-a-half months in intensive care the patient leaves the unit, having recovered all his cerebral functions, but no longer being independent.
The family's main concern has always been the quality of survival which can be offered to the patient. The daughter here being at the same time the family, the head of the nursing staff, and above all a nurse, is confronted with several successive logics; that of the nurse, seeing like her colleagues relentless prolongation of life on the part of the doctor, that of a relative, seeing justified therapeutic persistence on the part of the doctor, and that of an informed daughter, reacting in the interest of her father, with all professional logic forgotten. Dilemma: relentless prolongation of life, therapeutic persistence and response to the wishes of the family seem to be constantly incompatible elements, and even not beneficial to the patient because the quality of the survival becomes secondary.

1. From the standpoint of international law

No provision of international human rights law sees the concept of "quality of life" as the limit, though implicit, to the concept of "life" and the "right to live", the latter indeed being the basis for all other fundamental rights, as well as the fulcrum of the "hard core" of the ECHR (see Article 15 (2)) as well as the Covenant on Civil and Political Rights. On this subject see also the reply to case 91.

For the rest, the concept of the relentless prolongation of life seems to stem from the results obtained rather than being an a priori. This is the case here at least, since the patient has recovered all his cerebral functions, even though he has lost his autonomy.

In any event, the family's wishes (a concept not in fact defined in international human rights law) have no legal value.

As for the "physician's logic", see Articles 1, 2 and 4 of the BC.

2. From the ethical standpoint

If the nurse daughter is afraid that her professional conduct will be affected because of her family link with the patient she should, if possible, renounce her nursing role in this particular case.

3. From the standpoint of religious moralities

a. *Catholic*

"The right to live takes the form for the sick person in the terminal phase as a right to die in all serenity, in human and Christian dignity. This does not mean the power to contrive one's own death or have another do so, but rather to live one's death in a human and Christian fashion rather than trying to avoid it at any cost".[1]

Relentless prolongation of life goes against this logic because it consists in "the use of particularly exhausting and distressing methods to artificially prolong the agony".[2]

"This is contrary to the dignity of the dying person and to the moral duty of the acceptance of death and of the ultimate pursuit of its course."[3]

However, in this particular case there has been respect of the principle of proportionality of treatment, according to which the health professional, in evaluating the methods, "must make the appropriate choices, namely take the patient as the reference point and act in accordance with his true condition".[4]

"Earthly life is a fundamental but not an absolute good. This is why it is necessary to identify the limits of the obligation to maintain a person alive. The distinction – already defined – between "proportionate" measures which must never be renounced so as not to hasten or cause death, and "disproportionate" measures which one may, and in order to avoid slipping into relentless prolongation of life, should, renounce, is the ethical criterion for the identification of these limits. In this,

---

1. Charter of health personnel, No. 119.
2. John Paul II, Address to the participants at an international congress on assistance for the dying, in *L'Osservatore Romano*, 18 March 1992, No. 4.
3. Charter of health personnel, No. 119.
4. John-Paul II, Address to two working groups organised by the Academy of Sciences, 21 October 1985, in *Insegnamenti*, VII/2, p. 1082, No. 5.

the health agent finds a reassuring signification and indication for the solution of the complex cases entrusted to his responsibility."[1]

It is important to stress the necessity for normal care, for example alimentation and hydration, which must always be administered to the sick person.[2]

b. *Protestant*

The formulation of the dilemma speaks of "constantly incompatible elements, and even not beneficial to the patient", but it does not say what the latter, who has "recovered all his cerebral functions", thinks about what has happened. Generally speaking, it is clear that the quality of the survival is an important factor which needs to be taken into account in programming operations and treatment. But defining this quality is not easy and would require more than a few pages to set out.

c. *Jewish*

In this case we are not told the patient's age. It is always difficult to make a precise prognosis, so as long as there is still hope of a favourable outcome, everything should be attempted.

The word "euthanasia" arouses opposition in the traditional Jewish world, for which there can be no exception to, no derogation from, the respect of human life. Judaism refuses the idea of killing out of compassion to cut short the patient's suffering.

The legalisation of active euthanasia is the negation of the universal right to life. Administering a lethal injection with the intention of shortening life is an act forbidden by Jewish law. Hebraic law is against any form of decriminalisation of active euthanasia. The *Shulhan Arukh*, the code of Jewish law, is categorical on this subject: "When somebody is dying, he is considered as living in all respects. Thus it is forbidden to disturb him, and anybody who does so is considered a murderer. What can he be compared with? A guttering candle. As soon as anyone touches it, it goes out. Even if he remains in agony for a long time, resulting in great suffering for himself and his loved ones, it is still forbidden to hasten death." Legalising euthanasia would be opening the door to all abuses. People speak of mercy killing, killing out of pity. But pity is a dangerous and ambiguous concept. Often the compassion towards the sick person conceals motives less noble than might be thought. The psychiatrist Henri Baruk recalls that the word euthanasia in Hebrew is *hamatat hessed* (killing out of pity), but the word *hessed* has a double meaning in Hebrew:

---

1. Pontifical Council *Cor Unum*, "Some ethical questions relating to seriously ill and dying persons", 27 June 1981, in *Enchiridion Vaticanum*, No. 7, Official documents of the Holy See, 1980-1981, EDB, Bologna, 1985, p. 1143, paragraph 2.4.1.
2. See the Charter of health personnel, No. 120.

"pity", but also "opprobrium, excess of unthinking and abusive passion". The sentiment of pity and compassion, say the sages of the Talmud, should be supported by a concern for truth according to the classic expression *hessed vé émeth*.

On the other hand, relentless prolongation of life is not a moral duty. Helping a sick person to survive is a praiseworthy act, but maintaining a prolonged artificial survival for a dying person whose vital functions are irretrievably impaired, and this with the aid of sophisticated apparatus, is a scientific exploit but by no means a humanitarian action. The *Shulhan Arukh*, explains the Jewish position thus: "If there is any cause whatever which prevents the dying man from expiring, it is permitted to remove it; in this case, there is no direct action (which accelerates death), but only the removal of the cause (which is retarding death) without touching the dying man."

In the light of this text, it is legitimate to ask whether Judaism does not demand the right of the individual to die in dignity, calm and peace, without sterile recourse to leading-edge medical technology.

In any event the sick person must be provided with the four things essential to the survival of any person: food and drink, through drip or nasogastric tube, oxygen and if necessary blood transfusion.

"It is for the Jewish people, the people of 'Thou shalt not kill' and 'Thou shalt choose life', conscious of a twofold tradition of respect for life and the relief of the suffering of others, to find the difficult path which permits these two principles to be respected when, as is the case here, there is a patent contradiction. In Jewish ethics there are neither paths already traced nor doors wide open. There are simple lamps to light our way in a night where suffering, emptiness and death lie in wait" (See F. Rausky, in T.J. 1318 of 16 March 1995).

d. *Muslim*
The quality of life depends on the duty set out in the reply to case 87. Therapeutic insistence is an ethical rule.

e. *Buddhist*
This is another case concerned with the fine distinction between relentless prolongation of life and failure to assist a person in danger. In any event, the informed opinion of the family should prevail over any other decision.

4. From the standpoint of agnostic morality

Relentless prolongation of life cannot be justified by the wishes of the family. The treatment should be proportionate with the reasonable chance of dignified survival.

Family

A patient is taken in his bed to the radiology service. On his return he tells the nurse he was very afraid of dying in the waiting room after the examination and he had no possibility of calling anyone. The family was present when the porter came to collect him, but waited in the ward and then regretted not having accompanied the patient.

Dilemma: place of relatives in the care system; the patient's right to psychological support. Need to make members of the family understand that they can play an important role in helping a sick relative to cope with his illness and return to a better state of health.

1. From the standpoint of international law

See Article 5 of Recommendation R (80) 4 of 30.4.1980 concerning the patient as an active participant in his own treatment, in which the Committee of Ministers of the Council of Europe recommends the governments of member states to encourage "additional training for all team members in information techniques, educational non-directive communication techniques and health education".

For the rest there is no reply in international law now in force.

2. From the ethical standpoint

Satisfying the wishes of the patient and the family if this does not constitute an obstacle to care.

3. From the standpoint of religious moralities

a. *Catholic*

It is always necessary to bear in mind that an integral part of therapy is assistance to the patient also with regard to the anxieties he suffers in the critical moments of the illness: "beyond medical aid, what the sick person needs is love, human and supernatural warmth, which can and must be provided by all those close to him, parents and children, doctors and nurses".[1]

"In these cases the role of the families is irreplaceable."[2] As far as the family is concerned, their assistance should be encouraged within limits of the requirements of the service. To avoid having the family's concern ending up by increasing the

---

1. Congregation for the doctrine of the faith, Declaration on euthanasia, 5 May 1980, Part II.
2. John Paul II, *Evangelium Vitae*, 25 March 1995, No. 88.

patient's anxiety, it is necessary for the staff to make every effort to give a certain amount of advice to the families of people in hospital to ensure that everything they say or do really is for the good of the sick person.

b. *Protestant*

The answer is given by the formulation of the question: help is an essential part of the therapeutic process and the family can play an important role here. But it remains to be seen how this can be organised in practice.

c. *Jewish*

A sick person is a vulnerable one. He is generally worried because he does not know what tomorrow will bring. He needs to be reassured, helped and supported. He has the right to constant psychological and moral support. This forms an integral part of his therapy. It is therefore necessary to do everything to permit the family to play its role and help the sick relative to fight the disease and thus return to a better state of health. If the patient is afraid and needs a member of the family to accompany him to the X-ray unit, there should be somebody there who can do so.

d. *Muslim*

See the reply to case 87.

e. *Buddhist*

Everything which can help the patient, including the presence of his family, must be employed in the provision of care.

4. From the standpoint of agnostic morality

The presence of the family in this case would not disturb the proper functioning of the service or the quality of the care. On the contrary, a patient should not be left alone, or at least should always have the possibility of calling a member of the hospital staff.

412

Family

Mrs X, 72, lives with her son, a general practitioner. She goes into hospital for surgery, but when she has recovered and is ready to be discharged, the son insists that the surgeon should keep her in the active service in the hospital for some time yet. In fact the son can no longer have her in his home, she does not want to go into a retirement home, and in any case there is no room in the establishment closest to her son.
Dilemma: take action to make the doctor take account of the social status and dignity of the patient and take a concerted decision without interfering in the mother-son relationship, or should the nurse herself do this as part of her function, or say nothing?

1. From the standpoint of international law

If it is no longer necessary or useful to keep a patient in an active hospital service, respect for the right of others to health care means that the hospital bed should be freed (Articles 14 of the ECHR, 3 and 4 of the BC).

Furthermore, if the patient refuses to be placed in a retirement home, she cannot be installed in one against her will (Article 8 (1) of the ECHR: right to the respect of private life; Article 5 (1) of the BC, the concept of "intervention in the health field" being then understood as an intention performed for the purpose of rehabilitation), unless in the terms and under the conditions of Article 6 (3) of the BC (see also point 43 of the explanatory report).

2. From the ethical standpoint

Intervene as mediator.

3. From the standpoint of religious moralities

a. *Catholic*

Even though there are no explicit references in the magisterium of the Catholic Church, in the light of its general principles it is easy to say that it is not in conformity with the dignity of the person and his requirements of health and assistance to waste medical care resources to suit personal convenience and for non-medical reasons.

It is not right that thanks to the son's position this woman should occupy a bed which another may need more than she does.

b. *Protestant*

Strictly in terms of the case set out here, remaining in a hospital service can be only a provisional solution. It is therefore necessary to get down to the basic problem of the medium and longer term as soon as possible. Having done this, questions of "sutures" always arise, and always find a solution. For the rest, it seems above all that the doctor involved in the dilemma is embarrassed by the fact that one of the people involved is a colleague.

c. *Jewish*

If Mrs X does not want to go into a retirement home, it is important to determine the reasons for her refusal and then try to act accordingly. If she is sufficiently independent, the possibility should be envisaged of her living alone, with appropriate help from the social service department.

If she is not sufficiently independent for this, it would be necessary to convince her of the need to accept going into a retirement home, and if she still refuses persuade the son to take her back into his home.

In any event, if Mrs X is lucid she should participate in the decision.

d. *Muslim*

See cases 89 and 91.

e. *Buddhist*

The nurse should tell the son that she knows the psychological state of the patient and promote dialogue between them. This could be oriented towards a convalescent home, for example.

4. From the standpoint of agnostic morality

Encourage the son to make the necessary arrangements to be able to take his mother back. If this is absolutely impossible, the mother must be persuaded to accept temporary placement in a home some distance away.

Family

*Mrs X, 65, has cancer of the uterus. She is treated by anti-cancer chemotherapy.
She is supposed to be discharged to a convalescent home, but refuses, saying that
she still feels too weak, fatigued by the disease and no longer having any appetite.
The family agrees with her and asks for her to be kept in hospital for a while, after
which the family will look after her convalescence.*
*Dilemma: Mrs X can go into a convalescent home, her state of health does not
justify her being kept in hospital. Her and the family's opposition to leaving the
hospital are prejudicial to any improvement in her health.*

1. From the standpoint of international law

The medical opinion being that the patient should leave the active hospital service, not to be placed in the care of totally inexpert persons but to go on receiving
medical treatment in a convalescent home, only the consent of the patient is
required, the opinions or wishes of the family having no legal value.

In this sense, see Articles 4 and 5 of the BC, all the more so as a prolonged stay
in hospital would tend to oppose any improvement in the patient's state of health.
See also Article 6 (3) of the BC, as well as point 43 of the explanatory report.

2. From the ethical standpoint

Extend the hospitalisation to increase the chances of convincing the patient.

3. From the standpoint of religious moralities

a. *Catholic*

If the patient's state of health really does not justify the extension of her stay in
hospital, but leaving does not correspond with her own and the family's wishes,
then the staff should use all their psychology to try to make them understand the
necessity of leaving the hospital.

It is not right to prevent other people whose need is greater from having access
to hospital resources. "The health professional must take care in his relations with
the patient to ensure that his human qualities add weight to his professional action
and that his competence is more effective thanks to his understanding of the sick
person."[1]

---

1. Charter of health personnel, No. 104.

b. *Protestant*

"Mothering" is rarely an ideal therapeutic solution. In view of the patient's age and her ailment, going into a convalescent home would no doubt do a great deal of good. Psychological support and treatment could accompany this necessary convalescence.

c. *Jewish*

Hospitalism is a phenomenon frequently found. It is possible that this patient is suffering from it and it is therefore important to find the medical solution to her problem. If this is not the case, it would be necessary to try to reassure and calm her, explaining that her treatment can be continued only in a convalescent home.

It would also be necessary to explain the danger she runs in remaining in a hospital environment, where there is often the risk of additional infection by hospital germs.

In any event, it is important to tread carefully and try to avoid upsetting the patient, explaining the reasons for the decision.

d. *Muslim*

See cases 89 and 91.

e. *Buddhist*

It should be explained to the patient that her state of health could improve just as well in a more appropriate establishment such as a convalescent home as in the hospital, and she could also benefit from the presence of her family.

4. From the standpoint of agnostic morality

This patient should not be kept in hospital. Being fully informed, she can choose either to go into a convalescent home or to organise her convalescence with her children.

Family

Following the death of his father, an adolescent is hospitalised for massive hair loss. In the hospital an aerated wig is made available to him. He agrees to wear it, but his mother objects, fearing that the wig will hinder the regrowth of his hair. Dilemma: basic health education for families including an understanding of the role carers expect them to play to help improve the state of health of their sick relatives or the uninhibited expression of the families' anguish which carers have to deal with to the detriment of the dignity and interest of the patient, whatever his or her age.

1. From the standpoint of international law

The mother's opposition must come in second place according to Article 12 of the Convention on the Rights of the Child: "States Parties shall assure to the child who is capable of forming his or her own views the right to express those views freely in all matters affecting the child, the views of the child being given due weight in accordance with the age and maturity of the child. For this purpose, the child shall in particular be provided the opportunity to be heard in any judicial and administrative proceedings affecting the child, either directly, or through a representative or an appropriate body, in a manner consistent with the procedural rules of national law."

In the same sense, see Article 6 (2), second sub-paragraph, of the BC: "The opinion of the minor shall be taken into consideration as an increasingly determining factor in proportion to his or her age and degree of maturity, and point 45 of the explanatory report appended thereto.

2. From the ethical standpoint

The interest and desires of the patient must have priority.

3. From the standpoint of religious moralities

a. *Catholic*

Health personnel should try to inform patients' families about the basic principles of health education; they should help them to understand that they can make a very valuable contribution to improving the health of the person they love. "There is also preventive health care in the broad sense, in which the action of the health professional is but one component (...). Preventive action (...) requires the convergent harnessing of all the operational forces of society."[1]

---

1. Charter of health personnel, No. 52.

b. *Protestant*

The "dignity and interest of the patient" involved here are first of all his own affair. The role of the carers, especially in this case, is not to adopt a position but to favour the exchange between mother and son as much as possible, it being understood that "the one who has to wear the wig (or not)" will have the last word.

c. *Jewish*

Only the best interest of the patient should be taken into account. In this particular case the adolescent should wear the wig made available to him, to contribute to the improvement of his state of health.

On the other hand, the mother's concern must be understood, and an effort should be made to explain the reason for the treatment proposed. Basic health education is required for families, for they have a vital role to play in helping to improve the mental and physical health of their sick relatives.

d. *Muslim*

See cases 89 and 91.

e. *Buddhist*

Patient explanation is called for, to make the mother understand the advantage of the wig for her son's dignity and psychological equilibrium.

4. From the standpoint of agnostic morality

The interests and dignity of the patient must come first, regardless of his age.

Family

Mrs X, aged over 80, is in hospital and does not eat any more. The doctor prescribes the introduction of a nasogastric feeding tube. After she has removed this tube to which she objects several times, the nurses have to attach her hands by straps. The patient, nevertheless, manages to remove the tube by bringing her head down to one of her hands when in the wheelchair.

Her husband says he wants the tube kept in and any useful additional tests, such as scanner examination, should be made, knowing that the patient is tired of all this insistence and refuses care. The nurses are concerned about the situation. Dilemma: to die while being treated against one's will and with a great deal of suffering at the insistence of the family or to die in a chosen way, serenely and with one's dignity respected, receiving palliative care.

1. From the standpoint of international law

It is not clear in this case whether the "professional standards" referred to in Article 4 of the BC, already referred to many times, permit one or more solutions to the problem of feeding the patient, other than the nasogastric probe. If other possibilities are available, one should be chosen since the patient does not tolerate the probe.

This probe in fact should have been inserted with the patient's consent (Articles 7 of the Covenant on Civil and Political Rights; and 5 (1) and (2) of the BC, since this is a therapeutic intervention which is not a routine medical act for which consent is often implicit, provided that the patient has been fully informed (point 37 of the explanatory report appended to the BC). Being in fact an invasive treatment, express consent may be required (ibid.).

Point 67 of the same explanatory report states that even the exercise by the patient of the right not to know this or that fact concerning about his or her health "is not regarded as an impediment to the validity of his consent to an intervention" (in this connection see the reply to case 90 and point 65 of the explanatory report cited therein).

If according to the state of the art there are now other solutions to the problem of feeding the patient, i.e. to promote health and relieve pain, taking into account the psychological well-being of the patient, see the reply to case 88 and the professional obligations and standards in the country concerned (Article 4 of the BC and points 32 and 33 of the explanatory report).

It should be pointed out in passing that the international human rights law now in force has not yet tackled the problem of the boundaries between due care, relentless prolongation of life and passive euthanasia through the withdrawal of care; that the right to live constitutes the foundation *par excellence* of the "hard core" of the ECHR (Article 15 (2)) with respect to which any interference, infringement or limitation calls for very narrow and scrupulous interpretation in the established case-law of the Court, no derogation being admitted; that the fundamental principle of non-discrimination (Article 14 of the ECHR) imposes that no distinction should be made between the "right to live" of a young person and that of an old person; and that the problem of the "quality of life" as a limit to the right to life is at present unknown in positive international law.

For the rest, see once again the comments on cases 88 and 90, as well as the reply to case 14.

The wishes of the husband have no legal value.

If the patient suffers from impairment of her mental faculties, Article 6 (3) of the BC and the difference between this provision and Article 7 of the BC.

If the patient is incapable of giving an opinion on the intervention but has previously expressed her consent or opposition, at a time when she was capable of discernment, Articles 9 of the BC provides that "the previously expressed wishes relating to a medical intervention by a patient who is not, at the time of the intervention, in a state to express his or her wishes shall be taken into account", but they do not explicitly address the problem of the wish not to be treated or to cease to be treated.

2. From the ethical standpoint

Respect the desire of the patient. Do not leave the tube in place but insert it only for force-feeding.

3. From the standpoint of religious moralities

a. *Catholic*

"When called upon to give medical treatment to a patient, the health professional should be in possession of his express or tacit consent."[1] "The 'person', the one most responsible for his own life, should be the centre of all assistance; the others are there to help, not to replace him."[2]

If the patient is capable of understanding and expressing desires, and refuses the tube and any further examinations, then the staff must express their disagreement, because to let the patient die as she requests would be euthanasia. "Medical and paramedical personnel — faithful to their duty to be always at the service of life

---

1. Charter of health personnel, No. 72.
2. Pontifical Council *Cor Unum*, "Some ethical questions relating to seriously ill and dying persons", 27 June 1981, in *Enchiridion Vaticanum*, No. 7, Official documents of the Holy See, 1980-1981, EDB, Bologna, 1985, p. 1137, paragraph 2.1.2.

and to assist it to the end – cannot lend themselves to any form of euthanasia, not even at the request of the person concerned, and even less of his family. The fact is that no right is accorded to anybody with regard to euthanasia, because no right is given which permits one to dispose arbitrarily of one's own life. No health professional can therefore make himself the executive protector of a right which does not exist."[1] If the patient is not capable of expressing valid consent, "the health professional may, and in extreme situations, must, presume consent for therapeutic interventions which in all knowledge and conscience he considers necessary. In the case of temporary absence of consciousness and will, this is by virtue of the principle of therapeutic confidence, namely the original confidence which made the patient put himself in the professional's hands. In the case of permanent absence of consciousness and will, this is by virtue of the principle of responsibility in health care, which obliges the health professional to take charge of the patient's health."[2]

b. *Protestant*
The choice is clear: it is better to let the patient die in a chosen and serene fashion than to force her to have treatment she refuses. But is it certain that the husband is inaccessible to frank discussion of the matter?

c. *Jewish*
If the patient refuses the nasogastric feeding tube, it is necessary to envisage other possibilities for feeding her, after discussing the problem with her. Several alternatives are open to the doctor: the parenteral route, the use of microprobes or jejunostomy (method which involves an operation under local anaesthetic to enable the patient to be fed with the minimum of discomfort).

The fact of refusing the tube does not necessarily mean that the patient does not want to live.

It is necessary to evaluate her more or less deep depression (aid of a neuropsychiatrist) and try to convince her by giving a maximum of explanations, listening attentively and adopting an appropriate therapeutic approach.

d. *Muslim*
See the reply to case 90. The generalisation of euthanasia is prohibited in Islam. The doctor alone must act according to his conscience and in any event on a case-by-case basis.

---

1. Charter of health personnel, No. 148.
2. *Idem*, No. 73.

e. *Buddhist*

It is important to avoid relentless prolongation of life and to respect the patient's wishes to the end, so that she can die in peace.

4. From the standpoint of agnostic morality

Only the patient's wishes should be taken into account.

Rights of the individual

Mr X, 58, has been in hospital for some time and is cachectic. He has had a tracheotomy and has to have respiratory assistance. The doctor feels he cannot do anything more for him and decides to send him to a specialised centre. The doctor has not informed the patient for fear of his reaction, and when members of the family are informed after the transfer, they are annoyed. The patient dies a few hours later.

The carers who carried out the move regret it.

Dilemma: act with regret on medical orders after losing confidence in the doctor or take action to have the patient's and family's right to information respected before carrying out the orders.

1. From the standpoint of international law

The transfer of the patient from the hospital to a specialised centre in this case qualifies as a medical intervention according to all the provisions of the BC. As a result, in the terms of Article 5 (1) of this text, consent should have been obtained. This is so even though the doctor did not inform the patient about his condition for fear of his reaction (Article 10 (3) of the BC). In fact, point 67 of the explanatory report states that even the exercise by the patient of the right not to know certain information about his or her health "is not regarded as an impediment to the validity of his consent to an intervention". In this connection see the reply to case 90.

As regards the members of the family, they should have been informed that the patient was being transferred to another establishment, in order to respect the right to family life as stipulated in Article 8 (1) of the ECHR.

As regards the behaviour of the nurses, reference should be made to the professional obligation and standards in force in the country concerned, as per Article 4 of the BC.

2. From the ethical standpoint

If the patient is conscious, his consent must be obtained after he has been informed. If he is unconscious, the doctor must act in consultation with the family.

3. From the standpoint of religious moralities

a. *Catholic*

In this case the care team should take action to ensure respect of the "right of the person to be informed about his own state of health",[1] and the relevant therapeutic possibilities, rather than carrying out the doctor's orders without the knowledge of the patient and his family. The respect of this right expresses consideration for the patient and respect of his dignity as a person. In so doing, it must not be forgotten that "the duty of truth to the patient in the terminal phase requires discernment and human tact on the part of carers".[2] The right to be informed "does not disappear in the presence of a diagnosis and prognosis of an illness which will cause death, but other factors are also involved. The fact is that this information implies important responsibilities".[3]

b. *Protestant*
Another communication problem. Could the doctor not have been warned of the dangers of the path he was taking? In any event, it is not so much a matter of the right to information as of the need for the informed consent of the patient (and the family), which is fundamental and overrides any other consideration.

c. *Jewish*
Not informing the patient in this case may be understandable in view of his condition, but the doctor should have consulted members of the family and explained the reasons why he recommended this transfer. In no event can the doctor substitute his own conception of the quality of life for that of his patient. People cannot be treated arbitrarily. It is inexcusable not to inform the patient or the family.

In any event, the doctor should inform the nursing team of the reasons which made him act in this way. If the reasons are not satisfactory, the nurses could, if appropriate, speak to a colleague and see with him how the situation could be remedied.

d. *Muslim*
See the reply to case 97.

e. *Buddhist*
It is essential to respect the right to information of the patient and his family before taking any action whatever, through respect of the dignity of the person.

---

1. *Idem*, No. 125.
2. *Idem*, No. 126.
3. *Idem*, No. 125.

4. From the standpoint of agnostic morality

The patient's right to information should be respected.

Rights of the individual

A terminal phase cancer patient complains of not seeing her visitors and the excessive administration of sedatives which make her sleep too much.
The nurse tells the doctor of the patient's complaints and wishes but he refuses to modify the treatment.
Dilemma: make the doctor understand that a patient may choose other ways than isolation from the world and in particular his or her nearest and dearest, or point out that the right to health is not contrary to the right to have information and maintain social contacts.

1. From the standpoint of international law

According to the established case-law of the Court, the concept of "private life" as in Article 8 of the ECHR encompasses not only private life proper, but also relations with other persons (in particular those closest). Respect of the patient's private life would therefore imply that she should be able to receive visitors in hospital. On the other hand, it is for the doctor to decide, on the basis of his scientific knowledge and the professional obligations and standards applicable in the specific case (Articles 4 of the BC and point 32 of the explanatory report) to decide whether a different treatment can adequately ease the patient's suffering, any medical intervention having to be relevant and proportional to the aim pursued.

2. From the ethical standpoint

The patient's clearly expressed desire must be respected.

3. From the standpoint of religious moralities

a. *Catholic*

It is appropriate to invite the doctor to carefully evaluate whether there are other possibilities which, while still being good for the patient, do not cut her off completely from contact with the people around her and above all her loved ones. It is necessary to point out "the importance for man to end his days, so far as possible, in the integrity of his personality and the relations it maintains with his milieu, above all with his family (...). Given the conditions in which certain therapies are administered and the total isolation that they impose on the patient, it is not irrelevant to mention that the right to die as a human being and with dignity implies this social dimension."[1]

---

1. Pontifical Council *Cor Unum*, "Some ethical questions relating to seriously ill and dying persons", 27 June 1981, in *Enchiridion Vaticanum*, No. 7, Official documents of the Holy See, 1980-1981, EDB, Bologna, 1985, p. 1140, paragraph 2.2.2.

As regards the administration of analgesics, the principle of the informed consent of the patient still applies. The doctor in fact enjoys "no separate or independent right *vis-à-vis* his patient. In general, he can act only if the patient explicitly or implicitly (directly or indirectly) authorises it."[2]

b. *Protestant*

There is no real dilemma and the question is the following: how to make a doctor understand what the therapeutic relationship is? As for the "right to health" mentioned here (apparently conflicting with the right to information and to maintain social contacts), it appears to be more like the doctor's right to act as he wishes in authoritarian fashion. This "right" is not upheld by any kind of morality or by any legal text.

c. *Jewish*

A patient suffering from terminal cancer who is in constant pain would not be able to benefit from the visits of her loved ones.

In this case it is necessary to so arrange the treatment as to give her periods of consciousness, warning her that she will probably suffer more physically during these periods.

This arrangement can be made only after having explained the situation to the patient. The doctor's decision should be taken only after the patient has been informed.

d. *Muslim*

Concertation between several doctors and nurses is necessary. "In case of doubt, teaches the Prophet, seek other authorised opinions, even if this contradicts the Prophet."

e. *Buddhist*

The nurse should remind the doctor of the importance of the patient's being able to die consciously and in peace, surrounded by the affection of the family.

4. From the standpoint of agnostic morality

There is no dilemma. It is simply a matter of achieving a balance between palliative care and the patient being able to maintain contact with her nearest and dearest.

---

2. Pius XII, "Address to the doctors of the G. Mendel Institute", 24 November 1957, in AAS 49, 1957, p. 1031.

Rights of the individual

*Miss X, 19 and a drug addict, no fixed abode, is four months pregnant
(first pregnancy).
She is hospitalised to have the neck of the uterus tied because of the danger of
miscarriage. Among other examinations the doctor orders an HIV test, telling the
nurse to take the blood sample for this test without informing the patient.
The result is positive and this is confirmed by a second test.
As the patient's consent was not sought, she is not informed of the result
of the test. The doctor acts to maintain the pregnancy though there is a threat to
the life of both the patient and her child (falling T4 lymphocyte count).
A therapeutic abortion is not proposed to the patient. Knowing nothing of her
health problem, she wants to keep the child and agrees to the tying.
Dilemma: remain linked to the doctor in the illegal act of taking a blood sample
for an HIV test without the patient's knowledge, knowing of the doctor's
deliberate refusal to inform her and helping her to keep the child by means of
surgery, or refuse to co-operate, raising the problem of the future of mother
and child so that the patient can take an informed decision before any operation.*

1. From the standpoint of international law

The patient's consent to the HIV test is essential according to Articles 7 of the Covenant on Civil and Political Rights, and 5 (1) of the BC. Furthermore, since this is a therapeutic intervention which is not a routine medical act for which consent is often implicit, provided that the patient has been fully informed (point 37 of the explanatory report appended to the BC), express consent may be required (ibid.). The same applies regarding the communication of the results of the test (Articles 10 (1) of the ECHR and 10 (2) of the BC).

The patient has the right to freely decide for herself (Article 8 (1) of the ECHR) as regards her sex life and the continuation or termination of her pregnancy, the woman being, according to Commission decisions, the person most concerned.

2. From the ethical standpoint

A nurse, as well as a doctor, can invoke the conscience clause.

3. From the standpoint of religious moralities

a. *Catholic*
The doctor enjoys "no separate or independent right *vis-à-vis* his patient. In

general, he can act only if the patient explicitly or implicitly (directly or indirectly) authorises it."[1] In this particular case there is also violation of the "right of the person to be informed about his own state of health",[2] a right which is explained by the need to give the patient "a precise picture of his problem and of the therapeutic possibilities, as well as the risks involved, the difficulties and the likely consequences."[3] This principle applies regardless of the fact that the woman could be induced to have an abortion; it is, nevertheless, necessary to recall "the gravity of induced abortion", and that "what is eliminated is a human being who is starting to live" and "these reasons, however serious and tragic they may be, can never justify the deliberate suppression of an innocent human being."[4] The nurses should therefore invite the doctor to act so as to respect the rights of the woman and of the child, then favour the reconciliation between the truth of the diagnosis and safeguard of the life of the child to be born.

b. *Protestant*

One can but encourage the nurse to distance herself from the doctor's attitude and find a way of making him reconsider his decision or to inform the mother (or have her informed) of her true condition. There is also a further question upstream of the dilemma considered: by what right can an HIV test be made without the consent of the person concerned?

c. *Jewish*

It is important to know why the doctor considered it necessary to keep this child despite the risks.

Given the context, it is normal that the doctor should carry out an Aids test, but it is unacceptable not to inform the patient.

Even if he did not inform the patient that he was making the test, he should at least, once he had the results, explain these to her and the risks entailed for herself and for the child. Not informing this woman carries the risk of her having sexual relations with somebody else and thus transmitting the virus to her partner.

In any event, refusal on the part of the nurse is no solution. A fruitful dialogue should be established between the doctor and the nursing team. The nurses have the right to know the whys and wherefores of the treatments and examinations offered to patients.

---

1. Pius XII, "Address to the doctors of the G. Mendel Institute", 24 November 1957, in AAS 49, 1957, p. 1031.
2. Charter of health personnel, No. 125.
3. *Idem*, No. 72.
4. John Paul II, *Evangelium Vitae*, No. 58.

If the doctor persists in his refusal to inform and explain, it will be necessary to speak to another colleague. In the case of a serious breach of deontology or ethics, the nursing team can appeal.

d. *Muslim*

In principle, before the 120th day (according to a *hadith*, namely one of the rules of conduct decreed by the prophet Mohammed, the foetal body does not receive the *rouh* – the divine spirit which makes him human – until the 120th day, after three stages of 40 days of organisation of the receptacle) therapeutic abortion is not a murder, because according to Muslim law the foetus does not yet have human status. In this case the doctor's attitude requires a *shura*, or concertation.

e. *Buddhist*

It is the nurse's duty to inform her superiors and oppose the doctor's illegal attitude.

4. From the standpoint of agnostic morality

In this case the blood test is perhaps illegal but, nevertheless, justifiable.

However, the patient should be informed about her condition and about the risk to both herself and the child, so that she can make a free and informed choice about whether to be a mother or not.

Rights of the individual

When a nurse is trying to establish his case history, Mr X refuses to answer most of the questions, being suspicious of precipitate divulgence in the hospital and even of the processing of these data in the hospital.
Dilemma: how to treat a patient effectively if he has no confidence in the carers and fears the early divulgence of the information concerning him.

1. From the standpoint of international law

No reply in positive international law, except in the case where the fear is based on the fact that all personal data on patients is processed automatically.

In this case, reference is made to the Convention for the Protection of Individuals with Regard to the Automatic Processing of Personal Data (Council of Europe 28.1.1981-1.9.1982), Recommendation R (81) 1 of the Committee of Ministers of the Council of Europe on regulations for automated medical databanks (23.1.1981) and Recommendation R (83) 10 of the Committee of Ministers of the Council of Europe on the protection of personal data used for scientific research and statistics (23.9.1983). See also Article 10 (2) of the ECHR and Article 10 (1) of the BC.

2. From the ethical standpoint

The free choice of the patient must be respected and he should be given the possibility of turning to other carers.

3. From the standpoint of religious moralities

a. *Catholic*
It is important to make the patient understand that if he is to derive physical and mental benefit from treatment, he must have confidence in the hospital staff, even though there may be some reserve. In fact, "medical and health care activity is founded on an interpersonal relationship of a particular nature. It is the meeting between a 'confidence' and a 'conscience'".[1] The particular nature of this relationship means for the health personnel that they must be discreet about the private life of patients; this is a moral duty rather than a professional one. The nurse must make the patient understand this and win his confidence.

---

1. Charter of health personnel, No. 2.

b. *Protestant*

By trying to instil confidence in him, namely through trying to identify the reasons for his distrust and making him understand that his fears are groundless.

c. *Jewish*

The patient is not so very wrong. It is understandable that certain patients might refuse to always answer certain nurses, because they do not know the degree of confidentiality of the nurse establishing the medical history.

It is therefore necessary to seek the reasons why confidence is not established between this patient and the nurse.

On the other hand, if it is a doctor who is establishing the medical history, the situation is quite different. The patient has come to the hospital to be treated. It is necessary to clearly explain to him that the information requested will remain strictly confidential and is important for establishing his case history and for being able to give him the optimum treatment. It is therefore essential to win the patient's confidence, for if this confidence is not established, there is the risk of having problems, even as regards the treatment. It should not be forgotten that a good deal of the cure depends on the climate of confidence that the doctor succeeds in establishing with his patient.

d. *Muslim*

Medical secrecy should be stressed.

e. *Buddhist*

It is essential to win the patient's confidence, otherwise the therapeutic relationship is impossible.

4. From the standpoint of agnostic morality

The patient needs to be reassured. It should be explained that the quality of the treatment partly depends on the quality of the information, and that this information is protected by medical secrecy.

Rights of the individual

A father is worried about the fact that the family doctor seems to insist on vaccinating his children of 15 and 22 against hepatitis B. This vaccination is not compulsory, the majority of doctors do not suggest it, and he does not like the idea.
Dilemma: need to inform families of the real value of the care, treatment or medical act proposed, to ensure that they are well received.

1. From the standpoint of international law

One of the two children in this case is a minor (adolescent), assumed to be capable of discernment, while the other is an adult.

Under these circumstances it is the consent of the subjects concerned that counts; the opinion of the minor can and should be duly taken into consideration in view of his age and degree of maturity (Article 12 (1) of the Convention on the Rights of the Child; Article 6 (2) of the BC and point 45 of the explanatory report.

2. From the ethical standpoint

Agreed – no dilemma.

3. From the standpoint of religious moralities

a. *Catholic*

Health professionals should be capable of establishing a calm dialogue with those they see regularly, using the methods most appropriate to the particular case, so as to be able to give them the correct information on the importance of the medical act and what health care means, even at the level of prevention, for the good of either the individual or of society. "The safeguard of health commits the health professional above all in the field of prevention. Prevention is better than cure, either to avoid the inconvenience and suffering of sickness, or to spare society the costs, economic or other, of the treatment."[1]

b. *Protestant*

One of the children is adult, so it is for him to decide what to do. Since the other child too is old enough to have his own opinion, this should be taken into account.

---

1. Charter of health personnel, No. 50.

Furthermore, it is difficult to see how it is possible, ethically or practically, to "treat" a healthy person against his will.

c. *Jewish*

Vaccination against hepatitis B is not compulsory. It therefore cannot be imposed on anyone at all. Unless the doctor suspects something else.

The doctor must therefore explain the reasons for his proposing this vaccination.

Having said this, the field of vaccination is expanding all the time, and is prevention not better than cure?

d. *Muslim*

Reconsider the definition of preventive medicine.

e. *Buddhist*

The father should ask the family doctor for an explanation as to why he insists on this vaccination, and should approach other practitioners.

4. From the standpoint of agnostic morality

Families should be informed about the real benefits of vaccinations. The final decision must be taken by the family in the case of children who are still minor, otherwise by the children themselves.

Rights of the individual

In a general medical service, a young patient with hepatitis B is subject to therapeutic isolation because his blood is infectious. Contrary to the texts governing the precautions to be taken, there is a custom of pasting a red spot on the door to warn non-medical staff that they should be careful. The patient refuses to have this spot on his door.
Dilemma: discretion concerning diagnosis; education of non-medical staff and organisation of work.

1. From the standpoint of international law

Respect of the rights of health professionals requires that the people concerned should be informed about the infectious disease so that they can take appropriate precautions (Article 10 (1) of the ECHR). Nevertheless, the patient has the right not to have confidential information concerning his health divulged in such a way as to infringe his private life in the health field (Articles 10 (2) and 8 (1) of the ECHR and 10 (1) of the BC).

For the rest, no specific response in international law.

2. From the ethical standpoint

Respect the patient's wishes.

3. From the standpoint of religious moralities

a. *Catholic*
Discretion crowns the nurse's moral virtues. In the present case, the duty of social solidarity by which the hospital staff are bound can be observed by organising the work differently and, above all, through adopting measures which do not marginalise anyone. For the nurse, "the patient is never reduced to simply being a clinical case – he is not an anonymous individual to whom the results of one's own knowledge are applied – but always 'a sick man' towards whom one must adopt an attitude of true 'sympathy' in the etymological sense of the term".[1]

b. *Protestant*
The patient is right, and besides the reactions connected with his own sensitivity, he can argue on the basis of the confidentiality of the diagnosis and medical secrecy.

---

1. Charter of health personnel, No. 2.

Similarly, any kind of stigmatisation must be prohibited: there is no difference in nature between the "red spot" and the "yellow star".

c. *Jewish*

The fact that a red spot is stuck on the door to warn staff to take particular care is a practice contrary to the texts governing the precautions to be taken. It is therefore necessary to refuse this practice. It is also, and above all, necessary to communicate clearly to the patient and if appropriate his entourage the motives or reasons for his isolation and the protective measures this implies.

It is of course necessary to find a less glaring and less discriminatory way of protecting the staff. Note, for example, in the patient's file, the type of contagion and the precautions to take.

If the staff feel threatened, they should appeal to the legal institutions to get the law changed.

It is important of recall that isolation is not always aimed at protecting the medical team; sometimes the patient also has to be protected, especially if his immunity defences are impaired.

d. *Muslim*

Explain the collective responsibility to the patient.

e. *Buddhist*

It is essential that every person be respected.

4. From the standpoint of agnostic morality

An effort should be made to inform non-medical staff, and any mnemotechnical aids that may be used must in no case reveal a diagnosis.

Rights of the individual

Mr X, 92, was operated on for cancer a few months ago. At the time the family was told that if there was any further outbreak or complication the outlook would be very poor. As a result of a recent fistula with substantial hydric and ionic losses and a malaise, Mr X is again hospitalised in an intensive care unit. A few hours after his arrival he seems very much better, but has to remain in intensive care because of the fistula. Shortly afterwards he is operated on and transferred from intensive care to a single room in the surgical department where he will receive care until he dies.

Because of the explanations given at the time of the first operation, the family were prepared for bereavement soon after the patient had to go back into hospital. To their great surprise they found themselves faced with the demands of a patient who wants to go home after a few hours because he feels much better, then with the anxiety of a second, unexpected, operation, then the result of this second operation, then having to accompany a dying man after having thought that if there was a second operation this meant that he had a chance of recovery.

Members of the family feel trapped between the doctors' prognosis, having to lie to the patient when he felt restored to life, the prolonged agony of death after the second operation.

They are disoriented and complain to the nurses about the doctors' competence with respect to the following points:

– lack of sufficient information;

– lack of advice on the attitude to adopt vis-à-vis the patient;

– lack of sufficient information to be able to make appropriate arrangements (send for the children who live a long way away, stay at the patient's bedside or not, make arrangements for a funeral, etc.).

Dilemma: adoption of a technical view of the doctor's task, to the detriment of consideration of the human dimension of the patient and his family.

1. From the standpoint of international law

No reply in positive international law.

Article 4 of the BC stipulates that "any intervention in the health field, including research, must be carried out in accordance with relevant professional obligations and standards", and point 38 of the explanatory report states that "Doctors and, in general, all professionals who participate in a medical act are subject to ethical and legal imperatives. They must act with care and competence".

In its turn the lack of adequate information for the family (a concept which is not yet defined at international level however, reference always being made to national

437

law) to be able to take decisions based on the patient's state of health could constitute a violation of Article 8 (1) of the ECHR (respect of private and family life) and Article 10 (1) of the ECHR (right to information). Possible application by analogy of a number of Court decisions ruling that the right of parents and their children to live together and maintain stable relationships is without doubt a fundamental aspect of family life protected by Article 8 (1) of the ECHR. Thus the right of parents to visit children living with foster families or in homes remains fundamental (see Decision Nos. 120 and 121 of 8.7.1987 in cases *O. H. B. R. and W.* v. *United Kingdom,* and 307 B of 24.2.1995 in the *McMichael* case (*Commission* v. *United Kingdom*).

2. From the ethical standpoint

Agreed on the necessity to improve the quality of the relationship with the patient.

3. From the standpoint of religious moralities

a. *Catholic*

It is always necessary to bear in mind both the obligation to humanise care and hospitalisation and that of informing the patient's family.

"The doctor-patient relationship should again be based on a dialogue involving listening, respect and consideration; it should again be an authentic meeting between two free men or, as has been said, between 'confidence' and a 'conscience'."[1]

"The health professional is invited, either individually, or through associative forms of action, to think, while treating the patent, of the members of his family, doing what he can to inform, advise, guide and support them."[2]

b. *Protestant*

This case is complicated, not so much in its principle as in the many stages involved, but in any event we can but advocate the practice of a medicine which is not simply technical and does not disregard the human dimension and the patient's family.

c. *Jewish*

The role of the doctor is to do his best to relieve suffering and help patients live. In any new situation the doctor has to provide what he considers to be the most appropriate solution.

---

1. John Paul II, "Address to the participants in two congresses of medicine and surgery", 27 October 1980, in *Insegnamenti*, III/2, p. 1010, No. 6.
2. Charter of health personnel, No. 55.

The family knows the patient's situation very well. It is for them to make the necessary arrangements as they wish. An attempt is being made here to make the doctor responsible for a situation which is not of his making.

However, and despite what has just been said, the doctor should keep the family informed as the situation evolves and let them know the different eventualities. It is also the doctor's duty to complement this information, counsel them in all honesty, and try to guide the somewhat disoriented family.

d. *Muslim*

After seeking several opinions, inform the patient and/or the family and act as in case 89.

e. *Buddhist*

In any circumstance, even unforeseeable, the situation would be less painful if the patient were generally informed about his state and if the family were involved in the medical approach.

4. From the standpoint of agnostic morality

The patient's decision must be respected. In this case he did not refuse the operations and seems happy to have survived. The emotional strain for the family therefore has to take second place.

Rights of the individual

Mrs X, 86, is in hospital in an intensive care unit with a heart disorder. The patient wants to be left to die in peace. The family asks the carers not to relentlessly prolong life. The doctor prescribes reanimation in the case of cardiac arrest and insists that the nurses carry out his instructions to the letter. The nurses disagree with this order.
Dilemma: treatment without consensus and against the patient's wishes.

1. From the standpoint of international law

The problem of the legitimacy of the renunciation of the entitlement to and exercise of the right to life has not yet been addressed or resolved by international human rights law, and neither has the boundary been defined between due care, relentless prolongation of life and passive euthanasia through the withdrawal of care at the request of the patient.

As regards the BC, see the comments on cases 88, 90, 92, 97 and 98.

2. From the ethical standpoint

Relentless prolongation of life is contrary to medical ethics.

3. From the standpoint of religious moralities

a. *Catholic*

The respect of the entire person of the patient requires that "When they have to take medical action on a patient, health professionals should be in possession of his express or tacit consent (...). It is necessary to request informed consent from the patient."[1] The health professional cannot do what this patient requests: "sharing another person's suicidal intention and helping him realise it by what is known as 'assisted suicide' means that one becomes a collaborator, and sometimes an actor oneself in an injustice which can never be justified even if it responds to a request."[2]

b. *Protestant*

The duly informed opinion of the patient and family must come first.

---

1. Charter of health personnel, No. 72.
2. John Paul II, *Evangelium Vitae*, No. 66.

c. *Jewish*

The doctor is the sole authority empowered to decide the treatment to be given. If the doctor insists that the nurses reanimate the patient in the case of cardiac arrest, this means that the pathology offers a chance of recuperation. In this case, the doctor is but assuming his role, which is to privilege life. The nurses must in this case be the doctor's right hand. Their role is certainly to listen, but above all to ensure that the prescriptions are executed in accordance with the doctor's wishes. Refusing to execute the doctor's orders would risk creating anarchy in the service. It is necessary for them to be able to discuss things with the doctor and above all be able to ask to know the reasons for the prescribed treatment. Constant, open and fruitful dialogue should exist not only between the patient, the family and the medical team, but also within this team.

d. *Muslim*
Medical consensus.

e. *Buddhist*

The nurses should inform the doctor of the their disagreement and inform their superiors about this attitude.

4. From the standpoint of agnostic morality

The doctor must respect the patient's informed wishes and not impose relentless prolongation of life.

Rights of the individual

Mr X, 80, unmarried and with no family, is hospitalised because of the dislocation of an artificial hip joint. He refuses to eat and says he wants to die. A nasogastric feeding tube is inserted. The patient pulls it out. The carers disagree about this tube : some are for, others against.
Dilemma : therapeutic insistence or accompaniment for the dying man.

1. From the standpoint of international law

The problem of renouncing the entitlement to and/or the exercise of the right to life has not yet been resolved by international human rights law: reference should be made to the reply to case 97.

As regards the behaviour of the doctors and health care professionals in general, reference should be made to Article 4 of the BC.

2. From the ethical standpoint

The tube should not be left in place but should be inserted only for force-feeding.

3. From the standpoint of religious moralities

a. *Catholic*

It is always necessary to pay attention to the patient's wishes. In fact "the person, the one mainly responsible for his own life, must be the point of reference for any action to assist him. The others are there only to help him, not to take his place".[1]

However, it must not be forgotten that "alimentation and hydration, even artificial, should be classified as normal care always due to a patient if they are not dangerous for him. Their unjustified suspension could amount to veritable euthanasia".[2] Furthermore, their administration in no way amounts to therapeutic insistence but is a normal part of accompanying the dying person. Refusal on the part of the patient represents euthanasia and "Medical and paramedical personnel – faithful to their duty to be always at the service of life and to assist it to the end – cannot lend themselves to any form of euthanasia, not even at the request of the person

---

1. Pontifical Council *Cor Unum*, "Some ethical questions relating to seriously ill and dying persons", 27 June 1981, in *Enchiridion Vaticanum*, No. 7, Official documents of the Holy See, 1980-1981, EDB, Bologna, 1985, p. 1137, paragraph 2.1.2.
2. Charter of health personnel, No. 120.

concerned, and even less of his family. The fact is that no right is accorded to anybody with regard to euthanasia, because no right is given which permits one to dispose arbitrarily of one's own life. No health professional can therefore make himself the executive protector of a right which does not exist".[1]

b. *Protestant*

An attempt should be made to find out what underlies the patient's refusal to eat or be fed. But if it turns out that he really is prepared to face death, in the name of what should he be prevented?

c. *Jewish*

The fact of refusing the nasogastric tube does not necessarily mean that the patient wants to die. Perhaps he is uncomfortable and finds it difficult to bear the presence of this tube. A neuropsychiatrist could also help by determining the more or less serious state of depression of this patient and perhaps proposing medical treatment for it.

Because of the good prognosis for his physical condition and the possibility of good recovery, it is necessary to try to help this patient. It is therefore necessary to envisage other possibilities of feeding the patient, after having discussed it with him. Several alternatives are open to the doctor: the parenteral route, the use of microprobes or jejunostomy (method involving an operation under local anaesthetic to enable the patient to be fed with the minimum of discomfort).

d. *Muslim*

See the reply to case 89.

e. *Buddhist*

Dialogue is required to give the patient all the information concerning his state.

4. From the standpoint of agnostic morality

The patient's free decision must be respected. He should be given only the care he needs to be allowed to die in dignity.

---

1. *Idem*, No. 148.

Rights of the individual

Mr X, 62, has cancer of the bladder and has had two urethrotomies.
The doctor has told this patient that the disease is not serious, but the patient knows
that this cannot be true. He asks the nurses questions and does everything to discuss
his illness with them because he knows they know the truth and can help him.
Dilemma: take action to reduce the inconsistency between the care approach
and the medical approach so as to make the treatment more effective. Should the
doctor be brought face-to-face with the patient so that he has no choice and has
to speak to him on a level he can understand, or should the patient's questions be
ignored, knowing that not responding to a fundamental need for information
prejudices the effectiveness of the treatment and negates the dignity and humanity
of the patient.

1. From the standpoint of international law

According to Articles 10 (1) of the ECHR and 10 (2) of the BC everyone has the right to know any information collected about his state of health unless he has expressed the wish not to be so informed (Article 10 (2) of the BC): the right to know and the right not to know.

In his turn, the doctor – where a wish not to be informed has not been expressed – has to communicate this information to his patient, the only exception to the right and obligation of information in the health field being the "therapeutic exception", namely the case where informing the patient (for example of a fatal prognosis) would be likely to seriously harm the patient's health: it is for national legislation to establish this exception (Article 10 (3) of the BC). "In terms of point 67 of the explanatory report appended to the BC, the right (or necessity) not to know this or that fact concerning his health is not regarded as an impediment to the validity of the patient's consent to an intervention".

The problem of the boundaries between "silence" ("domestic law may justify the doctor in sometimes withholding information"), "delivering information with circumspection" (and "restraining the paternalist approaches which might ignore the wish of the patient" (see Article 5 of the BC and point 34 of the explanatory report, as well as point 65 of the latter) is not solved in Article 10(3) of the BC. Point 69 of the explanatory report stipulates in fact that "(...) In some cases, the doctor's duty to provide information which is also covered under Article 4 conflicts with the interests of the patient's health. It is for domestic law, taking account of the social and cultural background, to solve this conflict".

As regards the way the nurses should act *vis-à-vis* both the doctor and the patient, reference should be made once again to Article 4 of the BC.

2. From the ethical standpoint

Agree with the first part of the alternative.

3. From the standpoint of religious moralities

a. *Catholic*

"A person has a right to be informed about his own state of health. This right does not disappear in the presence of a diagnosis and prognosis of an illness which will cause death, but other factors are also involved. The fact is that this information implies important responsibilities which cannot be escaped. There are responsibilities connected with the treatment which has to be given with the informed consent of the patient."[1] The magisterium of the Catholic Church also recalls that the truth must be communicated with "discernment and human tact",[2] and that "it should be adjusted to the wavelength of love and charity".[3]

It is necessary to say first of all that the communication of the diagnosis is the duty of the doctor responsible for the treatment, not the nurse; in this particular case she should therefore invite the doctor to engage in a "relationship of sharing and communion"[4] with the patient, within which the doctor would find a way to communicate to the patient the necessary information on his state of health.

b. *Protestant*

Priority must always go to discourse, and to the dignity and humanity of the patient.

c. *Jewish*

If the doctor has decided to hide the truth from this patient, it is perhaps because he has serious reasons concerned with his physical or mental health. In this case, it is necessary to explain them to the nurses.

A constructive dialogue should be established between the doctor and the nurses in order to decide in common accord on the policy to adopt *vis-à-vis* this patient. It is necessary to determine together what type of information can be given, and how to give it.

What must be avoided above all is any discordance between the behaviour of the doctor and that of the nurses, because in this case the situation would become unmanageable. There would then be a risk of the patient no longer having confidence in either the doctor or the nurses.

---

1. Charter of health personnel, No. 125.
2. *Idem*, No. 126.
3. *Idem*, No. 126.
4. *Idem*, No. 127.

d. *Muslim*
See case 89.

e. *Buddhist*
The doctor should be placed face-to-face with the patient and speak to him on a level which he can understand.

4. From the standpoint of agnostic morality

The nurse must endeavour to reduce the incoherence between the care approach and the medical approach. In practice, she must try to convince the doctor that it is in the patient's interest that he should be informed, but if the doctor refuses to accept this argument she cannot take action in his place.

Rights of the individual

Mr X, 38, has a cancer with cerebral metastases. It is necessary to implant a chamber to continue the chemotherapy. Knowing nothing about his disease or its stage of evolution, the patient thinks he will soon be well again and asks the nurse why he has to have a chamber implanted now he has completed his treatment. Dilemma: reply by giving a false reason or give no reply because of the good mental state of the patient favourable to a better quality of end of life, reinforcing his illusion, or ask the doctor to explain the treatment so that the nurse can explain the true reason for the use of this technique in his precise case so that he can understand and manage what has happened and retain his dignity.

1. From the standpoint of international law

According to Articles 10 (1) of the ECHR and 10 (2) of the BC, the patient who asks to be informed about his health has the right to receive all information collected about his health, though account must be taken of the wording of Article 10 (3) of the BC, with respect to which reference should be made to the reply to case 107.

For the rest, according to Article 4 of the BC, all concerned must act in accordance with relevant professional obligations and standards, taking into account the psychological well-being of the patient.

2. From the ethical standpoint

The doctor has to decide between information and silence on the disease, taking care not to deprive the patient of his hope for a cure.

3. From the standpoint of religious moralities

a. *Catholic*

It is necessary to bear in mind both the "right of the person of be informed about his own state of health"[1] and the "right to informed consent"[2] for the treatment to be given.

As regards the first point, "This right does not disappear in the presence of a diagnosis and prognosis of an illness which will cause death, but other factors are also involved. The fact is that this information implies important responsibilities

---

1. Charter of health personnel, No. 125.
2. *Idem*, No. 72.

which cannot be escaped. There are responsibilities connected with the treatment which has to be given with the informed consent of the patient".[1]

As regards the second point, the Catholic Church stresses that in general: "In order that the choice should be made in all knowledge and freedom, it is necessary to give the patient a precise picture of his problem and of the therapeutic possibilities, as well as the risks involved, the difficulties and the likely consequences. That is, it is necessary to request informed consent from the patient."[2]

b. *Protestant*
Pretexts and refusal to answer questions should be prohibited. But are we always sure what a seriously ill patient really wants and can bear?

c. *Jewish*
Everything depends on the patient's personality and the way in which matters are discussed with him.

If the patient has to take precautions, it is necessary to tell him the truth in order to give the treatment the maximum chance of success and make sure he does nothing incompatible with his state of health.

In addition, the patient ought to make a will, but it is important to suggest this in a subtle kind of way, so that the patient cannot be sure of the prognosis.

In other cases, everything depends on the patient's psychology. The family entourage and the family doctor can help in the decision, because they know the patient's personality and way of reacting very well.

If it is decided to say nothing, it is necessary that all the medical personnel respect this decision, which is very difficult to ensure in a public hospital.

In other cases, it is better to leave the patient in ignorance. This counts among the white lies. One of the factors for a cure is the hope of survival. If this hope is dashed by revealing the cruel truth, it could have very negative repercussions for the patient.

A decision like this should never be taken by one person alone. It is necessary that it should be taken collectively, taking account of the entourage.

d. *Muslim*
Medical opinion.

e. *Buddhist*
The doctor should be asked to explain the treatment to the patient so that the nurse can then explain the use of this technique, appropriate to his case.

---

1. *Idem*, No. 125.
2. *Idem*, No. 72.

4. From the standpoint of agnostic morality

The nurse must tell the doctor about the patient's request for explanation and insist that he meet it.

Rights of the individual

Young C, 14 years old, 1.50 m tall and weighing 50 kg, is in a public health establishment specialising in psychiatry. He has previously had several stays in different psychiatric institutions for children because of behavioural problems (running away from home, backwardness at school, etc.).
His mother died six years ago. Since then it is known that the father has been sexually abusing the boy.
After two months in the hospital, marked by a period of intense excitation, C asks to return to his father's home. The children's judge raises no objection. The carers are always present for the whole of the father's visits.
Dilemma: the question is whether to remain with the alternative of putting the boy at risk by allowing him to return to his father or maintaining his isolation by keeping him in hospital, or to break out of it by establishing a process for changing the terms of father-son communication before considering discharging the boy from hospital.

1. From the standpoint of international law

The text does not state whether the boy's request to return to his father's home (a request to which the children's judge is not opposed) has resulted in family court proceedings. In the course of this procedure, the need for the child to continue psychiatric treatment in the hospital (or at least not to stay with his father) should have been presented to the judge by the medical team (Article 9 (1) of the United Nations Convention on the Rights of the Child), and the child should have been heard (Article 12, *idem*), since he is capable of forming his own views.

It also should be noted that according to Article 19 of this convention: "States Parties shall take all appropriate legislative, administrative, social and educational measures to protect the child from all forms of physical or mental violence, injury or abuse, neglect or negligent treatment, maltreatment or exploitation, including sexual abuse, while in the care of parent(s) (...). Such protective measures should, as appropriate, include effective procedures for the establishment of social programmes to provide necessary support for the child and for those who have the care of the child, as well as for other forms of prevention and for identification, reporting, referral, investigation, treatment and follow-up of instances of child maltreatment described heretofore, and, as appropriate, for judicial involvement."

If, on the contrary, the request has not led to legal proceedings, reference should be made to Article 20 of the Convention on the Rights of the Child, according to which "A child temporarily or permanently deprived of his or her family environment, or in whose own best interests cannot be allowed to remain in that environment, shall be entitled to special protection and assistance provided by the state (...). Such care should include, *inter alia,* foster placement, *Kafalah* of Islamic law, adoption of, if necessary, placement in suitable institutions for the care of children". For the rest, please refer to Article 4 of the BC and to points 28 and 32 of the explanatory report, according to which doctors and health care professionals in general have the essential task not only to heal patients but also to take the proper steps to promote health and relieve pain, taking into account the psychological well-being of the patient.

2. From the ethical standpoint

Agree with the second branch of the alternative.

3. From the standpoint of religious moralities

a. *Catholic*

Even though there are no explicit references in the magisterium of the Catholic Church, it can certainly be said that there is an obligation for the hospital staff to protect the boy from the sexual violence of the father even if he himself requests to leave the establishment and return home.

The nursing staff do not have the authority to decide, but have the obligation to inform the medical authorities of the danger which exists if the boy is allowed to leave the hospital and the necessity of informing the children's court; the latter may establish contact with the social services, in order to bring about a change in the father-son relationship.

b. *Protestant*

It should be possible to discuss the case with the children's judge, on whom various possible solutions depend (placement with a third person or institution, conditional custody for the father, etc.).

c. *Jewish*

If the judge considers that the child can go back to life with his father without danger, and if the doctor corroborates this view, I do not see why the nurses should oppose their decision.

The judge and the doctor are not going to put the boy's health in danger. They are aware of the family situation and it is for them to take the necessary decision.

The opinion of the nursing team obviously has to be taken into consideration and it is necessary to make the father very aware of the risks he runs if he should endanger the boy's physical or mental health.

It is also necessary to insist that the father agrees to undergo psychotherapy.

451

d. *Muslim*

Save the child.

e. *Buddhist*

It is preferable to establish a process of father-son dialogue and at the same time ensure that the father receives treatment.

4. From the standpoint of agnostic morality

The hospital staff have the obligation to inform the children's judge and the public prosecutor's office and to keep the boy until a placement solution can be found.

Rights of the individual

Mrs X, 96, is hospitalised in an orthopaedic service. When it comes to the operation, the surgeon chooses an unusual technique which increases the time spent under anaesthetic and hence the risk involved in the operation, and does so without informing either the patient or her family. The nurses do not agree with this choice.
Dilemma: expose the patient to a higher risk than normal without informing her or her family and against the opinion of the nurses, or act in collaboration with the nurses and with the consent of the patient, with the family being informed, respecting the dignity and wishes of the patient.

1. From the standpoint of international law

The right to information about one's health is one of the fundamental rights of the person concerned according to Articles 10 (1) of the ECHR and 10 (2) of the BC, all the more so as information is the necessary precondition for consent to or refusal of a medical intervention (Articles 7 of the Covenant on Civil and Political Rights, and 5 (1) and (2) of the BC). In this case in particular (see points 35 and 36 of the explanatory report appended to the BC) the information must be sufficiently clear and suitably worded for the layman. The patient must be put in a position, through the use of terms they can understand, to weigh up the necessity or usefulness of the aim and methods of the intervention against the risks and the discomfort or pain it will cause. This information must namely cover the risks involved in the intervention (or in alternative courses of action), i.e. it must cover not only the risks inherent in the type of intervention contemplated, but also any risks related to the individual characteristics of each patient, such as age or the existence of other pathologies. It should be noted that, in terms of point 37 of the explanatory report appended to the BC, invasive acts or treatments may require express consent.

For the rest, it is for the doctor to choose the form of intervention, taking account in particular of established scientific facts, professional obligations and standards and the rules of conduct applicable. The intervention must meet the criteria of relevance and proportionality between the aim pursued and the means used (Article 4 of the BC: a particular course of action must in fact be judged in the light of the specific health problem raised by a given patient (point 33 of the explanatory report appended to the BC). So far as previously expressed wishes are concerned, see Article 9 of the BC and point 62 of the explanatory report.

2. From the ethical standpoint

Everything depends on the doctor-patient relationship, which is a private matter in which the nurse cannot interfere. Agree with the second branch of the alternative.

3. From the standpoint of religious moralities

a. *Catholic*

In the case of operations which are not usual, "the good of the person, protected by ethical norms, requires the respect of preconditions essentially concerned with consent and risk".[1] This consent "must be informed as regards the experimentation, its objectives and the possible risks involved, so that the patient may give or refuse his consent in full knowledge and freedom. The doctor in fact has no rights over the patient other than the rights that the patient himself confers upon him".[2]

In any event, there must be "great respect of the patient in the application of new treatments still in experimental stage (...) where they still present a high level of risk".[3]

The surgeon may not subject the aged patient to greater risk by selecting a longer and experimental technique; this would be illicit even if the subject had given her consent (or, in the case of incapacity of the patient, her representatives).

The nurses, in the presence of a serious breach of ethics, have the duty to express their opposition to the surgeon himself and, if this has no effect, to the medical authorities: "Nursing staff do not consent to and do not co-operate directly in any act which is contrary to morality, especially an act which deliberately goes against human life or directly starts to diminish or destroy the physical or mental integrity of the patient's person".[4]

b. *Protestant*

Here again there is no real dilemma: it is clear that the second solution is to be preferred; but why does the doctor make this decision? Is he unthinking or does he have a technical reason not apparent to staff with less training?

---

1. Charter of health personnel, No. 76.
2. John Paul II, "Address to the participants in two congresses of medicine and surgery", 27 October 1980, in *Insegnamenti*, III/2, p. 1009, No. 5.
3. John Paul II, "Address to the participants of a course on 'human pre-leukaemia'", 15 November 1985, in *Insegnamenti*, VII/2, p. 1265, No. 5.
4. International Catholic Committee of Nurses and Medico-Social Assistants, Code of Deontology, 1972, Article 3.

c. *Jewish*

The presentation of this case does not tell us whether there are good reasons which necessitate the change of technique. In this case, the doctor is the only person authorised to decide the procedure to be used "Do not remain impassive before the blood of your neighbour", says Leviticus.

If it is a normal case, the doctor obviously has to give the patient the best chances for success. His vocation is to defend the physical and mental health of his patients and ease their suffering in the respect of life and of the dignity of the person. He must also inform all concerned. The nurses' opinion is certainly enlightening, but it is for the doctor alone to take the responsibility for the operation and to assume any consequences arising from it.

d. *Muslim*
Medical consensus.

e. *Buddhist*

It is necessary to act in concert with the nurses, with the consent of the patient and with her family being informed, out of respect for the patient's dignity.

4. From the standpoint of agnostic morality

Except in the case of unforeseen circumstances the surgeon should follow the technique that has been explained to the patient. If a change of technique is made, however, it is not for the nurse to pass judgment.

Satisfaction of the individual's basic needs

Mr X, 85, has been living in a retirement home for some years. He is paralysed on the left side and anorexic. He refuses the prescribed nasogastric feeding tube and clearly expresses his desire to die.
Dilemma: find the cause of the refusal to live and try to remedy this rather than forcing the patient to live against his will.

1. From the standpoint of international law

Reply in the first sense, while taking account of the fact that the patient's refusal to live has no legal value, the problem of the legitimacy of the renunciation of the entitlement and exercise of the right to life not having yet been resolved in international human rights law.

See the replies to cases 90 and 97.

2. From the ethical standpoint

If the patient is conscious, his desire must be respected. If not the answer is the same as in case 90 if he pulls the tube out.

3. From the standpoint of religious moralities

a. *Catholic*

Considering that "alimentation and hydration, even artificial, should be classified as normal care always due to a patient if they are not dangerous for him";[1] considering also that "When they have to take medical action on a patient, health professionals should be in possession of his express or tacit consent";[2] and lastly, considering that "human life is of a sacred and inviolable nature",[3] then in the present case a specialist psychiatrist should be called in to treat the patient for anorexia (a mental illness).

Force-feeding may be practised only if the patient is not capable of understanding and desiring because of a mental illness or if this intervention is in response to an emergency situation. It is then necessary to recommend the presence of the family and warm human assistance, for "the patient who knows he is surrounded by an affectionate, human and Christian presence does not sink into depression and

---

1. Charter of health personnel, No. 120.
2. *Idem*, No. 72.
3. John Paul II, Evangelium Vitae, No. 53.

anxiety like he who, on the contrary, feeling abandoned to his fate of suffering and death, requests an end to his life".[1]

b. *Protestant*
Same reply as in case 108.

c. *Jewish*
Refusing to have a nasogastric feeding tube inserted does not necessarily mean that the patient wants to die. It signals some malaise that the patient is suffering. It is therefore necessary to speak with him to see why he removes the tube and try to find some other, less uncomfortable, way of feeding him.

It is also necessary to call upon a neuropsychiatrist, members of the family and the family doctor to try to find the cause of this behaviour.

Above all, efforts should not be abandoned too quickly, because medicine implies in all circumstances the constant respect of life and human dignity.

d. *Muslim*
The main thing is to take care of the patient's morale, according to the teaching of Avicenna in *Urdjuza* and the tradition of the prophet (*Hadith*) in Bukhari.

e. *Buddhist*
It is necessary to find the cause of the refusal to live and try to alleviate it.

4. From the standpoint of agnostic morality

The patient should be helped to live, but in the final resort it is for him to decide whether he wishes to eat or not.

---

1. Charter of health personnel, No. 149.

Satisfaction of the individual's basic needs

Mr B, 50, former opera singer, operated on two years ago, has a tracheostomy for life. Occasionally meets his wife whom he says was attracted by the easy life when he was rich and handsome; no longer sees his children. Following a pneumonia complicated by septicaemia, he becomes an incontinent bedridden invalid, refuses all food and refuses to take care of his tracheotomy. After a period in which the nurses had to do everything, he is now capable of caring for the tracheotomy but deliberately refuses to recover his ability to communicate and look after himself. He is too young for definitive placement in an institution and it is impossible for him to return home. The nurse's diagnosis is loss of all hope associated with forced social isolation and uncertainty about the future. Dilemma: constrain the carers to find a humanitarian solution which is part of the task of any carer, admit the refusal to leave the hospital, allow him to be discharged on the pretext that he has a home to go to and once he has left the hospital the carers are no longer concerned.

1. From the standpoint of international law

No reply in international legal texts. Point 31 of the explanatory report appended to the BC does indeed state that "doctors and, in general, all professionals who participate in a medical act are subject to legal and ethical imperatives. They must act with care and competence, and pay careful attention to the need of each patient", but it does not define what should be done. The same is to say as regards point 32 of the explanatory report to the BC, which states that "it is the essential task of the doctor (and health care professionals) not only to heal patients but also to take the proper steps to promote health (...), taking into account the psychological well-being of the patient".

If it is thought that the refusal to take care of himself is due to a mental disorder of a serious nature, reference should be made to Article 7 of the BC and points 51 and 52 of the explanatory report: if an impairment of the person's mental faculties is observed, an intervention necessary to treat specifically these mental disorders may be permitted even if the patient does not consent, provided that the failure to intervene would result in a serious harm to the health of the individual (or to the health or safety of others). Point 53 of the explanatory report adds to it that "a number of member states (...) permit interventions for certain serious situations, such as the treatment of a serious somatic illness in a psychotic patient" but point 54 stresses that, unless serious harm is likely to result to the person's health (for example, where a person suffers from a suicidal tendency), treatment without consent is prohibited".

2. From the ethical standpoint

A psychiatrist should be called in.

3. From the standpoint of religious moralities

a. *Catholic*

Given the patient's depressive state, the nursing team should request the intervention of a psychiatrist or clinical psychologist and then, if necessary, the help of the social services for readaptation in the family: "certain malaises and illnesses of a mental nature can be approached and treated by means of psychotherapy. This technique embraces a variety of methods which permit the individual to help his fellow man to achieve a cure or at least an improvement in his condition".[1]

The patient cannot be abandoned nor can his refusal to communicate be accepted positively, nor can he be discharged with no guarantee of his being accepted by the family. This derives from two principles: that of respect of the patient as regards his "right to live in all human dignity"[2] and that of sociality-subsidiarity.

b. *Protestant*

The children must be brought face-to-face with their responsibilities.

c. *Jewish*

If it is known that outside the hospital, the patient risks endangering his life, it is necessary to keep him in the hospital environment until a humane alternative solution is found for him. It is not possible to get rid of a patient and escape responsibility for him on the pretext that the hospital staff are no longer concerned. The role of the doctor is not only to cure, but also, and above all, to prevent.

Among the possible solutions, it is certainly necessary to envisage the possibility of installing him at home with a nurse to look after him.

It is clear that the patient's wife and children have a duty to do everything possible to make life easy for their husband and father.

d. *Muslim*

The care team should inform the members of the family and place them before their responsibilities (assistance to a person in danger).

---

1. Charter of health personnel, No. 105.
2. *Idem*, No. 46.

e. *Buddhist*

The care team must be persuaded to adopt a humanitarian attitude.

4. From the standpoint of agnostic morality

The care team must see it as its duty to seek any humanitarian solution to help this man who is not capable of taking responsibility for himself.

Satisfaction of the individual's basic needs

Mrs X only asks to urinate when a carer offers to accompany her to the toilets.
She is very happy with this, but when the workload in the unit is too great the staff
apply a napkin; she is classified incontinent.
Dilemma: contributing to making a patient dependent to suit the organisation
of work, or adapt this organisation to the patient's needs even though she may be
the only one in the service who needs the organisation to be changed.

1. From the standpoint of international law

One of the guiding principles of international human rights law is the fact that the structures set up by people should be appropriate and adapted to the respect of the rights and dignity of other people. This is true in particular as regards the weakest or most disadvantaged individuals (the sick, women, children, old people, the handicapped, prisoners).

In the same sense, see Article 1 of the BC, in the terms of which "Parties to this Convention shall protect the dignity (...) of all human beings and guarantee everyone, without discrimination, respect for their integrity and other rights and fundamental freedoms with regard to the application of biology and medicine", and Article 2 of the BC, according to which "the interests and welfare of the human being shall prevail over the sole interest of society and science".

For the rest, no specific reply other than reference to Article 4 of the BC.

2. From the ethical standpoint

The patient's interest must come before the organisation of the service.

3. From the standpoint of religious moralities

a. *Catholic*
The dignity of each person requires that the entire hospital organisation should be oriented according to the needs of the patient; towards giving the most efficient and humane assistance possible. Health personnel "must do everything to ensure that patients are assisted as their dignity of persons 'made in the image of God' requires".[1]

---

1. John Paul II, "Address to the Catholic hospitals of the whole world", in *Insegnamenti*, VIII, 2, 1985, Libreria Editrice Vaticana, p. 1647.

b. *Protestant*

The answer is contained in the question: it would be better to find a form of organisation adapted to the case. But if this were really impossible, or too seldom possible, is it not worth talking about it with the patient herself so that she can be involved?

c. *Jewish*

If it is a question of organisation, it is necessary to do everything possible to suit this patient and adapt the organisation of the service to her needs.

If it is a question of resources, the community should also do everything possible to facilitate the optimum provision.

If it is question of priorities, the choice is sometimes difficult to make.

d. *Muslim*

Adapt to the patient's needs.

e. *Buddhist*

It is preferable to adapt the organisation to the patient's needs, if this is possible.

4. From the standpoint of agnostic morality

The organisation of the service should be adapted to the patient's needs in such a way as not to make her dependent.

Satisfaction of the individual's basic needs

A male patient is subject to repeated fits which are corrected by readjusting the doses of medication. He has another fit while his wife is there. She calls the nurses who ask her to leave the room while they do what is necessary. Called back a few moments later she finds that her husband has died. The nurses learn only some time later that she has never got over being absent when her husband died after keeping him company day and night throughout his stay in hospital. Dilemma: understanding the process of accompanying a dying person and of bereavement. Not excluding the nearest and dearest.

1. From the standpoint of international law

No specific reply in international law, though account should be taken of the wording of Article 8 (1) of the ECHR, which stipulates the right to respect of private and family life and Article 4 of the BC.

2. From the ethical standpoint

Yes, to the extent that the family's presence does not hamper nursing care.

3. From the standpoint of religious moralities

a. *Catholic*

The person whose life is becoming increasingly precarious and difficult because of illness "is a person in need of humane and Christian accompaniment; doctors and nurses are called upon to give him their skilled and inalienable support".[1]

The family, on the one hand, plays a very important role from the standpoint of support for the patient and communion with him, but on the other is itself afflicted by suffering and in its turn needs comfort, especially in the face of death.

In the case under consideration, the wife should have been called before her husband's death and not marginalised at such a delicate and tragic moment of her life.

There is also the moral obligation to help the relatives, in this case the wife, to cope with the bereavement.

---

1. Charter of health personnel, No. 115.

b. *Protestant*

Two factors are involved here: accompanying the dying person, in which those close to him should be involved as much as possible – though without trying to turn this into a panacea – and coming to terms with bereavement, something the wife in question has obviously been unable to do. But is this the concern of the carers alone?

c. *Jewish*

It is true that it is extremely frustrating for the wife to have been absent at the moment when her husband died after having kept him company day and night throughout his hospitalisation.

If the nurses ask the wife to leave the room while administering treatment, they have good reasons to do so. They need to be free to do their job, and they perhaps wanted to spare the wife from distressing scenes which might have traumatised her for life.

It is certainly important that this lady should meet the nurses to talk about things.

In cases where treatment can be administered in the presence of the family without it interfering with the work in any way, the family's wishes should certainly be met.

d. *Muslim*

The patient's nearest and dearest should not be excluded in what is deemed medically to be the terminal phase.

e. *Buddhist*

It is most important that the close family be present at the moment of death.

4. From the standpoint of agnostic morality

The nearest and dearest must not be prevented from accompanying a dying person.

464

Satisfaction of the individual's basic needs

Two hospital patients share a room. One of them refuses to wash, to the point where the air is unbreathable. The other does not complain. In line with the philosophy which guides the real nursing role, the desired nursing role, which is to take care of people, the status of the human being, the conception of health and the limits of the nursing function with respect to those of the other health professions, the nurse invites the patient to go to the shower, use it as much as he wishes and explains why it is necessary to wash. The patient still refuses. Dilemma: health education (and perhaps here this is the patient's way of saying that he wants a single room).

1. From the standpoint of international law

No reply in international law. See, however, Recommendation R (80) 4 of the Committee of Ministers of the Council of Europe concerning the patient as an active participant in his own treatment, and in particular paragraph F, points 2 to 5: "Innovations should be promoted at the training stage to enable professionals to be receptive to patients' needs and to facilitate the patients' co-operation in their own treatment. Training curricula for students and all professionals which are geared to society's need for improvement of primary health care should envisage the earliest possible contact with practice in primary care and the psycho-social problems of the patients involved. Subsequent and vocational training should be integrated and related to practice, not only with hospital patients, but also with patients of general practitioners. This should include appropriate training in prevention, prophylaxis, early diagnosis and health education. This will prepare them for future co-operation in health care teams. Training programmes for medical, nursing and paramedical staff should include information on all patient associations to encourage them to inform their own patients or relevant associations. Additional training for all team members in information techniques, education in non-directive communication techniques and health education should be encouraged."

2. From the ethical standpoint

Agreed.

3. From the standpoint of religious moralities

a. *Catholic*

Even though there are no explicit references in the magisterium of the Catholic Church, it can certainly be said that in a hospital personal hygiene is of the utmost importance and a lack of it may be seriously detrimental to the health of the person concerned and others.

Before proceeding to compulsory treatment, for which it is necessary to have the due authorisations, the intervention of the psychologist should be requested, to discover the reason for the refusal to wash. It is necessary, nevertheless, to bear in mind that "in these cases preventive intervention is the priority remedy, and the most effective (...). It requires the convergent harnessing of all the operational forces of society".[1]

b. *Protestant*

One person's freedom stops where another's begins. This also applies in a hospital ward. However, the refusal to wash may indeed be the method adopted to get a single room. Several questions then arise: should this desire be acceded to? Should it be dismissed simply because it has been "improperly" formulated? If it is acceded to and the patient continues not to wash, then what? It may also be considered that a good shower never did anyone any harm.

c. *Jewish*

The fact that the room-mate does not complain excludes the hypothesis that the patient who does not wash is trying to say he wants a single room.

It is therefore necessary to try to convince this patient to wash, for his own sake and for his entourage. If he refuses, the nurses should give him a bed bath or oblige him to take a shower if they can.

d. *Muslim*
See case 111.

e. *Buddhist*

It is necessary to talk to the patient and evoke the respect of his room-mate and of the medical team, and to stress the importance of respecting the rules of the establishment.

4. From the standpoint of agnostic morality

The role of the nurse is to ensure that hygiene is respected.

---

1. Charter of health personnel, No. 52.

Satisfaction of the individual's basic needs

A child is born with a double coil of umbilical cord around the neck. He has several circulatory arrests and is reanimated each time. There is brain damage and he has convulsions. Serious sequels are to be expected. The doctor tells the nurses to go on reanimating the baby in the case of any further circulatory arrests.
Dilemma: should the child receive all the palliative care required by his condition while nature is allowed to take its course, or should he be reanimated simply to maintain a vegetative life which will ruin the lives of the parents?

1. From the standpoint of international law

The concept of the "quality of life" as a limit to the right to life is totally unknown in international human rights law, in which life represents an absolute value (and right) (see Articles 2 (1) and 15 (2) of the ECHR; 6 (1) of the Covenant on Civil and Political Rights; and 6 (1) of the Convention on the Rights of the Child).

Also to be noted is the wording of Article 6 (2) of the Convention on the Rights of the Child: "States Parties (...) shall ensure to the maximum extent possible the survival and development of the child".

Since in the terms of Articles 2 (1) of the ECHR and 6 (1) of the Covenant on Civil and Political Rights "no one shall be deprived of his life intentionally", the patient should be given all necessary and essential care according to the state of scientific knowledge to which refers also Article 4 of the BC.

2. From the ethical standpoint

In the case of a disagreement between doctor and nurse on the prognosis there is nothing to say that the nurse must be right.

3. From the standpoint of religious moralities

a. *Catholic*

In view of the fact that the circulatory arrests are due to a secondary cause and that children's nerve tissue is characterised by considerable plasticity, in the present case the reanimation of the child respects the principle of proportionality of treatment. "It is certain that the moral obligation to treat oneself and to have oneself treated exists, but this obligation must be seen in relation to specific situations; that is it is necessary to determine whether the therapeutic resources available are objectively in proportion to the prospects for improvement".[1]

---

1. John Paul II, *Evangelium Vitae*, No. 65.

b. *Protestant*

Generally speaking, the Protestant view stresses the fact that life is not simply a biological process but implies quality and relationships. These last may admittedly be found where they are least expected, but in this particular case it is difficult to see any reason not to "let nature take its course".

c. *Jewish*

The role of the doctor must always be to give life. He has the duty to save this child if the medical prognosis is not catastrophic and if he considers that there is a possibility of saving it. "You must not remain impassive before the blood of your neighbour" says Leviticus.

If, on the other hand, he considers that the situation is hopeless and there is nothing more to be done, it is necessary to give this baby all the comfort care required by his state, while letting nature take its course.

d. *Muslim*

Respect medical opinion.

e. *Buddhist*

Human life is respected if there is no relentless prolongation of life.

4. From the standpoint of agnostic morality

The baby should be given palliative care while allowing nature to take its course.

Satisfaction of the individual's basic needs

The nurses in an intensive care unit are convinced after talking together that a patient in phase II coma is lost, but they have to go on applying reanimation procedures instead of accompanying care.
Confronted by the same patient in phase III coma, the nurses feel guilty about having prolonged the agony and say: "If nature had been allowed take its course when this patient was admitted, he would have died long ago and we would have spared him a good deal of suffering".
In a hospital service the treatment of the patient is seen by the nurses as being relentless prolongation of life, and what is more their questions to the doctor remain unanswered. For this reason a nurse (or even all the nurses in a service) finds herself in an awkward position between what the doctor says to the family and her professional conscience which says she should be accompanying the patient and the family. She has to find a solution acceptable to her conscience.
Dilemma: reanimation procedures while remaining in the comfortable role of simply obeying orders, or accompaniment for a dying person, or both while preserving her dignity and reducing the intensity of useless suffering for the patient.

1. From the standpoint of international law

Since the concept of relentless prolongation of life is still extremely vague from the legal standpoint there is no reply in international law.

Article 4 of the BC in fact, while being concerned with legal and professional obligations and standards, and competent administration of treatment, and not only what is done but also how it is done (points 30, 31 and 32 of the explanatory report), does not define what is to be done in a case like this one, the only certain thing being that it is an essential task of the doctor not only to heal patients but also to take the proper steps to (...) relieve pain, taking into account the psychological well-being of the patient" and that "the intervention must meet the criteria of relevance and pro-portionality between the aim pursued and the means used" (point 33).

Concerning relations between the nurses and doctors involved, reference should be made to the laws and codes of conduct in force in the country concerned.

If the patient had expressed his wishes when he was capable of discernment, see Article 9 of the BC, cited in the reply to case 97, to which reference should be made.

2. From the ethical standpoint

Agree with the third proposed attitude, otherwise the same answer as in case 118.

3. From the standpoint of religious moralities

a. *Catholic*

"Conscious of being neither the master of life nor the master of death", the health professional "has to make the appropriate choices, namely base himself on the patient, and act as a function of his real condition".[1] He is thus called upon to apply the principle of proportionality of treatment which in this case is respected, because phase II and III comas represent acute crises of the central nervous system but do not yet constitute imminent death. Only "in the imminence of inevitable death despite the methods employed, is it permissible, in all conscience, to take the decision to renounce treatments which would bring only a precarious and painful reprieve, though without interrupting the normal care due to a patient in such a situation. The doctor could not then reproach himself for non-assistance to a person in danger".[2]

b. *Protestant*

Same answer as in the previous case. The fact that the question is asked shows how useful it would be to have places of reflection where these problems could be approached in a spirit of co-operation and discussed dispassionately.

c. *Jewish*

The doctor is the only authority capable of taking the necessary decisions. He also assumes full responsibility for them.

If the doctor does not tell the whole truth to the family, this is because he hopes to reanimate the patient. He thinks that in this case his duty is to try to be reassuring.

It is then necessary to promote communication between doctors and nurses in the interest of the patient and of the service.

d. *Muslim*

"Letting nature take its course" is a view rejected by the teaching of Islamic medicine (*Averroes*). The Koran requires that each individual be responsible for others and combats evil acts and recommends good action, hence necessary concertation.

e. *Buddhist*

The dignity of the patient must be preserved and unnecessary suffering avoided.

---

1. Charter of health personnel, No. 120.
2. Congregation for the doctrine of the faith, Declaration on euthanasia, 5 May 1980, in AAS 72, 1980, p. 551.

4. From the standpoint of agnostic morality

The nurse must fulfil her subordinate role as best she can.

Satisfaction of the individual's basic needs

A woman patient of 30 in a psychiatric hospital has a scalp wound as the result of a fall. The duty doctor sutures the wound without using any local anaesthetic. The patient moans.
Dilemma: easing suffering is one of the raisons d'être *of the nurse, and there is no medical reason for not using a local anaesthetic.*

1. From the standpoint of international law

See Article 5 (1) of Recommendation R (83) 2 of the Committee of Ministers of the Council of Europe concerning the legal protection of persons suffering from mental disorder placed as involuntary patients: "A patient put under placement has a right to be treated under the same ethical and scientific conditions as any other sick person and under comparable environmental conditions. In particular, he has the right to receive appropriate treatment and care."
In the same sense, see Article 4 of the BC.

2. From the ethical standpoint

The doctor assumes full and entire responsibility for his acts.

3. From the standpoint of religious moralities

a. *Catholic*
The use of analgesics is not only permissible, but is even obligatory in the case of very painful operations, unless the patient refuses them or the urgency of the situation does not permit the time to administer any anaesthetic.
"Sometimes the use of analgesic and anaesthetic drugs and techniques cause the suppression or diminution of consciousness and the use of the higher faculties. To the extent that such interventions are not directly aimed at the loss of consciousness and freedom but of sensitivity to pain, and are contained within strict limits of clinical needs alone, they must be considered ethically legitimate."[1]

b. *Protestant*
The doctor's behaviour is to be denounced.

---

1. Charter of health personnel, No. 71.

c. *Jewish*

The role of the doctor is to relieve suffering and to treat sickness. Nobody has said it is necessary to suffer. There is therefore no reason to justify the behaviour of this doctor who stitches a wound without any local anaesthetic, leaving the patient to moan in pain.

Suffering is ethically intolerable. Every effort must be made to avoid having a patient suffer physically or mentally. Judaism is opposed to calm resignation in the case of pain. Judaism prohibits leaving a living creature, man or animal, to suffer. It calls for action and solidarity when another is suffering; there can be no excuse for idleness disguised as pity. Doctors who try to ease the suffering of others perform a *mitswa*, an action of great religious and moral value.

d. *Muslim*
See case 117.

e. *Buddhist*
If there is no medical reason for opposing the use of a local anaesthetic, then of course one must be given so that the patient will not suffer.

4. From the standpoint of agnostic morality

The fact is that a few stitches in the scalp are generally made without any local anaesthetic as the intervention is no more painful than giving a local anaesthetic.

Satisfaction of the individual's basic needs

Mr X, 55, has a slipped disc. He is in hospital for an operation the date of which has been fixed. Despite his state of pre-operation agitation connected with chronic alcoholism, the operation takes place as planned. The agitation persists in the post-operation phase. He is strapped to his bed.
Dilemma: take action before the operation so that the patient will be calm in the post-operation phase, or disregard the true conception of nursing care in order to maintain peace among the carers.

1. From the standpoint of international law

No reply in positive international law. As regards the BC, reference should be made once again to Article 4, namely to scientific knowledge, technical competence, legal rules and professional obligations and standards applicable in the country concerned.

2. From the ethical standpoint

The post-operative consequences in an alcoholic patient are unpredictable in the case of withdrawal. This raises a complex psychiatric question to which nurses can hardly give the answer.

3. From the standpoint of religious moralities

a. *Catholic*

"The alcoholic is a sick person who requires medical treatment and support in the form of solidarity and psychotherapy. Entirely humane rehabilitation methods should be implemented for him."[1] Thus the respect of the patient requires that before performing the operation action must be taken to calm his agitation, both to avoid possible negative influences on the operation and to avoid having to take coercive measures which offend against the dignity of the person.

b. *Protestant*

The formulation of the dilemma is not very clear. It is obviously necessary above all to use methods which cause the least suffering possible to the patient.

---

1. Charter of health personnel, No. 98.

c. *Jewish*

It is obviously necessary to take action before the operation to ensure that the patient will be calm in the post-operation phase. If he is alcoholic, it is necessary to give him a preventive treatment to avoid any danger and any discomfort for the patient, especially as we know that simple and effective treatments exist.

d. *Muslim*

See cases 99 and 117.

e. *Buddhist*

It is necessary to take action before the operation to ensure that the patient will be calm in the post-operation phase, to avoid having to attach him to the bed, which is a form of aggression.

4. From the standpoint of agnostic morality

The doctor who will be responsible for the patient after the operation must intervene before it to ensure that the patient is calm and relaxed.

Satisfaction of the individual's basic needs

Mr X, 60, had his right leg amputated some time ago.
He uses a wheel chair and has had his flat fitted out as a function of his handicap.
Because he suffers a lot of pain due to arthritis and infected wounds in his left leg
and the frequent hospitalisation this entails, he asks for this leg to be amputated
too.
The surgeon does not envisage such an amputation.
The nurses think it is desirable, all the more so because the patient has requested
it and he suffers too much.
Dilemma: despite their disagreement, should the nurses give way to the doctor,
who wants the patient to keep his leg as long as possible because the hospital is
there to calm the pain when it becomes unbearable, or try to convince the doctor
that he should do as the patient wishes, knowing that this will release him from
pain and give him a decent quality of life, for which he is prepared and for which
his home is already equipped.

1. From the standpoint of international law

See the wording of Article 1 of the BC, according to which "Parties to this Convention shall protect the dignity (...) of all human beings and guarantee everyone, without discrimination, respect for their integrity".

Reference should also be made to the scientific knowledge and professional obligations and standards in force in the country concerned, as provided for in Article 4 of the BC.

2. From the ethical standpoint

This is a question to be settled in consultation with another specialist in the same field.

3. From the standpoint of religious moralities

a. *Catholic*

In this case we are confronted with the problem of "therapeutic mutilation". It is necessary to consider the conditions of the case. "For the patient to recover his health, it may be necessary in the absence of other remedies, for operations which involve the modification, mutilation or ablation of organs. Therapeutic manipulation of the organism is justified here by the principle of totality, defined as a principle of therapy",[1] which governs the obligatory nature of the medico-surgical interventions.

---

1. Charter of health personnel, No. 66.

In addition to the patient's consent, "three things condition the moral acceptability of an operation with involves anatomical or functional mutilation: first, that the maintenance of functioning of a particular organ in the organism as a whole provokes serious damage in the latter or constitutes a threat; second that this damage cannot be avoided or at least significantly reduced other than by the mutilation in question and the efficacy of the latter is well assured; finally, that it can reasonably be expected that the negative effect, namely the mutilation and its consequences, will be compensated by the positive effect of eliminating the danger for the entire organism, easing pain, etc."[2]

In this case not all the conditions justifying the mutilation are fulfilled, because the pain in the left leg can be treated and because the quality of life after the amputation of the second leg would not be better.

b. *Protestant*

The patient can always be advised to consult another doctor and/or decide with those around him what it would be best to do.

c. *Jewish*

The doctor should consider whether it is possible by means of medicaments to alleviate the suffering enough to avoid the amputation, which requires major surgery. The doctor should try to avoid the amputation through creating an acceptable quality of life.

If the doctor is really unable to relieve the pain sufficiently, and the patient asks for it, it will perhaps be necessary to envisage this amputation, since the patient is already in a wheelchair and his flat is adapted to this new situation.

d. *Muslim*
See the Shura.

e. *Buddhist*

A second medical opinion should be sought, given the importance of saving the patient's leg.

4. From the standpoint of agnostic morality

In the interest of the patient the nurse can express her opinion to the doctor in all conscience.

---

2. Pius XII, "Address to the participants at the 26th Congress organised by the Italian Urological Society", 8 October 1953, in *Discorsi e Radiomessaggi di Sua Santità*, Pio XII, Vol. XV, Tipografia Poliglotta Vaticana, 1969, pp. 373-374.

Medical glossary

Cases

1. *Azoospermia*: Absence, temporary or permanent, of spermatozoids in the semen.
2. *Tubal obstruction*: Obstruction of the fallopian tube (musculo-membranous duct forming part of the female reproductive system) where fertilisation of the ovule by a spermatozoid takes place.
3. *Post abortum*: After termination of pregnancy, deliberate or otherwise.
   Tubal ligation: Ligation (tying) of the fallopian tube in the female reproductive system, preventing any fertilisation.
6. *Vas deferens*: A duct (of about 40 cm) which carries the sperm from the end of the epididymis to the urethra.
8. *Downs syndrome or trisomy 21*: Accidental chromosomal anomaly in which an extra, third chromosome is present at the 21st pair, causing varying degrees of mental and physical disability (mongolism).
9. *Amniotic fluid*: Liquid surrounding and protecting the embryo, then the foetus, throughout gestation, contained in the placenta.
   Spina bifida: Congenital malformation of the vertebral column: instead of fusing, the vertebral arches remain separate and the spinal canal is left open at the back, leading to paralysis and serious functional nervous anomalies.
14. *Amyotrophic lateral sclerosis or Charcot's disease*: A rare disease of the spinal cord accompanied by degeneration of the cerebrospinal tract (nerve fibres running from the spinal bulb to the lower end of the cord, governing the motor functions of the lower limbs) and atrophy of the anterior horn cells (gradual paralysis).
15. *Metastasis*: Development of a secondary (cancerous) tumour, mostly malignant, at a point in the body other than the site of the primary tumour.
16. *Hydrocephalus*: Dilation of the cranium in a new-born or young child as a result of an abnormal accumulation of cephalo-spinal fluid.
    Myeclocytic leukaemia: The most widespread leukaemia. A cancerous disease of the blood, characterised by the abnormal proliferation of white corpuscles, particularly polymorphonuclear leucocytes.
21. *Heterozygous twins*: Twins originating with two different fertilised ovules, attached to the same placenta.
27. *Peritoneal and pleural metastases*: Peritoneum: serous membrane covering

the walls of the abdominal cavity and the organs it contains; pleura: double layer of tissue enclosing the lungs.

28. *Teratogenic substance*: Substance likely to cause congenital malformation.

32. *Genome*: A person's genetic material made up of all the genes, coding or not, carried by the chromosomes and present in each nucleus of his cells.

33. *Huntingdon's chorea or chronic hereditary chorea*: Rare neurological disease of genetic origin (1/10 000) leading ineluctably to death between 30 and 40 years of age following dementia and cachexia.

35. *Adam Stokes syndrome*: Syndrome characterised by cardio-circulatory syndrome and nervous accidents of varying degrees of severity, such as a momentary arrest of the cerebral circulation or an extremely slow pulse (bradycardia).

42. *Lumbar sympathectomy*: Surgical removal of a lumbar nerve (along the spinal column) indicated for certain arterial diseases.

44, 47, 48

Prostatectomy: Surgical resection of the prostate.

Aids: Acquired immune deficiency syndrome.

HIV: Retrovirus causing human immune deficiency.

Seropositive: A person in whom the presence of HIV antibodies has been shown by tests. This person, who does not necessarily show the symptoms of Aids, may transmit the virus by means of blood and sexual contact.

59, 60, 66

IVF: *in vitro* fertilisation;

ZIFT: zygote intra-fallopian transfer.

76. *Phase 1 experimentation*: Evaluation of the tolerance to the product administered and the reproducible organic and functional modifications induced by it.

77. *Mesencephalic tissue*: Tissue from the middle brain, containing in particular dopaminergic neurones.

Parkinson's disease or shaking palsy: A progressive chronic disorder of the central nervous system characterised by impaired muscular co-ordination and tremor.

78, 92.

Haemodialysis: The use of an "artificial kidney" to filter circulating blood through a semi-permeable membrane to remove waste products.

82. *Recombinatory human erythropoiteine*: Substance producing red corpuscles in the bone marrow.

91. *Sarcoma*: Malignant tumour arising from connective tissue.

92. *Septicaemia*: "Blood poisoning".

93. *MAP*: Medically assisted procreation.

98, 112.

    Tracheotomy: Surgical incision into the trachea ("windpipe") in the case of obstruction of the upper air passage.

107.   *Ureterostomy*: Joining the ureter to the skin.

111.   *Hemiplegia*: paralysis of one side of the body.

    Anorexia: Neurosis causing refusal of food.

112.   *Cachexia*: Generally weakened condition.

117.   *Phase II coma*: Light coma with some reflexes retained.

    Phase III coma: Deep coma. Total absence of reflexes.

Definitions

In the context of the principles applicable to patients' rights in Europe, the terms below are to be understood in the sense of the definitions provided:

Discrimination: Distinction made between persons in similar situations on the basis of race, sex, religion, political opinion, national or social origin, association with a national minority or personal antipathy.

Health care: Medical, nursing and similar acts and services performed by care providers and establishments.

Care providers: Doctors, nursing staff, dentists and other members of health professions.

Medical act: Any form of examination, therapy or intervention carried out for diagnosis, preventive care, treatment or rehabilitation by a doctor or any other care provider.

Care establishment: Any institution providing health care, such as a hospital, nursing home or an establishment for people with handicaps.

Patient: Any person, sick or not, resorting to health services.

Palliative care: Care given to a patient who has reached a stage where the prognosis for his disease can no longer be improved with the therapeutic resources available; this expression also applies to the care given when death is imminent.

List of abbreviations

ACHR	Inter-American Convention on Human Rights
CIOMS	Council for International Organisation of Medical Sciences
Commission	European Commission of Human Rights (Council of Europe)
Court	European Court of Human Rights (Council of Europe)
BC	Convention for the Protection of Human Rights and Dignity of the Human Being with regard to the Application of Biology and Medicine: Convention on Human Rights and Biomedicine
ECHR	European Convention on Human Rights (Council of Europe)
ECOSOC	Economic and Social Council
EEC	European Economic Community
EU	European Union
ICRC	International Committee of the Red Cross
NECTAR	Network of European CNS (Central Nervous System) Transplantation and Restoration
OAS	Organisation of American States
OAU	Organisation of African Unity
UD	Universal Declaration of Human Rights (UN)
UN	United Nations
WMA	World Medical Association
WPA	World Psychiatric Association

Sales agents for publications of the Council of Europe
Agents de vente des publications du Conseil de l'Europe

AUSTRALIA/AUSTRALIE
Hunter publications, 58A, Gipps Street
AUS-3066 COLLINGWOOD, Victoria
Fax: (61) 33 9 419 7154

AUSTRIA/AUTRICHE
Gerold und Co., Graben 31
A-1011 WIEN 1
Fax: (43) 1512 47 31 29

BELGIUM/BELGIQUE
La Librairie européenne SA
50, avenue A. Jonnart
B-1200 BRUXELLES 20
Fax: (32) 27 35 08 60

Jean de Lannoy
202, avenue du Roi
B-1060 BRUXELLES
Fax: (32) 25 38 08 41

CANADA
Renouf Publishing Company Limited
5369 Chemin Canotek Road
CDN-OTTAWA, Ontario, K1J 9J3
Fax: (1) 613 745 76 60

CZECH REPUBLIC/RÉPUBLIQUE TCHÈQUE
USIS, NIS Prodejna
Havelkova 22
CZ-130 00 Praha 3
Fax: (420) 2 242 21 484

DENMARK/DANEMARK
Munksgaard
PO Box 2148
DK-1016 KØBENHAVN K
Fax: (45) 33 12 93 87

FINLAND/FINLANDE
Akateeminen Kirjakauppa
Keskuskatu 1, PO Box 218
SF-00381 HELSINKI
Fax: (358) 9 121 44 50

GERMANY/ALLEMAGNE
UNO Verlag
Poppelsdorfer Allee 55
D-53115 BONN
Fax: (49) 228 21 74 92

GREECE/GRÈCE
Librairie Kauffmann
Mavrokordatou 9, GR-ATHINAI 106 78
Fax: (30) 13 23 03 20

HUNGARY/HONGRIE
Euro Info Service
Magyarország
Margitsziget (Európa Ház),
H-1138 BUDAPEST
Fax: (36) 1 111 62 16
E-mail: euroinfo@mail.matav.hu

IRELAND/IRLANDE
Government Stationery Office
4-5 Harcourt Road, IRL-DUBLIN 2
Fax: (353) 14 75 27 60

ISRAEL/ISRAËL
ROY International
17 Shimon Hatrssi St.
PO Box 13056
IL-61130 TEL AVIV
Fax: (972) 3 546 1423
E-mail: royil@netvision.net.il

ITALY/ITALIE
Libreria Commissionaria Sansoni
Via Duca di Calabria, 1/1
Casella Postale 552, I-50125 FIRENZE
Fax: (39) 55 64 12 57

MALTA/MALTE
L. Sapienza & Sons Ltd
26 Republic Street
PO Box 36
VALLETTA CMR 01
Fax: (356) 233 621

NETHERLANDS/PAYS-BAS
InOr-publikaties, PO Box 202
NL-7480 AE HAAKSBERGEN
Fax: (31) 53 572 92 96

NORWAY/NORVÈGE
Akademika, A/S Universitetsbokhandel
PO Box 84, Blindern
N-0314 OSLO
Fax: (47) 22 85 30 53

POLAND/POLOGNE
Głowna Księgarnia Naukowa im. B. Prusa
Krakowskie Przedmiescie 7
PL-00-068 WARSZAWA
Fax: (48) 22 26 64 49

PORTUGAL
Livraria Portugal
Rua do Carmo, 70
P-1200 LISBOA
Fax: (351) 13 47 02 64

SPAIN/ESPAGNE
Mundi-Prensa Libros SA
Castelló 37, E-28001 MADRID
Fax: (34) 15 75 39 98

Llibreria de la Generalitat
Rambla dels Estudis, 118
E-08002 BARCELONA
Fax: (34) 343 12 18 54

SWITZERLAND/SUISSE
Buchhandlung Heinimann & Co.
Kirchgasse 17, CH-8001 ZÜRICH
Fax: (41) 12 51 14 81

BERSY
Route d'Uvrier 15
CH-1958 LIVRIER/SION
Fax: (41) 27 203 73 32

UNITED KINGDOM/ROYAUME-UNI
TSO (formerly HMSO)
51 Nine Elms Lane
GB-LONDON SW8 5DR
Fax: (44) 171 873 82 00

**UNITED STATES and CANADA/
ÉTATS-UNIS et CANADA**
Manhattan Publishing Company
468 Albany Post Road
PO Box 850
CROTON-ON-HUDSON, NY 10520, USA
Fax: (1) 914 271 58 56

STRASBOURG
Librairie Kléber
Palais de l'Europe
F-67075 STRASBOURG Cedex
Fax: +33 (0)3 88 52 91 21

Council of Europe Publishing/Editions du Conseil de l'Europe
Council of Europe/Conseil de l'Europe
F-67075 Strasbourg Cedex
Tel. +33 (0)3 88 41 25 81 – Fax +33 (0)3 88 41 39 10
E-mail: publishing@coe.fr – Website: http://book.coe.fr